Rehabilitation Outcomes

Rehabilitation Outcomes
Analysis and Measurement

edited by

Marcus J. Fuhrer, Ph.D.
Baylor College of Medicine
and
The Institute for Rehabilitation and Research

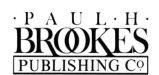

Baltimore • London

Paul H. Brookes Publishing Co.
Post Office Box 10624
Baltimore, Maryland 21285-0624

Typeset by Brushwood Graphics Inc., Baltimore, Maryland.
Manufactured in the United States of America by
The Maple Press Company, York, Pennsylvania.

Library of Congress Cataloging-in-Publication Data

Rehabilitation outcomes.

   Includes bibliographies and index.
   1. Rehabilitation—Evaluation.   2. Social service—
Evaluation.   I. Fuhrer, Marcus J., 1933–
[DNLM: 1. Outcome and Process Assessment (Health Care)
2. Rehabilitation. WB 320 R3457]
RM930.R365   1987   362.1'786   87-894
ISBN 0-933716-77-X

Contents

Contributors

Deborah A. Allen, Ph.D., Department of Sociology-Anthropology-Psychology at the American University in Cairo, 113 Kasr el Aini Street, P.O. Box 2511, Cairo, Arab Republic of Egypt.

Deborah A. Allen is an associate professor in the Department of Sociology-Anthropology-Psychology at the American University in Cairo, Egypt. She was formerly on the faculties of Psychiatry and Pediatrics at the University of Connecticut School of Medicine and was Director of Research for the University of Connecticut Research and Training Center for Pediatric Rehabilitation. Her research and publications have been primarily in the field of early intervention. She has also been active in consultation and evaluation concerned with early childhood programs.

Al Alquist, M.S., Department of Rehabilitation Medicine, University of Washington, RJ-30, Seattle, WA 98195.

Al Alquist is an exercise physiologist within the Department of Rehabilitation Medicine at the University of Washington. His research interests include the effects that exercise has on elderly people, and the effects of exercise on the immune system. He has developed several fluorometric enzyme assays for assessing skeletal muscle functional capacity. His most recent work includes evaluating the effects of exercise on tumor initiation and promotion in mice. Currently he is conducting research to measure functional aerobic capacity/impairment in major burn patients, multiple sclerosis subjects, and amputees fitted with various prosthetic devices.

William A. Anthony, Ph.D., Center for Psychiatric Rehabilitation, Boston University, Sargent College, 1019 Commonwealth Avenue, Boston, MA 02215.

William A. Anthony is director of the Center for Psychiatric Rehabilitation and a professor in the Department of Rehabilitation Counseling at Boston University. He has worked in various roles in the field of psychiatric rehabilitation and has been honored for his performance as a clinician (U.S. Army Commendation Medal, 1970), research (Mary Switzer Fellow, 1979), and educator (Sargent College Dr. Evelyn Kirrane Award, 1981). He is a past president of the National Association of Rehabilitation Research and Training Centers. His 10 books include *Principles of Psychiatric Rehabilitation, The Skills of Helping,* and *The Art of Health Care.* He has also authored six book chapters and more than 50 journal articles. He is co-editor of the *Psychosocial Rehabilitation Journal.*

Yehuda Ben-Yishay, Ph.D., New York University Medical Center, RIRM, 345 East 24th Street, NY 10010.

Yehuda Ben-Yishay is an associate professor of clinical rehabilitation medicine at NYU School of Medicine. He is currently Assistant Chief of Division of Behavioral Sciences, and Director of the Head Trauma Program of the NYU Medical Center, Rusk Institute. Between 1974 and 1984 he was also visiting director of the Israel National Institute for The Rehabilitation of the Brain Injured (Rekanaty Center). In 1976 he received the Howard A. Rusk Award, and in 1982 the William F. Caveness Award, for distinguished contributions in the field of head injury. He edited the NYU Monograph Series, *Working Approaches to Remediating Cognitive Deficits in Brain Damaged Persons,* has authored and co-authored numerous chapters and papers, and has been responsible for numerous presentations and workshops on various aspects of the neuropsychologic rehabilitation of brain injured persons. Currently, he serves on the editorial boards of *The Journal of Head Trauma Rehabilitation* and of *Brain Injury.*

Brian Bolton, Ph.D., Arkansas Research and Training Center in Vocational Rehabilitation, West Avenue Annex, University of Arkansas, Fayetteville, AR 72701.

Brian Bolton is a research professor at the University of Arkansas. He is a Fellow of the American Psychological Association (Evaluation and Measurement in Rehabilitation Psychology) and of the Society for

Personality Assessment. In 1986, he received the Burlington Northern Foundation Award for Excellence in Research at the University of Arkansas. His books include the *Psychology of Deafness for Rehabilitation Counselors, Psychosocial Adjustment to Disability, Vocational Adjustment of Disabled Persons,* and the *Handbook of Measurement and Evaluation in Rehabilitation* (2nd ed.). He has contributed to the *Eighth* and *Ninth Mental Measurements Yearbooks*, Volumes 1–6 of *Test Critiques*, the *Encyclopedia of Clinical Assessment*, Volumes 2 and 4 of the *Annual Review of Rehabilitation, Functional Psychological Testing, Psychology for Health Science Students*, and the *Handbook of Multivariate Experimental Psychology* (2nd ed.). He was previously editor of the *Rehabilitation Counseling Bulletin* and is currently advisory editor to College-Hill Press and serves on the editorial boards of four journals.

Michael Boltwood, M.S.W., School of Education and Counseling Psychology, Stanford University, Palo Alto, CA 94305.

Michael Boltwood earned a bachelor's degree in sociology from the University of California at Los Angeles and a master's degree in social work from the University of Washington. Shortly after receiving his master's degree, he joined the University of Washington Burn Center at Harborview Hospital in Seattle as its clinical social worker. In 1983 he also became a co-principle investigator in the Department of Rehabilitation Medicine's 3-year project studying the recovery of patients after suffering a major burn injury. He is the co-author of a book chapter on social work in a trauma care setting and has made several presentations to the American Burn Association regarding factors relating to the quality of recovery after a major burn. He is currently in the doctoral program in counseling and health psychology at the School of Education, Stanford University.

Carolyn M. Brunner, M.D., Arthritis Rehabilitation Unit, Box 412, University of Virginia Medical Center, Charlottesville, VA 22908.

Carolyn M. Brunner is a professor of medicine in the Division of Rheumatology at the University of Virginia School of Medicine. Since 1983 she has been director of the Arthritis Rehabilitation Unit in the Rehabilitation Research and Training Center for Arthritis and Low Back Pain at the University of Virginia, which is supported by the National Institute on Disability and Rehabilitation Research. She is a Fellow of the American College of Physicians and of the American Rheumatism Association. She is interested in research concerning methods of maintaining persons with arthritis at work, and is developing a program for arthritis patients with the State of Virginia Department of Rehabilitative Services.

Julia F. Costich, Ph.D., Department of Rehabilitation Medicine, University of Kentucky Medical Center, Lexington, KY 40536.

Julia Costich is administrative manager of the Department of Rehabilitation Medicine, University of Kentucky College of Medicine, affiliated with Cardinal Hill Hospital. She has published in the areas of health services research and medical education. In addition to presentations at national rehabilitation meetings, she has organized and chaired symposia on literature and medicine.

Paul Decelles, M.S., Return to Work Center, The Menninger Foundation, Jayhawk Tower, 700 Jackson, 9th Floor, Topeka, KS 66603.

Paul Decelles, is a Research Associate at the Menninger Foundation. His research interests include analysis of disability-related statistics and population modeling. He is co-author of many of the Return to Work Center publications on workers who become disabled.

Gerben DeJong, Ph.D., National Rehabilitation Hospital, 102 Irving Street, N.W., Washington, DC 20010.

Gerben DeJong is the director of research at the National Rehabilitation Hospital (NRH). Prior to coming to NRH in 1985, he served as senior research associate and associate professor with the Department of Rehabilitation Medicine at Tufts University School of Medicine in Boston. He is the author of more than 80 papers on health and disability issues ranging from the epidemiology of disability to medical rehabilitation outcomes. His works have appeared in diverse publications such as *Business and Health, Scientific American, Stroke,* and the *Journal of Health Politics, Policy, and Law*. His works have appeared in more than seven different languages. In 1985, he received the Licht Award for Excellence in Scientific Writing from the American Congress of Rehabilitation Medicine. He is a frequently invited speaker both in the United States and abroad. In 1984, he was a Fulbright Scholar in the Netherlands.

Barbara J. deLateur, M.D., Department of Rehabilitation Medicine, University of Washington, RJ-30, Seattle, WA 98195.

Barbara deLateur received her bachelor's degree (Philosophy) from St. Louis University in 1959, Doctor of Medicine from the University of Washington in Seattle in 1963, and master of science in 1968, also from the University of Washington. Following a rotating internship (1963–1964), Dr. deLateur completed a 3-year residency in Physical Medicine and Rehabilitation under the tutelage of Justus F. Lehmann, M.D. at the University of Washington. She has been chief of the Rehabilitation Medicine Service at Harborview Medical Center, a major trauma and burn center in Seattle, since 1970. Her research interests include exercise physiology, biophysics of heat, biomechanics of gait and orthotics, pain management, and assessment of outcome of various disorders such as stroke, head injury, and burns. She is a professor of Rehabilitation Medicine, University of Washington School of Medicine.

Donald J. Dellario, Ph.D., Medfield State Hospital, 45 Hospital Road, Medfield, MA 02052.

Donald J. Dellario is the Executive Director of Program and Organizational Development at Medfield State Hospital, and adjunct associate professor in the Department of Rehabilitation Counseling at Boston University. He has worked in various roles in rehabilitation services, research and education, and is licensed as a psychologist in Massachusetts. He is the former Associate Director of Research at the Boston University Center for Rehabilitation Research and Training in Mental Health and Director of Rehabilitation Education and Training at the University of Hawaii. He has published numerous articles, book chapters, and presentations concerned with rehabilitation topics. He sits on the editorial board of the *Rehabilitation Counseling Bulletin*, and has served as a reviewer for other rehabilitation journals.

Leonard Diller, Ph.D., Rusk Institute of Rehabilitation Medicine, New York University Medical Center, 400 East 34th Street, New York, NY 10016.

Leonard Diller is a professor of Clinical Rehabilitation Medicine at New York University Medical Center. He is Director of the Research and Training Center in Head Trauma and Stroke, and Chief of the Behavioral Science section of the Rusk Institute of Rehabilitation Medicine. He is a diplomate of the American Board of Examiners in Professional Psychology, a Fellow of the American Psychological Society, past president of the Division of Rehabilitation Psychology, former chairman of the Easter Seal Research Foundation, and currently vice-president of the American Congress of Rehabilitation Medicine. He is the author of more than 100 journal articles or chapters in books. He recently served as co-editor of *Neuropsychological Rehabilitation*. He is on the editorial board of six journals in the field of rehabilitation psychology, neuropsychology, and rehabilitation.

Gabriel R. Faimon, M.P.A., Return to Work Center, The Menninger Foundation, Jayhawk Tower, 700 Jackson, 9th Floor, Topeka, KS 66603.

Gabriel R. Faimon is director of the Rehabilitation Research and Training Center in the Menninger Return to Work Center. He served as administrator of the Kansas Vocational Rehabilitation Agency for nearly 5 years, preceded by more than 5 years of service in state administrative positions in employment and training programs. He has chaired or served as a member of numerous state and national committees related to vocational rehabilitation or employment and training activities. He has made more than 30 presentations related to work and disability to a wide variety of organizations, including legislative committees, employer groups, and the 1986 National Forum on Disability Policy.

Marianne Farkas, Sc.D., Center for Psychiatric Rehabilitation, Boston University, Sargent College, 1019 Commonwealth Avenue, Boston, MA 02215.

Marianne Farkas is the Director of Graduate Specialization Programs at the Center for Psychiatric Rehabilitation. She is also an assistant professor in the Department of Rehabilitation Counseling at Boston University where she directs graduate programs in psychiatric rehabilitation. She has worked as consultant, trainer, and researcher across the United States, Canada, and Europe on the development of psychiatric rehabilitation practitioners, programs, and systems. She has co-authored training packages and videotapes in psychiatric rehabilitation. She had contributed chapters to *Principles of Psychiatric Rehabilitation, Functional Assessment in Rehabilitation, Clinical, Legal, and Administrative Issues in Psychiatric Disability* and authored or co-authored articles in the area of training, program development, and research in psychiatric rehabilitation.

Stephen Forer, M.A., Santa Clara Valley Medical Center, 751 South Bascom Avenue, San Jose, CA 95128.
Stephen Forer is currently the rehabilitation services manager at Santa Clara Valley Medical Center and is responsible for providing program direction, coordination, and management of the 70-bed Rehabilitation Center. He is co-chairperson of the American Congress of Rehabilitation Medicine Task Force on Developing a Uniform Data System for Medical Rehabilitation; a member of the American Hospital Association Working Party on Alternative Payment Systems for Rehabilitation; a member of the Board of Directors and chairperson of the Data Sharing Committee for the California Association of Rehabilitation Facilities; a member of the Advisory Committee for the Health Care Financing Administration's Prospective Payment Project; and a member of the Prospective Payment Task Force of the National Association of Rehabilitation Facilities. He has given numerous professional and scientific presentations in the areas of program evaluation, functional assessment, and management information systems, and has over 29 publications to his credit.

Marcus J. Fuhrer, Ph.D., Department of Rehabilitation, Baylor College of Medicine, 1333 Moursund Avenue, Houston, TX 77030.
Marcus J. Fuhrer is a professor in the Department of Rehabilitation of Baylor College of Medicine, and vice-president for research of The Institute for Rehabilitation and Research (TIRR). He is director of the Research and Training Center for the Rehabilitation of Persons with Spinal Cord Dysfunction at Baylor College of Medicine and of the ILRU Research and Training Center on Independent Living at TIRR, both supported by the National Institute on Disability and Rehabilitation Research. He is a past president of the American Congress of Rehabilitation Medicine and of the National Association of Rehabilitation Research and Training Centers. He co-edited *Functional Assessment in Rehabilitation* and edited *Selected Research Topics in Spinal Cord Injury*. His research and writing have been concerned predominantly with medical rehabilitation outcomes, the federal support of rehabilitation research, cognitive processes in the Pavlovian conditioning of human autonomic responses, and the characteristics of peripheral sympathetic activity following transection of the human spinal cord.

J. Martin Giesen, Ph.D., Rehabilitation Research and Training Center on Blindness and Low Vision, Mississippi State University, P.O. Drawer 6189, Mississippi State, MS 39762.
J. Martin Giesen is the research director of the Rehabilitation Research and Training Center on Blindness and Low Vision, and a professor of Psychology at Mississippi State University. He has extensive training and experience in research methods, computer applications, and multivariate statistics. He is a member of the Society of Experimental Social Psychology and the American Psychological Association. He currently serves on the editorial board of the *Journal of Non-Verbal Behavior* and the *Annual Review of Social Psychology*. He has over 30 publications and over 20 research presentations in behavioral science/psychology and rehabilitation.

Carl V. Granger, M.D., Department of Rehabilitation Medicine, Buffalo General Hospital, 100 High Street, Buffalo, NY 14203.
Carl V. Granger is head of Rehabilitation Medicine at Buffalo General Hospital, and a professor of Rehabilitation Medicine, State University of New York at Buffalo. He is the project director with Byron B. Hamilton as principal investigator for the project entitled, "Development of a Uniform Data System for Medical Rehabilitation," funded by the National Institute on Disability and Rehabilitation Research. He is a member of the American Medical Association, the American Congress of Rehabilitation Medicine, past president of the American Association of Electromyography and Electrodiagnosis, past president of the American Academy of Physical Medicine and Rehabilitation, past president of the International Federation of Physical Medicine and Rehabilitation, and a member of the Medical Advisory Board of the National Multiple Sclerosis Society. He has over 60 publications among which is *Functional Assessment in Rehabilitation* (1984), edited with G.E. Gresham.

William H. Graves, Ed.D., Rehabilitation Research and Training Center on Blindness and Low Vision, Mississippi State University, P.O. Drawer 6189, Mississippi State, MS 39762.
William H. Graves is the director of the Rehabilitation Research and Training Center on Blindness and Low Vision and a professor of Counselor Education at Mississippi State University. He is a past president of the National Council on Rehabilitation Education, and a Mary E. Switzer Fellow. He chairs the Personnel Preparation Division of the Association for the Education and Rehabilitation of the Blind and Visually Im-

paired. He has been an officer and has held other leadership positions on the Board for Rehabilitation Certification and the National Rehabilitation Counseling Association. He has served on the editorial boards of the *Journal of Applied Rehabilitation Counseling* and *Journal of Rehabilitation Administration*; he currently serves on the editorial board of *Rehabilitation Education*. He is the co-editor of *Placement Services and Techniques*, and has published more than 25 journal articles.

Andrew S. Halpern, Ph.D., Clinical Services Building, University of Oregon, Eugene, OR 97405.

Andrew S. Halpern is the director of the Rehabilitation Research and Training Center in Mental Retardation, and a professor in the Division of Special Education and Rehabilitation at the University of Oregon. He has worked in a variety of positions during his career, including direct client service, university teaching, research, and agency administration. He has served as past president of the National Association of Rehabilitation Research and Training Centers, and as consulting editor to the *American Journal of Mental Deficiency*, the *Rehabilitation Counseling Bulletin, Career Development for Exceptional Individuals*, and the *Australia and New Zealand Journal of Developmental Disabilities*. A major focus of his research has been on instrument development and program evaluation, specifically in the areas of transition and community adjustment for adolescents and adults with disabilities. His publications include 3 books, 12 chapters in books, 4 test batteries, 1 set of curriculum materials, and approximately 30 journal articles.

Byron B. Hamilton, M.D., Ph.D., State University of New York at Buffalo, 462 Grider Street, Buffalo, NY 14215.

Byron B. Hamilton is a clinical associate professor of Rehabilitation Medicine, State University of New York at Buffalo. He is principal investigator of the project entitled, "Development of a Uniform Data System for Medical Rehabilitation," funded by the National Institute on Disability and Rehabilitation Research. He is a member of the National Task Force to Develop a Uniform Data System for Medical Rehabilitation. He was previously director of research at the Rehabilitation Institute of Chicago, and director of research for the NIDRR Rehabilitation Research and Training Center for Brain Injury and Stroke, Northwestern University, Chicago. His research interests and publications focus on evaluation of rehabilitation services.

Edward J. Hester, Ph.D., Return to Work Center, The Menninger Foundation, Jayhawk Tower, 700 Jackson, 9th Floor, Topeka, KS 66603.

Edward J. Hester received his doctorate in industrial psychology and psychometrics from Loyola University of Chicago. For the last 25 years he has been involved in rehabilitation program development, service delivery, and research. Dr. Hester is the inventor of the first computer-assisted vocational evaluation system. He is currently director of research of the Rehabilitation Research and Training Center in the Menninger Return to Work Center. Dr. Hester has been named a Switzer Scholar for 1986.

Mark V. Johnston, Ph.D., Office of Research, The New Medico Head Injury System, 78 Maplewood Shops, Northampton, MA 01060.

Mark V. Johnston is the senior research manager of The New Medico Head Injury System, where he specializes in computer management information systems, program evaluation, statistical analysis, and research on matters related to cost-effectiveness and cost-benefits in rehabilitation. He is chairman of the Ad Hoc Committee on Program Evaluation of the American Congress of Rehabilitation Medicine. In the past years he has served as director of program evaluation and development for rehabilitation and mental health at Glendale Adventist Medical Center, and consulted with rehabilitation facilities across the country. Recent publications include *Cost-Effectiveness of the Medicare Three-Hour Regulation* (1986), *Early Rehabilitation for Stroke Patients* (1983), *The Cost-Benefits of Stroke Rehabilitation* (1981), and *The Cost-Benefits of Medical Rehabilitation: Review and Critique* (1983).

Nicholas G. LaRocca, Ph.D., Medical Rehabilitation Research and Training Center for Multiple Sclerosis, The Albert Einstein College of Medicine, 1300 Morris Park Avenue, Bronx, NY 10461.

Nicholas G. LaRocca is an assistant professor of neurology (psychology) at The Albert Einstein College of Medicine. He holds a doctorate in clinical psychology, and is licensed for the practice of psychology in New York State. Dr. LaRocca coordinates research programs for the only Research and Training Center devoted exclusively to multiple sclerosis. He has contributed numerous chapters and articles on assessment in MS and on the psychological aspects of the disease. He coordinated the national field trials of the *Minimal Record of*

Disability, and co-edited the most recent revision. Dr. LaRocca is a frequent reviewer for the *Journal of Neurologic Rehabilitation*, and serves on the editorial boards of the *MS Quarterly Review* and *Rehabilitation Report*.

Margaret A. Nosek, Ph.D., Independent Living Research Utilization, 3233 Weslayan, Suite 100, Houston, TX 77027.

Margaret A. Nosek is an assistant professor in the department of rehabilitation, Baylor College of Medicine, and director of research for the ILRU Research and Training Center on Independent Living at The Institute for Rehabilitation and Research. She has published monographs, book chapters, articles, and conference reports on topics related to independent living. Specific topics included program models, philosophy, outcome assessment, program management, program evaluation, attendant services, and relationships with rehabilitation systems. She has also spoken and written on health maintenance and physical fitness for persons with disabilities. In the area of policy development, she researched and co-authored the *Long Range Plan for Texans with Disabilities* and the *National Policy for Persons with Disabilities*. She is a reviewer for *Rehabilitation Counseling Bulletin*, and was honored as a Switzer Scholar in 1985. Dr. Nosek has personal experience with disability, and a broad background in the independent living movement and in local, state, national, and international disability rights advocacy organizations.

Kent A. Questad, Ph.D., Department of Rehabilitation Medicine, University of Washington, RJ-30, Seattle, WA 98195.

Kent A. Questad received a bachelor of science degree in psychology from the University of Washington in 1975. He was subsequently employed as a research assistant and psychometrist in the Department of Rehabilitation Medicine of the University of Washington medical school where he worked on projects studying the needs of severely disabled persons and the activities of chronic pain patients. He completed a doctoral program in Rehabilitation Psychology at the University of Wisconsin, Madison, in 1983. He has published articles on topics ranging from chronic pain behavior to cognitive rehabilitation after brain injury. In 1983 he became a co-principle investigator in a 3-year project funded by the National Institute of Handicapped Research that studied the comprehensive recovery of patients after receiving a major burn injury.

Diana H. Rintala, Ph.D., Department of Rehabilitation, Baylor College of Medicine, 1333 Moursund Avenue, Houston, TX 77030.

Diana H. Rintala is an assistant professor of psychology at Baylor College of Medicine. She is director of the Behavioral Ecology Research Project that is involved in several studies regarding the rehabilitation outcomes and service needs of spinal cord injured persons after initial rehabilitation. Her other research interests include functional assessment methodology and treatment team functioning. She co-authored a chapter for *Functional Assessment in Rehabilitation*, and has written several research articles in rehabilitation journals. Her training as a social psychologist and subsequent work have involved considerable experience with statistics and research design.

Frances S. Sherwin, M.A., School of Health Related Professions, 435 Stockton Kimball Tower, State University of New York at Buffalo, 3435 Main Street, Buffalo, NY 14214.

Frances S. Sherwin is an assistant dean, School of Health Related Professions, SUNY at Buffalo. For the past 20 years, she has served as a technical writer and editor of numerous articles, grant proposals, and books on research in the areas of epidemiology, health services organization, nurse practitioners, allied health, orthopaedics, otolaryngology, and most recently, functional assessment in rehabilitation medicine.

Cynthia A. Stabenow, O.T.R., Arthritis Rehabilitation Unit Box 426, University of Virginia Medical Center, Charlottesville, VA 22908.

Cynthia A. Stabenow is an instructor in the division of rheumatology at the University of Virginia School of Medicine. Since 1983 she has been the coordinator of the Arthritis Rehabilitation Unit in the Rehabilitation Research and Training Center for Arthritis and Low Back Pain at the University of Virginia. She edited a chapter, "Physical Disabilities—Chronic Progressive Diseases," in Kielhofner's *A Model of Human Occupation* (1985). She was a member of the task force that developed *The Role and Function of Occupational Therapy in the Management of Patients with Rheumatic Diseases* approved by the Representative Assembly of the American Occupational Therapy Association (1986). She has presented several workshops on the role of occupational therapy in the evaluation and management of rheumatic disease patients.

John S. Tashman, M.S., 33 Amityville Road, Sound Beach, NY 11789.

John S. Tashman is a medical student at the State University of New York at Stony Brook. He has worked as a computer hardware and software consultant, and as a co-researcher in the departments of Rehabilitation Medicine at the Buffalo General Hospital and the Veterans Administration Medical Center, both located in Buffalo, NY. His research interests include development of software for a data-based system of evaluation for rehabilitation medicine; application of numerical optimization theory to human physiological systems; and digital acquisition, analysis, and control of data relating to those systems. His master's thesis in mechanical engineering is entitled "Constrained Optimization of the Electrically Induced Flexion Reflex of the Hemiplegic Via the Interior Penalty Function Formulation."

Karen A. Wagner, Ph.D., Department of Rehabilitation, Baylor College of Medicine, 1333 Moursund Avenue, Houston, TX 77030.

Karen A. Wagner is an assistant professor in the department of rehabilitation of Baylor College of Medicine. She is vice-president for education at The Institute for Rehabilitation and Research in Houston, and director of training in the Research and Training Center for the Rehabilitation of Persons with Spinal Cord Dysfunction at Baylor College of Medicine, supported by the National Institute on Disability and Rehabilitation Research. Her 15 years of professional experience include work in rehabilitation as director of rehabilitation counseling, and in acute medical care as a coordinator of research in neurosurgery. She has published in areas of head injury, spinal cord injury, and outcomes. She co-edited and contributed chapters to *Neurotrauma: Management, Rehabilitation and Related Issues, Volume I* (1986) and *Volume II* (1987).

Stephen T. Wegener, Ph.D., Department of Orthopedics and Rehabilitation, University of Virginia, Charlottesville, VA 22908.

Stephen T. Wegener is an assistant professor of orthopedics and rehabilitation and behavioral medicine and psychiatry. He is a clinical psychologist with research interests in chronic illness and pain management. He co-authored a monograph for the Arthritis Foundation, "Coping with Chronic Arthritis Pain," and has contributed to the *Chronic Pain Workbook*. He has published in *PAIN* and served as a reviewer for psychology and behavioral medicine journals.

Gale G. Whiteneck, Ph.D., Craig Hospital, 3425 South Clarkson Street, Englewood, CO 80110.

Gale G. Whiteneck is the director of research for Craig Hospital in Englewood, Colorado. Prior to specializing in spinal cord injury research, he was trained as a social science methodologist, and spent the early part of his career in applied research, program evaluation, and management information system design for a wide variety of health, education, and welfare programs. His recent spinal cord injury research has focused on functional assessment, handicap measurement, long-term outcomes, aging, and the cost of comprehensive life-time service delivery. In 1986, he received the Award for Excellence in Spinal Cord Injury Research from the American Spinal Injury Foundation for coordinating *A Collaborative Study of High Quadriplegia.*

Maria Zielezny, Ph.D., Department of Social and Preventive Medicine, SUNY at Buffalo, Buffalo, NY 14214.

Maria Zielezny is an associate professor of biostatistics in the department of social and preventive medicine, School of Medicine, State University of New York at Buffalo. She has over 20 years of experience as a statistical consultant for medical research at various medical school departments and health agencies. She is the author or co-author of over 40 research papers and book chapters. Her research includes developments and applications of multivariate statistical analysis, particularly in medicine and public health.

Preface

The conceptualization and measurement of rehabilitation outcomes warrant the utmost attention of rehabilitation service providers, administrators, researchers, educators, and policy analysts. The consideration of outcomes leads directly to questions about the very purposes of rehabilitation efforts and about grounds for our accountability as service providers. Additionally, there are factors operating currently that intensify the importance of thinking clearly about rehabilitation outcomes. One factor is the explosive growth of rehabilitation technologies, services, and techniques, each with its own rationale, advocates, and, typically, dearth of evidence for its effectiveness and efficiency. Another factor is looming change in how rehabilitation services are financed. Most observers agree that traditional, cost-based reimbursement will be replaced by other methods, perhaps involving prospective payment, that lend themselves more to cost containment objectives. It is widely feared that these changes will be associated with a decline in both the quality and outcomes of rehabilitative care. When the new reimbursement methods materialize, we will need to call on an armamentarium of tested research methods to document how client outcomes are being affected.

This volume encompasses outcome analysis in the areas of medical rehabilitation, vocational rehabilitation, psychiatric rehabilitation, the habilitation of persons with mental retardation, and independent living services. Thus, the book's design bucks the trend toward specialization and subspecialization in the human services generally, and in rehabilitation in particular. Its design reflects the conviction that there is a common core of values, attitudes, concepts, and practices that run throughout the different areas of rehabilitation. That commonality makes it likely that many problems and problem solutions pertaining to one area also apply to others.

Deficiencies in the quality of existing evidence regarding the effectiveness and efficiency of services surely emerge as a widely shared problem in rehabilitation. Common complaints include failure to employ research designs permitting causal inference, underspecification of the services provided, expedient study samples, unjustifiably brief follow-up intervals, and, above all, a paucity of formal studies of any kind. In view of this generally bleak state of the art, it is important to highlight occasional advances that occur in the conceptualization or investigation of rehabilitation outcomes. An example is development of the International Classification of Impairments, Disabilities, and Handicaps, supported by the World Health Organization (1980). It clarifies the focus of rehabilitation efforts and distinguishes them from other approaches to assisting persons with disability. A pan-rehabilitation view of outcome analysis is also potentially valuable for influencing research priorities by major sponsors (e.g., the National Institute of Handicapped Research[1]). That agency, as well as funding sources in the private sector, cannot be expected to elevate the importance assigned to rehabilitation outcome analysis unless the field itself subscribes to the import of that priority.

Many of the chapters dealing with applications of outcome analysis to particular impairment groups emerged from presentations at the May, 1985, annual conference in Washington, D.C., of the National Association of Rehabilitation Research and Training Centers. The choice of the conference theme, "Rehabilitation Outcome—How to Get It; How to Measure It; Implications for Policy," attests to current interest in the topic. The opportunity to recruit authors from among the presenters was important for two reasons. First, it was possible to achieve a reasonably comprehensive overview of the outcome topic because the 37 centers, spon-

---

[1]In the 1986 amendments of the Rehabilitation Act of 1973, the National Institute of Handicapped Research was renamed the National Institute on Disability and Rehabilitation Research. The former designation is retained throughout the text of this book because most of the editing had been completed before the renaming occurred.

sored by the National Institute of Handicapped Research, span much of the rehabilitation field. Second, the contemporaneity of the information was assured because the center's research typically represents the leading edge in their respective areas. Several chapters present findings that are unreported elsewhere.

This book has not been designed to compete with "how to" guides for conducting outcome analysis. Several detailed guides are available in the literature of health and human services, among the best being *Evaluation of Human Services* (Attkisson, Hargreaves, & Horwitz, 1978), *Evaluating the Impact of Health Programs* (Borus, Buntz, & Tash, 1982), *An Introduction to Program Evaluation* (Franklin & Thrasher, 1976), *Evaluation of Health Care* (Holland, 1983), *Evaluation Concepts and Methods: Shaping Policy for the Health Administrator* (Nutt, 1981), *Program Evaluation* (Posavac & Carey, 1980), *Health Program Evaluation* (Shortell & Richardson, 1978), and *Evaluation Research* (Weiss, 1972). Instead, the goal of the book is to promote the astute application of the principles and practices of outcome analysis to assessing the impacts of rehabilitation services. The writing is at a level appropriate for rehabilitation professionals and for graduate students preparing for careers in rehabilitation practice, administration, or research. Rehabilitation professionals are expected to find the material useful as a reference guide in planning outcome analysis or in critiquing the research of others. It also can serve as supplemental reading in graduate courses dealing with rehabilitation program management or research. The numerous disciplines for which the book is relevant include rehabilitation counseling, physiatry, special education, nursing, occupational therapy, physical therapy, psychology, and social work.

The book is organized in four sections. But first, Chapter 1 serves as an introduction by defining basic terms, distinguishing the principal purposes and types of outcome analysis, and discussing the design of outcome studies and the choice of measures. The chapter concludes by delineating a number of especially problematic issues in rehabilitation outcome analysis. The first section, Chapters 2 through 6, then reviews outcome analysis in the separate areas of medical rehabilitation, the habilitation of persons with mental retardation, psychiatric rehabilitation, vocational rehabilitation, and independent living. In each domain, information is provided about the nature of service interventions and target groups, kinds of outcomes and how they are operationalized, time frames within which outcomes are assessed, and additional research that warrants priority.

The next section, comprising Chapters 7 through 10, is concerned with methodological topics in outcome analysis that are pertinent to many different areas of rehabilitation. Chapter 7 deals with the choice of experimental designs, statistical analyses, and measures, and Chapter 8 examines the role of economic analyses. The authors of both chapters avoid a "cookbook" approach in favor of highlighting controversial issues and recommending solutions. Chapter 9, in contrast, provides abundant practical information about planning, executing, and reporting outcome studies in the context of operating rehabilitation programs. Chapter 10 concludes this section by describing development of an assessment tool potentially useful in standardizing the documentation of medical rehabilitation outcomes by facilities throughout this country.

The third section describes applications of outcome analysis to specific rehabilitation target groups. Included are persons with multiple sclerosis (Chapter 11), arthritis (Chapter 12), and burns (Chapter 13). The focus then shifts to infants and young children (Chapter 14) and to vision-impaired clients of state vocational rehabilitation agencies (Chapter 15). The section concludes with attention to persons with head injury (Chapter 16) and spinal cord injury (Chapter 17).

The policy implications of assessing rehabilitation outcomes are considered in the final section. Chapter 18 provides an illustration of how outcomes for persons with chronic mental illness are influenced by relationships between mental health and vocational rehabilitation agencies. Chapter 19 describes a policy-oriented study that emphasizes the importance of intervening while the disabled worker is still employed, instead of providing services after employment has been terminated. Chapter 20 illuminates ways in which policy changes of a major sponsor of services, the federal government, have an impact on rehabilitation services by influencing the care that patients receive before they are referred for rehabilitation. The book's last chapter considers how pending changes in health care policy and financing are likely to affect medical rehabilitation services and approaches to outcome analysis.

I want to acknowledge with deep appreciation the expert contributions of Carol A. Howland, who served as a consulting editor, and of Barbara Pascaretta, who assisted with the word processing and preparation of the manuscript.

REFERENCES

Attkisson, C.F., Hargreaves, W.A., & Horowitz, M.J. (Eds.). (1978). *Evaluation of human services*. New York: Academic Press.

Borus, M.E., Buntz, C.G., & Tash, W.R. (1982). *Evaluating the impact of health programs: A primer.* Cambridge, MA: MIT Press.

Franklin, J.L., & Thrasher, J.H. (1976). *An introduction to program evaluation*. New York: John Wiley & Sons.

Holland, W.W. (Ed.). (1983). *Evaluation of health care*. New York: Oxford University Press.

Nutt, P.C. (1981). *Evaluation concepts and methods: Shaping policy for the health administrator.* New York: SP Medical & Scientific Books.

Posavac, E.J., & Carey, R.G. (1980). *Program evaluation*. Englewood Cliffs, NJ: Prentice-Hall.

Shortell, S.M., & Richardson, W.C. (1978). *Health program evaluation*. St. Louis, MO: Mosby.

Weiss, C.H. (1972). *Evaluation research: Methods for assessing program effectiveness*. Englewood Cliffs, NJ: Prentice-Hall.

World Health Organization. (1980). *International classification of impairments, disabilities, and handicaps: A manual of classification relating to the consequences of disease*. Geneva: World Health Organization.

Dedicated with affection
to
William A. Spencer, M.D.

Rehabilitation Outcomes

Chapter 1

Overview of Outcome Analysis in Rehabilitation

Marcus J. Fuhrer

All sectors of rehabilitation are being buffeted currently by powerful winds of change. Important new components such as independent living and rehabilitation engineering services have been added relatively recently even while pressures for reducing overall service costs have increased. Traditional professional roles are being questioned in the face of mounting emphasis on self-help approaches administered by disabled persons themselves. These and other tensions are resulting in a reexamination of the basic premises of rehabilitation, including its purposes and justifications. Outcome analysis is at the forefront of such concerns because it encompasses the central question of what rehabilitation services ought to achieve for the persons receiving them. In turn, that question raises the issue of what rehabilitation actually achieves for service recipients and how those achievements can be identified and measured.

This chapter deals with many fundamental considerations involved in analyzing rehabilitation program outcomes. An objective is development of a framework to facilitate appreciation of subsequent chapters and of their interrelationship. A number of concepts are discussed, including rehabilitation program outcomes, impairment, disability, and handicap. The role of inferential logic in designating rehabilitation outcomes is emphasized. Four major purposes of rehabilitation outcome analyses are described, and two types of outcome analysis are differentiated. Approaches to designing outcome studies and selecting measures are then considered. The chapter concludes by identifying several major issues that characterize contemporary efforts to specify the impacts of rehabilitation programs.

CONCEPTUALIZING OUTCOMES, REHABILITATION, AND REHABILITATION OUTCOMES

In the literature of evaluation research, outcomes are understood to result from defined interventions. Interventions may range from being a specific service with readily delineated procedures and anticipated effects to being a program comprised of multiple services that are orchestrated to produce a complex, aggregate effect.

We are concerned in this book with programs that bear the designation "rehabilitation." *Rehabilitation outcomes* may be defined as changes produced by rehabilitation services in the lives of service recipients and their environment. The weakness of this definition is that no consensus exists about what is meant by "rehabilitation." This is due in part to the enormous diversity of interventions, target groups, and program goals to which the term is applied. As a result, most definitions of rehabilitation are notoriously

Preparation of this chapter was supported partially by the Research and Training Center for the Rehabilitation of Persons with Spinal Cord Dysfunction at Baylor College of Medicine and at The Institute for Rehabilitation and Research (National Institute of Handicapped Research Grant No. G008300044).

vague. For example, *Stedman's Medical Dictionary* (1982) defines rehabilitation as "restoration, following disease, illness, or injury, of ability to function in a normal or near normal manner." The meanings of "ability to function" and "in a normal or near normal manner" are elusive at best.

A definition of rehabilitation may be developed in one of two ways. The first, a "minimalist" approach, articulates the least common denominator underlying multifarious uses of the term in the health and social services. The definition quoted from *Stedman's* is an example. An alternative approach is to define rehabilitation in its fullest sense by attempting to state the meaning of "comprehensive rehabilitation." It may be defined as an individualized array of coordinated services aimed primarily at forestalling, minimizing, or reversing the occurrence of handicap, disability, and impairment. Essential service components of comprehensive rehabilitation are medical rehabilitation, psychosocial rehabilitation, and independent living services.

One of the strengths of this definition is its reliance on the *International Classification of Impairments, Disabilities, and Handicaps* (ICIDH) for assigning reasonably definite meaning to three salient characteristics of rehabilitation service recipients. According to the ICIDH, a development of the World Health Organization (WHO, 1980), *impairment* is "any loss or abnormality of psychological, physiological, or anatomical structure or function." Impairments are subclassified as intellectual, psychological, language-related, aural, ocular, visceral, skeletal, disfiguring, or "generalized sensory and other." The manner in which an impairment arises and the disease processes underlying it are not, in a formal sense, defining properties of that impairment. *Disability* is "any restriction or lack (resulting from an impairment) of ability to perform an activity in the manner or within the range considered normal for a human being" (WHO, 1980). As expressed by Wood and Badley (1980, p. 15), "disability is concerned with the restriction of compound integrated activities . . . such as represented by tasks, skills and behaviors." Subcategories of disability include communication, personal care, locomotion, and dexterity.

Handicap is "a disadvantage for a given individual, resulting from an impairment or disability, that limits or prevents the fulfillment of a role that is normal (depending on age, sex, social and cultural factors) for the individual. . . . Handicap thus represents socialization of an impairment or disability, and as such, reflects the consequences for the individual—cultural, social, economic, and environmental, that stem from the presence of impairment or disability" (WHO, 1980). The kinds and degree of handicap are shaped by the values, attitudes, and expectations comprising the individual's social environment. Among the dimensions of handicap specified are orientation, physical independence, mobility, occupation, social integration, and economic self-sufficiency.

To understand the potential role of rehabilitation services in having an impact on impairment, disability, and handicap, it is important to understand how these aspects of disablement may influence one another (Wood & Badley, 1980). Impairment contributes to the occurrence of disability, and both tend to produce handicaps of one kind or another. The sequence is merely probabilistic, however, so exceptions must be taken into account. For instance, the presence of impairment does not necessarily imply occurrence of disability or handicap. An individual with bilateral lower limb amputation is impaired, and may have locomotor disability, but may not be handicapped (e.g., disadvantaged in work or family roles). Stated more generally, severity at one level may not be commensurate with severity at other levels. A person with moderate facial disfigurement may exhibit little or no disability but be severely handicapped in some social situations. Nor is the direction of causation strictly one of impairment followed by disability followed by handicap. A succession of defeats in one's social role performance may result in a loss of morale reflected by inattention to personal care. If this happens to an individual with spinal cord injury, the result may be failure to practice self-management skills, associated with increased disability and development of pressure sores (an impairment).

To flesh out the definition of comprehensive rehabilitation, characterization of each of its three principal service components remains.

Medical rehabilitation may be understood as being an interdisciplinary medical activity, usually physician coordinated, that is provided to persons with chronic, physical disorders. It is aimed at ameliorating physical impairment, preventing the development of medical complications, and preserving and restoring functional capability needed for purposeful activity. As discussed more fully by Wagner (Chapter 2), medical rehabilitation stresses prevention of physiological or behavioral complications that tend to develop in association with the primary pathology and that are capable of producing impairment and disability. For some stroke patients, for example, preventable complications include physical deconditioning resulting from bedrest and passivity regarding self-care. Medical rehabilitation is sometimes termed "restorative medicine" to distinguish it from preventative and curative medicine.

As discussed by Alexander and Fuhrer (1984), *psychosocial rehabilitation* is an interdisciplinary process, principally educational in nature, intended to facilitate behavioral and psychological adaptation to impairment and disability and to enhance the person's performance in appropriate social roles, for example, as worker, student, and family member. Pertinent services include vocational counseling, social skills training, and family counseling.

Independent living services help persons with disability meet the demands of community life by providing assistance in recruiting and training personal care attendants, locating and maintaining appropriate housing, finding suitable transportation, obtaining financial support, and providing personal adjustment counseling, among other things. Although some of these services are provided by several different types of community agencies, they are provided most comprehensively by independent living programs (discussed by Nosek in Chapter 6).

Three remaining distinctions are worth making with regard to the definitions of rehabilitation and outcomes offered above. First, the terms in which rehabilitation is defined generally apply to the concept of *habilitation*. The principal difference is that rehabilitation refers to reacquiring lost ability; habilitation pertains to acquiring ability not possessed previously. The principal features of habilitative services for persons with mental retardation are described by Halpern (Chapter 3). Second, rehabilitation services are not restricted to persons with impairment, disability, or handicap. Authors such as Allen (Chapter 14) emphasize the importance of services directed to families that contain a disabled individual. The goal is not only better support of the disabled family member but also normalizing the lives of other family members. Third, the rehabilitation literature contains another usage of the term *outcomes* that is different from the proposed one and that is not associated with a particular intervention. For example, a chapter in a volume concerning the rehabilitation of patients with head injury contains a section entitled "Outcome" (Rimel & Jane, 1983). Among the topics discussed are mortality rates, the duration of coma, and the employment and financial status of these individuals 3 months after injury. Similar to discussions in the medical literature of the "natural history" of a disease, "outcome" is viewed implicitly as representing the cumulative impact of the individual's entire personal history following onset of the condition, and not solely as the result of a defined intervention.

REHABILITATION OUTCOMES AS INFERENCES

A rehabilitation outcome is never directly observed. One *can* observe improvements in clients' self-care skills following rehabilitation or the transformation from unemployment to employment. However, these changes per se are not rehabilitation outcomes. They become so only if we infer that the changes resulted from the services provided. In doing so, we directly confront the philosophical problem of causal attribution, that is, assigning the locus and extent of responsibility for observations made following an intervention. Imputations of causality are always fallible since they rest on a variety of assumptions, tacit understandings, and provisional hypotheses. Furthermore, two or more competing inferences about causation can almost always be drawn from a given set of observations.

There are two principal reasons why results of rehabilitation outcome studies are often equivocal. First, we know relatively little about *how* our interventions produce changes in service recipients. Therefore, we are unable to argue cogently why a given change should have been observed. Second, a multiplicity of factors can produce the changes that are observed. Postrehabilitation improvements on measures of impairment or disability may, for example, be due to remission of the underlying disease process and not to the services provided. Alternatively, a technologically sophisticated intervention may benefit patients because of the attention and social stimulation that therapists provide and not because of the intervention's technical features. Ambiguities of interpretation can be minimized, but not eliminated, by choosing outcome variables that are reasonably specific to the intervention being studied and by designing studies to neutralize the influence of factors other than the services provided. These strategies are discussed in a later portion of this chapter.

PURPOSES OF OUTCOME ANALYSIS

Rehabilitation outcome studies may have different purposes reflecting the interests of program managers, sponsors of the studies, outcome analysts themselves, or the perceived needs of audiences for which the information is intended. Most of these purposes fall into one of four groupings: 1) contributing to improved management of the program commissioning the study; 2) fulfilling quality assurance requirements of the program, 3) producing a foundation of generalizable knowledge for the rehabilitation disciplines, or 4) meeting the needs of policymakers. Although these four purposes are not mutually exclusive, studies reflecting one or the other tend to be different in focus, scope, and resourcing.

Management-Oriented Studies

To appreciate the role of outcome analysis in enhancing rehabilitation program management, one must understand the importance of program evaluation as an integral aspect of the management process. Evaluation of one kind or another

pervades each component of the management cycle. During program planning and design, evaluation is concerned principally with whether or not the proposed services are needed. Once the program is underway, monitoring is required to establish whether program procedures are working in the intended manner. Effective control requires answers to other questions dealing with program results. Do they conform with established goals for the program? Are the apparent results really attributable to program activities? In all of these instances, evaluation activities are intended to be at the service of management decision making of one kind or another.

There is an enormous literature discussing the principles and methods of program evaluation. An entree to that literature can be gained by reading any one of the references cited in the preface to this book.

Numerous classifications have been advanced to identify the principal foci of program evaluation. Suchman (1967) provided a particularly influential one, which follows:

"Effort"—The quality and quantity of program inputs, e.g., number of clients and kinds of sponsorship;

"Process"—The manner in which the program produces its outcomes;

"Performance"—Assessment of program outcomes;

"Efficiency"—Comparisons of program performance with costs that are incurred; and

"Adequacy"—The degree to which program performance meets existing needs.

For present purposes, this breakdown is important in making clear that program evaluation includes, but is not limited to, a focus on outcomes.

Rehabilitation program managers tend to be ambivalent about the imperativeness of conducting outcomes research in connection with evaluation. On the one hand, they subscribe to the importance of better standards of evidence regarding the effectiveness of their programs. Dependence on secondhand reports from clinical personnel or on occasional testimony by program recipients is recognized as being substandard compared to well-designed studies of the kind, amount, and durability of changes produced in service recipients. On the other hand, they recognize that obtaining the latter information entails considerable costs and that, even under the best circumstances, the information will not be available for a relatively long time after the service encounters that produced the outcomes. Consequently, managers usually require compelling reasons to undertake outcomes studies. Often these reasons pertain to sponsors' skepticism about the need for a current service or to the decision to introduce a costly new service. A wealth of practical information about conducting evaluation research within a particular rehabilitation setting is provided by Forer (Chapter 9).

Quality Assurance–Oriented Studies

Quality assurance procedures are designed to identify and correct deficiencies in the appropriateness and adequacy of client services. In connection with the delivery of health care services, quality assurance efforts changed in the 1950s from being voluntary to being required, first by the Joint Commission on the Accreditation of Hospitals and later by the federal government in connection with Medicare, Medicaid, and the community mental health program.

Donabedian (1966) first articulated a triad of concepts—structure, process, and outcome—that continue to encompass the thrust of quality assurance efforts. The structural approach involves an examination of program features that include the physical plant, characteristics of the staff, and administrative practices such as recordkeeping. The process approach is concerned with the degree to which client services conform with criteria indicative of acceptable care. Outcomes are understood very much in the sense used in this chapter.

Quality assurance procedures are implemented mostly by service providers themselves. Process and outcome determinations rely principally upon reviewing individual client records against consensually derived norms or mandated standards of care. Reports are generated documenting deficiencies and recommending correctives that, for the most part, are to be undertaken by the clinical staff. In practice, quality assurance efforts have placed less emphasis on outcomes than on process considerations. This seems to be changing, however, because of the realization that the character of outcomes is not guaranteed by the quality of the services provided (Baker, 1983; Green & Attkisson, 1984).

Discipline-Oriented Studies

The many disciplines contributing to rehabilitation share the goal of producing a body of theory, empirical generalizations, and systematic data to understand why rehabilitation services have the effects they do and to develop improved services. A derivative goal, one shared with other scholarly communities, is to enlarge understanding of the nature and implications of disability and handicap.

Many discipline-oriented outcome studies conform to a research model comprised of five classes of variables pertaining to: 1) service recipients, 2) service recipients' environment, 3) rehabilitation interventions, 4) time, and 5) observed results. Service recipient variables may pertain to the types and severity of impairments, disabilities, or handicaps as well as to age, economic status, educational attainment, or intelligence. Environmental factors may include degree of family support, ethnic background, availability of transportation, or status of the local economy. Rehabilitation interventions deal with the nature and intensity of the services provided. Time, a frequently overlooked consideration, may involve a variety of different intervals, such as between the occurrence of impairment and admission to a rehabilitation program or between discharge and follow-up. As suggested by the definition offered for rehabilitation outcomes, observed results may be classified according to whether they deal with service recipients' impairments, disabilities, or handicaps. A good deal of current rehabilitation research is devoted to understanding how results are influenced by varying an intervention and holding constant the other classes of variables. Other research holds constant the service being provided and attempts to learn how outcomes can be predicted by characteristics of service recipients or their environment. The study by Giesen and Graves (Chapter 15) of vocational rehabilitation

outcomes for visually impaired clients exemplifies the latter kind of investigation.

Policy-Oriented Studies

Outcomes research may be undertaken to illuminate public policy options regarding the rehabilitation system and the status of disabled persons.
Such studies are frequently instigated by federal
or state agencies responsible for the organization,
delivery, and financing of services for disabled
persons. Examples are studies of the state-federal
vocational rehabilitation program (Bolton, Chapter 5) and the Centers for Independent Living
Programs (Nosek, Chapter 6), both administered
by the Rehabilitation Services Administration.
Investigator-instigated outcome studies of a pol-
icy-analytic nature are rare in the rehabilitation
literature, a notable example being DeJong's
(1981) investigation of outcomes for persons with
spinal cord injury.

There are a number of hallmarks of policy-rel-
evant outcomes research. Perhaps most important, the research is expressly designed to answer
a policy question. Research undertaken for other
reasons may have policy implications, but the results are often too equivocal to influence policy.
The timeliness of policy-oriented information is
frequently paramount because the decisions to be
clarified are embedded in fast-moving events.
Particular emphasis is placed on independent
variables that are—or can become—a reflection
of public policy, such as different ways of financing services or defining service eligibility. Consistent with the intimate relationship between
policy research and practical politics, results
often need to be interpreted from multiple perspectives of different interest groups, within both
the rehabilitation community and the public at
large. In disseminating results, a premium is often
placed on face-to-face communication with decision makers or, more frequently, with members
of their staff, supplemented by comparatively
brief written reports in nontechnical language.

TYPES OF OUTCOME ANALYSIS

There are two basic kinds of outcome analyses,
those bearing on an intervention's effectiveness

and those dealing with its efficiency. A program
is effective to the extent that its performance is
congruent with expectations. Efficiency is concerned with the relationship between an intervention's outputs and inputs. It involves consideration, therefore, of an intevention's effectiveness
with respect to the resources consumed by it.

The distinction between analyses of program
effectiveness and program efficiency is not
meant to imply that studies of effectiveness must
ignore resource and cost considerations. Some
program goals may well be concerned with resource utilization, stating, for instance, that
charges be at or below competitors' or not exceed
a maximum level specified by sponsors. However, as discussed below, efficiency analyses are
distinctive for emphasizing a systematic treatment
of outcomes in relation to costs so that competing
programs can be compared.

Analyses of Effectiveness

A program's effectiveness depends upon how
closely its performance conforms with expectations. Many but not all of those expectations concern the outcomes to be achieved. Outcome expectations may be drawn from statements
describing program goals or from a more or less
explicit conceptual model of the program articulated by individuals either inside or outside of it.
Each of these sources of outcome expectations is
discussed in turn.

Goal Statements   The commonsense notion that outcome expectations for a program can
be extracted from its explicit goal statements is
often contradicted by experience. All too frequently, the language in which goals are expressed is ambiguous or clouded in rhetoric
intended for fund raising or mobilizing constitu-
ency support. In other instances, idealized long-
range aims are substituted where more concrete,
nearer term objectives are called for. In addition,
although managers may agree on a program's
several goals, they frequently disagree about the
relative importance of the separate goals.

Several different systematic procedures can be
used to promote greater consensus about program goals and their relative importance (Nutt,
1981). One of these, the Delphi process, is a mul-
tistage procedure that is adaptable in a number of

ways. For instance, participants such as upper-level management personnel and trusteeship members can be asked first to list what they believe are appropriate goals for the program. This material is then edited to obtain a representative, nonredundant listing of possible program goals. An indication is also provided of the frequency with which each goal was mentioned. That information is returned to participants to obtain an indication of goal statements to which they subscribe. In a subsequent stage, participants may be asked to rate the importance they assign to the more widely endorsed goals.

Program Modeling Outcome expectations also may emerge from efforts to model conceptually how a particular program appears to be working. The model attempts to characterize key features of a program, for example, its clientele, referral sources, and clinical operations. An effort is also made to specify causal linkages among program features and to articulate the rationale for those linkages so their plausibility can be assessed. In short, the model is a kind of mini-theory about how the program operates that allows one to deduce expectations about what the program's impacts should be.

The model of an operating program may point to outcomes that are negative in connotation. Undesirable outcomes are imaginable and they are not constituted merely by failure to achieve desired results. A novel vocational rehabilitation program may, for example, not only fail to place clients in remunerative employment, but also foster dependence on professional intercession at the expense of client initiative. Many commentators have urged that outcome studies be capable of revealing both the good and the bad news about a program. They fault studies that are limited solely to evaluating whether or not a program has achieved its expressed goals because goals are usually expressed exclusively in terms of benefits for service recipients.

Other Characteristics of Outcome Expectations A number of considerations should be kept in mind in formulating rehabilitation outcome expectations, whether as part of goal statements or a program model.

Impacts of a program may be viewed from quite different perspectives involving different value systems. The value perspectives of the disabled individual, society, and sponsors are three examples. The outcomes that each cherish are by no means the same. As voiced by the independent living movement, disabled persons emphasize outcomes consistent with their maintaining control over their own lives. Society's traditional concern is for the vocational and avocational productivity of its adult members, including those with disability. For sponsors, the overarching concern is minimization of total costs. Important potential benefits of a program may be overlooked if only some of these value perspectives are considered.

Value considerations also may clash if viewed separately from the standpoint of disability or handicap. For example, dependency may be permitted in everyday activities in order to diminish the handicap. Thus, persons with upper extremity weakness who are relatively slow dressing themselves may accept assistance in dressing if that dependency facilitates being on time at work.

Outcome expectations may be ordered on the grounds of logic, theory, or experience. The fact that some expectations may be formulated concretely and others abstractly makes it possible on logical grounds to subsume some expectations under others. Ability to use a motorized wheelchair is highly concrete; this ability as well as ambulation can be subsumed under the concept of mobility. Expectations also can be ordered in terms of presumed or demonstrated causal connections. For example, becoming employed may be expected to result in increased personal income, reduced transfer payments, and a likely increase in service recipients' satisfaction with their own lives. In designing a study, it is important to identify such logical relations among potential outcomes so that redundancy of measurement is avoided and gaps are covered.

Program outcomes can be ordered according to whether they are susceptible to short- or long-term realization. Demonstrable familiarity with self-care procedures or achievement of remunerative employment are examples of relatively proximate rehabilitation outcomes. Outcomes such as near-normal life expectancy or sustained job satisfaction can only be documented long after program completion. The distinction is a significant one because it is certainly possible for an intervention to produce its intended short-term outcomes but to have minimal long-term impacts.

The effects of rehabilitation may be expected to reverberate well beyond immediate service recipients. Consider the implications of successfully enhancing an individual's self-care skills and mobility. According to Hammerman and Maikowski (1981), such achievements may result in reducing demands on family members who are assisting the recipient, allowing them a greater opportunity to earn and to participate in community affairs. Increased self-care and mobility is also expected to allow the individual to participate more fully in community affairs, and that in turn is expected to contribute to improving community attitudes toward disabled persons.

Outcome expectations may be expressed in monetary or non-monetary terms. Increased earnings following rehabilitation is an example of a monetary variable; enhanced quality of life exemplifies a non-monetary one. Important alternatives exist between such obvious extremes. Being rehospitalized following medical rehabilitation is not a monetary outcome, although there are distinct monetary implications to rehospitalization. According to Johnston (1983), the duration of rehospitalization correlates very highly with total hospital charges, and those charges comprise the largest portion of direct disability costs. Reducing the incidence and duration of rehospitalization is thus one of the intended outcomes of medical rehabilitation. This is not to say, however, that reducing rehospitalization is important on monetary grounds alone. The setbacks that occur to patient and family morale and the discontinuities that occur in work and schooling are no less real (Meyers et al., 1985).

Analyses of Efficiency

We live in a world in which available resources are patently insufficient to pursue all of society's laudable goals. Resources devoted to one program are unavailable for another. The reality of scarcity underscores the imperative that costs be considered in deciding to undertake or sustain a program. Even demonstrably successful programs should be subject to having their efficiency scrutinized because it is possible that other programs can produce the same benefits at lower costs.

Programs consume many kinds and amounts of resources in the course of producing outcomes. Analyses of efficiency relate measures of program effectiveness to program costs. The fundamental question is, "Are the outcomes worth it?" That question can be addressed from either of two standpoints: benefit–cost analysis or cost-effectiveness analysis. Each in turn is discussed briefly below, and extended discussion is provided by Johnston (Chapter 8).

Benefit–cost analysis represents an attempt to designate all the benefits and costs of a program in monetary terms so they can be compared. The goal is to estimate return on investment considered as the ratio of benefits to costs or as net benefits, that is, benefits minus costs. Viewed by itself, a program is deemed successful if the benefit–cost ratio exceeds unity or if net benefits are positive. More typically, benefit–cost analysis is conducted to compare the ratios of different programs that are competing for resource allocations.

The principles of benefit–cost analysis are readily communicated, but their realization is plagued by a number of difficulties. One problem is the need to assess comprehensively both the benefits and costs of competing programs. Underrepresenting one program's costs or ignoring some of the benefits of a competing program assures an inequitable comparison of benefit–cost ratios. Another problem is that, for human services generally and rehabilitation especially, some program benefits, such as greater social participation by service recipients, are not directly expressable in monetary terms. Although means have been developed to express the equivalent monetary value of such benefits (e.g., Cardus, Fuhrer, & Thrall, 1981), the methods require assumptions to be made that may not be widely shared.

Cost-effectiveness analysis is an attractive alternative to benefit–cost analysis because it relaxes the constraint that benefits and costs be expressed in the same metric. Instead, benefits may be formulated in any one of a variety of terms, such as improvement in functional status or fewer episodes of ill health, and only costs need be expressed in monetary terms. The intent of cost-effectiveness analysis is to compare interventions having the same goal but different means of attaining it. For instance, two medical rehabilitation programs treating patients with the same condition might be compared in terms of which produces more average improvement in functional status per dollar charged. Cost-effectiveness comparisons can be problematic because rehabilitation programs are typically quite complex in the sense of having manifold objectives. Even programs sharing the same general goal and focusing on the same target groups are likely to differ in some of their specific objectives. At some point, those differences become numerous enough to conclude that the programs are not comparable in their goals. That is a difficult judgment to make, but it must be made to avoid invidious applications of cost-effectiveness analysis.

STRATEGY AND DESIGN OF OUTCOME STUDIES

The design of an outcome investigation involves a host of decisions, including criteria for enrolling subjects into the study, the number of subjects, the composition of groups whose data will be compared, and the occasions on which data will be acquired. An optimal design is one that uses the minimum amount of resources (e.g., number of subjects and amount of staff time) in providing the least equivocal answer to the question being posed.

The manifold questions that may be addressed by a rehabilitation outcome study include the following:

1. Do changes observed in service recipients after the intervention meet expectations or predesignated standards?
2. Are the changes better than those produced by the best established alternative intervention?
3. Which features of the intervention contribute to the outcomes?
4. Can even better changes be produced by altering one or more of those features?

5. Are changes observed for some types of service recipients better than those obtained for others?
6. What characteristics of service recipients at admission predict the amount of change the intervention will produce?

Choosing Study Questions

The salience of particular questions may be influenced by three considerations: the type of program, its developmental status, and the assumptions study designers are willing to make.

Many different program typologies are offered in the program evaluation literature. For present purposes, it is sufficient to emphasize the difference between a program intended to generate evaluation data and an established program for which management-relevant information is sought. The former is exemplified by service demonstration projects intended to show the feasibility and effectiveness of an innovative idea. Funding agencies generally will not support such demonstrations unless they embody a strong outcome study plan. Investigation of whether observed effects are causally attributable to the service innovation is often part of the plan. The question of causality is typically less prominent in management-oriented studies conducted by established programs. In these studies, questions are more likely to concern whether a change in a component service or the addition of a new service is producing the client changes that are expected.

The question a study is designed to answer also may reflect a program's developmental status. Early in a program's evolution, outcome studies may be postponed altogether in favor of process-oriented investigation intended to confirm that the program is operating as originally envisioned. Initial outcome studies may simply describe postintervention changes in service recipients and compare those changes with expectations. Studies designed to answer whether client changes are attributable to program operations are subject to postponement until those operations are judged to be stable. Stability of operation is no less a prerequisite for answering many of the other outcome questions listed above (Cronbach et al., 1980).

Finally, the choice of study questions also reflects the questioner's perspective, experience, and assumptions. Rehabilitation program managers who witness performance of their programs each working day may be satisfied that observed client changes are attributable to the services being provided. Their questions may simply be whether those changes are occurring to a satisfactory degree for an acceptable proportion of clients. On the other hand, policymakers interested in fostering such a program nationally may be unwilling to take for granted the program's causal significance and may insist upon a properly controlled study to resolve that uncertainty.

A sense of a program's purposes, developmental status, and the assumptions that reasonably can be made about it are all bases for developing a strategy of outcomes investigation tailored to a particular situation. In such a strategy, projected studies are ordered either in parallel or sequentially so that results of one interdigitate with the others. Failure at the onset to devise a prudent overall strategy may result in overloading the initial study with more questions than can be satisfactorily resolved or in calling for such extensive resources that launching the study is jeopardized.

Selecting a Design

Rintala (Chapter 7) reviews many of the study designs that are available to address particular outcome issues. She shares the viewpoint of prominent methodologists such as Campbell and Stanley (1966) and Cronbach (1978) that there is no such thing as the "best" design independent of the question being posed. There is a definite role, for example, for the simple "pre–post" design in which the same measures are obtained before and after an intervention, with no control group being involved. Results of such a study may be entirely appropriate for deciding whether average changes in service recipients are congruent with management expectations. The venerated random assignment control group design should be reserved principally for situations in which the question is whether or not the intervention is responsible for the changes observed.

When causation is the issue, there are important alternatives to the random assignment control group design. Designated "quasi-experimental designs" by Campbell and Stanley (1966), they do not involve the thorny problems of randomly assigning subjects to treatment and control groups. Quasi-experimental designs are often more feasible to undertake, but they cannot rule out as wide a range of competing explanations of observed results.

To this point, the discussion has focused upon a design's "internal validity," that is, the degree to which causal explanations are ruled out other than ones pertaining to the intervention. Another characteristic of designs is their "external validity" (Campbell & Stanley, 1966). Externally valid findings are those that can be generalized across settings, persons, dependent variables, or time. External validity is threatened, for example, when results depend importantly on a service provider's specific practice style or upon particular historical events associated with the intervention. The external validity of many rehabilitation outcome studies is jeopardized by the common practice of acquiring data solely from service recipients involved in a particular program. Instead of being due simply to the intervention itself, the results of such a study also may be attributable to characteristics of the clients that led them to be referred to the program or to seek it out. There is no assurance that the results would apply to groups free of such selection biases. The correctives—replication of an initial study or cooperative studies in which samples are drawn from multiple sites—are rarely employed.

Taking Time into Account

Time considerations loom large in designing rehabilitation outcome studies for at least two reasons. First, the consequences of a service may require some time to become apparent. For example, Farkas and Anthony (Chapter 4) cite evidence that the likelihood of a successful vocational rehabilitation outcome increases with time elapsed since the completion of services. Second, the durability of changes produced by rehabilitation services is a major consideration in weighing their efficacy. Although some rehabilitation interventions are expected to have lifelong impacts, the common practice is to document outcomes at a single follow-up contact relatively soon after the termination of services. The hazards of this practice are illustrated by results of a study by Garraway, Akhtar, Hockey, and Prescott (1980). They investigated effects of an occupational therapy program for stroke patients and found that, 3 months after discharge, the treated group exceeded a control group in levels of independence. One year later, however, the treated group decreased in independence while the control group increased. Contrary evidence also exists. Forer (Chapter 9) cites several studies indicating that the functional status of patients continues to improve following discharge from an inpatient rehabilitation program.

CRITERIA AND MEASURES

Designating Criteria for Outcome Expectations

An outcomes study may be impeccably designed and implemented, but fail miserably because the data collected about program participants are tangential to the outcome expectations of interest. The fault often lies with the fact that the outcome expectations were formulated too abstractly to suggest how they should be measured, resulting in measures being chosen arbitrarily. Disappointments of this kind are less likely if an additional planning step is interjected between formulating outcome expectations and selecting measures. That step involves developing criteria applicable to each program expectation. The criteria are such that, when they are fulfilled, the outcome expectation is considered to have been accomplished. The emphasis is upon operationally defining the criteria to facilitate the choice of measures.

The sequence of generating outcome expectations, operationally defining criteria, and choosing pertinent measures is exemplified by DeJong's (1981) study of independent living outcomes for persons with spinal cord injury. After explicitly defining what was meant by "independent living," two pertinent criteria were stipulated: restrictiveness of the individual's living arrangement and the individual's level of productivity. Measurement scales were developed by identifying 7 different living arrangements and 12 kinds of productivity, which were separately rank ordered and weighted by a panel of judges.

Choosing Measures

The research literature is replete with measures pertinent to criteria associated with various rehabilitation outcome expectations. Consequently, planning an outcomes study is most often a matter of selecting from among available measures rather than devising new ones.

There are many different sources and techniques of data collection. Data sources include existing service records of the program itself, program staff, program participants, persons outside the program who are knowledgeable about service recipients, and outcome study staff members. Data collection techniques include questionnaires, interviews, behavioral observations (including ratings and unobtrusive measures), and tests. Each source and technique has its distinctive assets and liabilities. The many tradeoffs involved are discussed at length in the program evaluation literature (e.g., Franklin & Thrasher, 1976; Posavac & Carey, 1980; Shortell & Richardson, 1978), in the rehabilitation research literature (e.g., Granger & Gresham, 1984; Halpern & Fuhrer, 1984), and in this book as well (Rintala, Chapter 7; Forer, Chapter 9). The discussion that follows is admittedly selective, reflecting the author's experience in choosing outcome measures.

One's first inclination may be to exploit available clinical or administrative records for clients served by the program under study. Overall costs of using such data are relatively low, notwithstanding expenses in retrieving the information and organizing it into a useful form. However, there are numerous pitfalls in attempting to use such data. For example, functional scales used by clinicians to track patients' progress may be of uncertain reliability and may be much more detailed than needed for outcome studies. Because record keeping has a relatively low priority within service programs, the data also suffer frequently from incompleteness and inaccuracy.

If the decision is made to acquire specialized data, self-administered questionnaires or telephone interviews are relatively low-cost alternatives. Questionnaires are particularly indicated when the information to be obtained is highly structured, for instance, is amenable to a multiple-choice answer format. Potentially disappointing rates of return of mailed questionnaires can be largely avoided by using reminder letters or follow-up phone calls. Telephone interviews are being used increasingly to obtain data from clients who have completed a rehabilitation program and returned to the community. Queries need not be structured to the extent necessary for self-administered questionnaires, although more open-ended questions put a considerable burden on subsequent effort to analyze content and code the answers.

For longitudinal studies tracking patients over the course of inpatient rehabilitation and thereafter in the community, a difficult choice is whether to assess functional status in terms of capability or actual performance. Capability, for example, in dressing or self-feeding, is assessed typically by a staff person who defines the task for the patient using standardized instructions and who then rates the amount of assistance the patient requires to perform the task. Actual performance can be documented simply by asking the patient how those activities were undertaken that day or during a typical day in the recent past. Proponents of assessing actual performance argue that a foremost objective of rehabilitation is to impact the service recipient's performance in daily life. Advocates of assessing capability point out that actual daily performance is greatly influenced by circumstances (e.g., availability of helpers or the time pressures of a particular day's schedule) and that documenting capability at least establishes the person's performance possibilities. In most outcome studies, functional status is assessed in terms of capability while the individual is a rehabilitation inpatient and in terms of self-reported typical performance after the person has returned home. This practice confounds two potential influences on functional status scores, one pertaining to staff-member observation versus self-report, the other pertaining to the

assessment of capability versus typical performance.

Considering the different sources and techniques of data collection highlights the fact that each has distinctive advantages, disadvantages, and indications for appropriate use. When possible, it is desirable to use more than one source or technique, especially for outcome expectations of particular importance in the given study. When the results of different measures converge, conclusions are strengthened. When they diverge, otherwise premature interpretation can be avoided.

OTHER SELECTED ISSUES IN REHABILITATION OUTCOME ANALYSIS

The subsequent discussion touches on several especially problematic features of rehabilitation outcome analysis that warrant additional comment.

The Ambitiousness of Expectations

Rehabilitation service providers may demonstrate considerable ambivalence in attempting to articulate expected outcomes of their programs, especially those that are relatively more comprehensive in character. On the one hand, there is a desire to express expectations that are very general and long range, for example, restoration of the individual to the highest possible level of independence and productivity. Narrower goals such as increasing self-care skills or obtaining employment are perceived as falling short of meeting the client's total needs and as understating the societal relevance of rehabilitation services. More broadly formulated, far-reaching goal statements are valued because they provide a basis for defining program standards, highlighting resources needed to provide more effective services, and indicating lines along which new service developments should proceed. On the other hand, rehabilitation providers are troubled by the affirmation of global, long-range goals, the accomplishment of which depends on many factors outside the control of their programs. These factors include clients' access to other community services, a supportive family, and a sound local economy. If these influences are working against clients, even the best conducted rehabilitation program is vulnerable to not meeting its goals.

Integrating the individual rehabilitation program into a coordinated system of other programs is one way to resolve the dilemma posed by cherished long-range rehabilitation goals and sharply constrained resources. A coordinated system of services is one in which clients' changing needs are anticipated and timely referrals are made to appropriate services as needs change. The potential importance of a systems approach to organizing services is emphasized by Farkas and Anthony (Chapter 4) for psychiatric rehabilitation, by Halpern (Chapter 3) for the habilitation of persons with mental retardation, by Diller and Ben-Yishay (Chapter 16) for persons with head injury, and by Whiteneck (Chapter 17) for persons with spinal cord injury. For individuals sustaining acute onset of a severe physical impairment such as spinal cord injury or multiple amputation, such a system may include acute care hospitalization to stabilize the individual medically; medical rehabilitation services to restore health and teach self-care skills; independent living services to provide assistance with housing, attendant care, or transportation; and vocational rehabilitation to facilitate career development. Globally defined outcome expectations involving maximization of health, independence, productivity, and quality of life seem appropriate for evaluating such service systems, while more narrowly delineated expectations seem appropriate for assessing the component services.

Documenting Program Processes

A major weakness of many rehabilitation outcome studies is insufficient data about the nature of the program intervention. It becomes impossible, therefore, to pinpoint features of the program to which the observed effects are attributable. One cannot depend wholly on program descriptions provided by administrators or on a program's stated goals because actual operations frequently depart from the intentions of managers or planners. Objective data need to be provided regarding, for example, the composition of the professional staff, the manner in which individual client services are coordinated, the nature and duration of the services provided, and sources of client sponsorship. Without this information, the investigator is at risk of attributing outcomes, either positive or negative, to a program that never actually existed. Efforts to generalize results to other programs are jeopardized, as are opportunities to replicate the program elsewhere.

Lack of Theory

References to theory are lacking in most studies of rehabilitation outcomes. As much as anything else, this omission reflects unavailability of well-elaborated theories of rehabilitation and disablement. The paucity of theory makes it difficult to organize knowledge in the field of rehabilitation into a coherent framework (Brown, Gordon, & Diller, 1983). Another result is inability to arrive deductively at well-formulated hypotheses regarding new, potentially effective interventions. Consequently, the development of new treatment methods becomes a matter of trial and error based on informed speculation. Relationships among problems encountered during service provision are not made explicit, so attempted solutions tend to be piecemeal.

The absence of sound theory also impairs both the formulation and interpretation of outcome studies. Since rehabilitation services are typically comprised of a large number of component interventions, it is difficult, without theory, to distinguish service components that are necessary conditions for achieving desired effects from those that are merely facilitative.

The ICIDH affords a promising, albeit partial, foundation for a satisfactory theory of disablement and the rehabilitation process. The constructs of impairment, disability, and handicap are cogently formulated, amenable to operationalization, and potentially comprehensive from the standpoint of rehabilitation program goals. A theory constructed on that conceptual foundation would explain, for example, why there are such prominent individual differences in the severity of disability, despite similar kinds and degrees of impairment. A parallel effort will be required to model essential characteristics of the rehabilitation process as they impact impairment, disability, and handicap. Noteworthy in that regard are the promising notions outlined by Brown et al. (1983).

An adequate theory of disablement and rehabilitation will also emphasize the importance of environmental features—social, material, and attitudinal—that impinge on the individual with impairment to moderate the occurrence or degree of disability and handicap. Although rehabilitation professionals pay lip service to the tenet that behavior results from the interaction of factors within both the individual and the environment, the causal significance of environmental influences is repeatedly neglected in formulating the goals of rehabilitation services, selecting interventions, and assessing outcomes. This neglect is due in part to the unavailability of a classification system and related measures for delineating environmental features and operationalizing pertinent variables (e.g., DeJong, 1981; Trieschmann, 1980). Only a smattering of relevant research developments has been reported. One example is the Environmental Negotiability Survey developed as part of the Longitudinal Functional Assessment System (Rintala et al., 1984). The survey quantifies the proportion of objects within the living setting that can be used by the individual without the aid of someone else.

CONCLUSION

The future of rehabilitation outcome analysis in terms of its volume and direction will continue to mirror changes in the climate within which rehabilitation services are provided. The sheer number of studies can be expected to increase as rehabilitation accommodates to the value systems of its practitioners, the public at large, spokespersons for disabled persons, and sponsors of service. The criteria for successful rehabilitation embedded in those value systems are likely to re-main inconsistent, if not outright contradictory. Spokespersons for interests of the general public will continue to assign highest priority to maximizing the social productivity of disabled persons, regarding both their vocational and avocational activity. Third-party sponsors who are not liable for the individual's lifelong disability costs will emphasize the cheapness of the immediate services for which they are responsible. Sponsors with longer term responsibility are less likely to view immediate service costs in isolation and are more likely to emphasize minimization of long-range, total costs associated with illness and dependency. Advocates for disabled persons will endorse the concern for eliminating dependency, although with qualification, because some degree of personal assistance is essential if many severely disabled persons are to retain options that make their lives fulfilling. Such diverse priorities will put a premium on designing multipronged studies that encompass the variety of outcome measures necessary to address these differing criteria of successful rehabilitation.

An increasing emphasis on formal outcome research will both contribute to and reflect adoption of a higher standard of evidence for judging the merits of current rehabilitation services and the promise of service innovations. In a bygone era in which the costs of innovations could be passed on almost automatically to sponsors, decisions to introduce new interventions into routine practice often reflected the viewpoint, "If it seems promising, let's do it." Now, in the prevailing climate of concern for reducing service costs, proposals to introduce new services are met with the challenge, "Show me that it works and that it's cheaper." The cost-effectiveness studies needed to address that challenge will serve the dual purpose of helping us weigh the effectiveness of contemporary practices as well as assess the potential benefits of newly developed ones. A proliferation of such studies will signify an important maturational milestone for the field as a whole.

REFERENCES

Alexander, J. L., & Fuhrer, M. J. (1984). Functional assessments of individuals with physical impairments. In A. S. Halpern & M. J. Fuhrer (Eds.), *Functional assessment in rehabilitation* (pp. 45–60). Baltimore: Paul H. Brookes Publishing Co.

Baker, F. (1983). Quality assurance and program evaluation. *Evaluation and the Health Professions, 6,* 149–160.

Brown, M., Gordon, W. A., & Diller, L. (1983). Functional assessment and outcome measurement: An integrative review. In E. L. Pan, T. E. Backer, & C. L. Vash (Eds.), *Annual Review of Rehabilitation* (pp. 93–120). New York: Springer-Verlag.

Campbell, D. T., & Stanley, J. C. (1966). *Experimental and quasi-experimental designs for research.* Chicago: Rand McNally.

Cardus, D., Fuhrer, M. J., & Thrall, R. M. (1981). Quality of life in benefit-cost analysis of rehabilitation research. *Archives of Physical Medicine and Rehabilitation, 62,* 209–212.

Cronbach, L. J. (1978). *Designing educational evaluations.* Palo Alto, CA: Stanford University.

Cronbach, L. J., Ambron, S. R., Dornbusch, S. M., Hess, R. D., Hornik, R. C., Phillips, D. C., Walker, D. F., & Weiner, S. S. (1980). *Toward reform of program evaluation.* San Francisco: Jossey-Bass.

DeJong, G. (1981). *Environmental accessibility and independent living outcomes: Directions for disability policy and research.* East Lansing: Michigan State University, University Center for International Rehabilitation.

Donabedian, A. (1966). Evaluating the quality of medical care. *Millbank Memorial Fund Quarterly, 44,* 166–206.

Franklin, J. L., & Thrasher, J. H. (1976). *An introduction to program evaluation.* New York: John Wiley & Sons.

Garraway, W. M., Akhtar, A. J., Hockey, L., & Prescott, R. J. (1980). Management of acute stroke in the elderly: Follow-up of a controlled trial. *British Medical Journal, 281,* 827–829.

Granger, C. V., & Gresham, G. E. (Eds.) (1984). *Functional assessment in rehabilitation medicine.* Baltimore: Williams & Wilkins.

Green, R. S., & Attkisson, C. C. (1984). Quality assurance and program evaluation. *American Behavioral Scientist, 27,* 552–582.

Halpern, A. S., & Fuhrer, M. J. (Eds.). (1984). *Functional assessment in rehabilitation.* Baltimore: Paul H. Brookes Publishing Co.

Hammerman, S., & Maikowski, S. (Eds.). (1981). *The economics of disability: International perspectives.* New York: Rehabilitation International.

Hunter, J., & Cornes, P. (1985). Work, disability and rehabilitation in perspective. In P. Cornes & J. Hunter (Eds.), *Work, disability and rehabilitation.* East Lansing: Michigan State University, University Center for International Rehabilitation.

Johnston, M. V. (1983). The costs and effectiveness of stroke rehabilitation: Measurement and prediction. *Dissertation Abstracts International, 45,* 507B. (University Microfilms No. AAD-84-11913)

Meyers, A. R., Feltin, M., Master, R. J., Nicastro, D., Cupples, A., Lederman, R. I., & Branch, L. G. (1985). Rehospitalization and spinal cord injury: Cross-sectional survey of adults living independently. *Archives of Physical Medicine and Rehabilitation, 66,* 704–708.

Nutt, P. C. (1981). *Evaluation concepts and methods: Shaping policy for the health administrator.* New York: SP Medical & Scientific Books.

Posavac, E. J., & Carey, R. G. (1980). *Program evaluation.* Englewood Cliffs, NJ: Prentice-Hall.

Rimel, R. W., & Jane, J. A. (1983). Characteristics of the head-injured patient. In M. Rosenthal, E. G. Griffith, M. R. Bond, & J. D. Miller (Eds.), *Rehabilitation of the head injured adult* (pp. 9–21). Philadelphia: Davis.

Rintala, D. H., Uttermohlen, D. M., Buck, E. L., Hanover, D., Alexander, J. L., Norris-Baker, C., Stephens, M. A., Willems, E. P., & Halstead, L. S. (1984). Self-observation and report technique (SORT): Description and clinical applications. In A. S. Halpern & M. J. Fuhrer (Eds.), *Functional assessment in rehabilitation* (pp. 205–222). Baltimore: Paul H. Brookes Publishing Co.

Shortell, S. M., & Richardson, W. C. (1978). *Health program evaluation.* Saint Louis, MO: Mosby.

Stedman's Medical Dictionary (24th ed.). (1982). Baltimore: Williams & Wilkins.

Suchman, E. (1967). *Evaluative research.* New York: Russell Sage Foundation.

Trieschmann, R. B. (1980). *Spinal cord injuries: Psychological, social and vocational adjustment.* New York: Pergamon Press.

Wood, P. H. N., & Badley, E. M. (1980). *People with disabilities—Toward acquiring information which reflects more sensitively their problems and needs.* New York: World Rehabilitation Fund.

World Health Organization. (1980). *International classification of impairments, disabilities, and handicaps: A manual of classification relating to the consequences of disease.* Geneva: Author.

SECTION I

Rehabilitation Area Reviews

Chapter 2

Outcome Analysis in Comprehensive Medical Rehabilitation

Karen A. Wagner

The notion of examining outcomes of patients who have received comprehensive medical rehabilitation is not a new one. Follow-up clinic visits and home visits have long been part of rehabilitation practice, not only to identify new problems but also to evaluate results of services provided. In recent years, however, the climate in which outcome analysis is done has changed. The motivation to document outcomes has shifted from being generated principally by rehabilitation professionals to originating also from service recipients and, even more so, from sponsors. At stake is the continued willingness of third-party sponsors, both federal and private, to view comprehensive rehabilitation services as necessary and affordable. As described by DeJong (Chapter 21), health maintenance organizations (HMOs), prospective payment systems based on the use of diagnostic related groups (DRGs), preferred provider organizations (PPOs), and the rapidly increasing number of self-insured companies are emerging economic influences that are likely to shape the future of medical rehabilitation. A variety of old questions are being asked with new insistence. What are the benefits of comprehensive medical rehabilitation? Can fewer services be provided while maintaining an acceptable outcome level? Can fundamental agreement be reached among third-party payors, taxpayers, professionals, and disabled persons about acceptable outcome levels? All of these questions are in the domain of outcome analysis.

This chapter first provides a working definition of comprehensive medical rehabilitation and its outcomes. There follows a review of outcome measures. Finally, special issues and problems are discussed that are encountered in assessing outcomes of comprehensive medical rehabilitation services.

DEFINING COMPREHENSIVE MEDICAL REHABILITATION

Comprehensive medical rehabilitation is not consistently or clearly defined in the literature. As a result, one is not sure just what should be assessed when questions arise about the effectiveness of comprehensive medical rehabilitation services.

"Comprehensiveness" in the present context alludes to the scope of patient needs addressed and to the variety of services provided. Comprehensive medical rehabilitation[1] may be defined, therefore, as the provision of medical and psychosocial services to persons with chronic

Preparation of this chapter was supported in part by the Research and Training Center for the Rehabilitation of Persons with Spinal Cord Dysfunction at Baylor College of Medicine and at The Institute for Rehabilitation and Research (National Institute of Handicapped Research Grant No. G008300044).

[1]This term is different from but related to "comprehensive rehabilitation" and "medical rehabilitation" as defined by Fuhrer (Chapter 1).

physical disorders in order to minimize impairment, disability, or handicap. (The latter three terms are defined in Chapter 1 in accord with the *International Classification of Impairments, Disabilities, and Handicaps* [ICIDH]; World Health Organization [WHO], 1980). Services are also afforded family members in an effort to normalize their lives so that they can play a supportive role in the life of the individual.

Some of the disorders addressed by comprehensive medical rehabilitation services have sudden onset, such as traumatic brain injury, spinal cord injury, amputation, stroke, or burns. Also included are conditions that have a gradual onset and that tend to be progressive, such as multiple sclerosis, muscular dystrophy, rheumatoid arthritis, or cancer.

Medical rehabilitation services are seldom relevant to altering impairments, such as paralysis or amnesia, that are associated with the primary condition, such as brain injury. The major concern of the therapies is to ensure that secondary conditions do not arise that produce additional impairment and disability. For example, spinal cord–injured patients are turned every 2 hours or so to guard against skin breakdown, and urine is monitored to minimize the occurrence of urinary tract infection that can result in kidney damage. Therapeutic interventions directed at minimizing disability include muscle strengthening to facilitate mobility and participation in activities of daily living (ADL). Mobility training consists of such activities as walking in parallel bars, stair climbing, or learning to transfer from a wheelchair to an automobile. Examples of ADL include eating, dressing, using the telephone, and preparing a meal. When impairments cause defects in cognitive abilities, therapies may include efforts to increase short- and long-term memory skills, develop problem-solving strategies, and maintain attention to a task.

Needs at the level of disability and especially handicap are addressed by psychosocially oriented services. These services are an essential element in ensuring that medical rehabilitation services are comprehensive. Adjustment counseling assists patients to understand how their disability impacts on themselves or their families. Counseling and education assist the individual to deal with issues surrounding sexual identity and interpersonal relationships. Vocational and avocational counseling focus either on resumption of previous activity or redirection of plans consistent with interests and abilities.

The determination of which services to provide and when to provide them is shaped by the perception of patients' changing needs over time. DeLoach, Wilkins, and Walker (1983) described four stages of medical rehabilitation: 1) acute medical care, 2) physical restoration, 3) intensive medical rehabilitation, and 4) follow-up services.

Acute medical care is the initial stage in the treatment process. Emphases are on assuring the individual's survival and physiological stability. The focus shifts then to preventing secondary medical complications such as contractures or pressure sores. The patient is, for the most part, a passive recipient of services during this stage of care.

The physical restoration stage focuses on assessing the individual's rehabilitation potential and on devising and implementing some kind of rehabilitation plan. For conditions such as stroke, head injury, or spinal cord injury that may involve muscular paralysis, therapists periodically assess patients' residual voluntary control of individual muscles, the strength of those muscles, and the range of motion of particular joints. Treatment focuses on optimizing physiological recovery and on teaching self-care skills. During this stage, the patient becomes an active participant in the care process. As DeLoach et al. (1983) pointed out, "In medical rehabilitation programs with minimal staff, stage two frequently marks the conclusion of effective medical rehabilitation efforts because services that might allow severely disabled people to reach their optimum levels of independent functioning are not available" (p. 106).

During the intensive medical rehabilitation stage, a variety of trained staff members are available to meet a wide array of emerging patient needs. The specific disciplines involved depend on the disabling condition. Typically represented are a physiatrist, rehabilitation nurse, physical therapist, occupational therapist, speech therapist, psychologist, social worker, rehabilitation counselor, and recreational therapist. Patient needs also may dictate the services of other specialist physicians, a prosthetist, orthotist, audiologist, neuropsychologist, or rehabilitation engineer. These and other professionals work together as an interdisciplinary team to provide the disabled person with the training and equipment necessary to optimize function. As DeLoach et al. (1983) stated, "the emphasis begins to shift from primarily physical restoration efforts to efforts aimed at role restoration—efforts, that is, that are intended to help patients cope with the demands of living outside a sheltered setting" (p. 109). In short, psychosocial issues at the level of handicap become a primary focus of care.

Services comprising the follow-up service stage assist the individual to maintain a satisfactory level of independence and health after returning to the community. Notwithstanding the need for such services, they materialize for only a minority of patients, even a minority of those discharged from comprehensive medical rehabilitation facilities. The distance between the facility and many patients' residences as well as the unavailability of sponsorship are frequently cited reasons for follow-up services not taking place.

UNDERSTANDING OUTCOMES

There is confusion in the medical rehabilitation literature concerning what is meant by the term *outcome*. Two usages are involved, one describing a group's status at some point following onset of disease or trauma, and the other describing a group's response to a particular intervention.

Status-oriented outcome studies are intended to document how a particular disease or injury affects patients in any one of a number of ways—medically, behaviorally, or socially. Such studies may focus, for example, on a cohort of patients who have had a condition such as traumatic brain injury for a specified period of time. Alternatively, the study may have a longitudinal design with data collection beginning when a condition such as multiple sclerosis is diagnosed and continuing at successive intervals. The purpose of such studies is strictly descriptive. Although determinants that shape the results cannot be decisively known, the studies are useful for providing epidemiological information or for assessing patient needs.

Intervention-oriented outcome studies, the focus of this chapter, are intended to establish the effects of defined intervention on a specific patient group. A causal relationship between the intervention and the observed results is either assumed or the paramount focus of the investigation. In that spirit, Brown, Gordon, and Diller (1983) stated, "An outcome is defined as a change in some aspect of the service recipient's world, where the changes are strongly enough associated with the provision of rehabilitation services so that it is typically (though not necessarily statistically) causally attributed to service provision" (p. 95). Similarly, Luker (1981) stated, "Outcome . . . refers to the end result of care in terms of its effect on the patient/client" (p. 92). The Commission on Accreditation of Rehabilitation Facilities (CARF, 1979) also maintains that outcome studies of patients served in inpatient medical rehabilitation facilities must be done in a way that allows the observed results to be related to the services provided.

OUTCOME ANALYSIS MEASURES

For the discussion that follows, measures are distinguished in four ways according to: 1) the ICIDH constructs of impairment, disability, and handicap; 2) intended users—a single facility or multiple facilities; 3) intended target groups—a single diagnostic group or multiple ones; and 4) the kind of behavior recorded—capability or typical performance.

ICIDH Arrayed Measures

Impairment Instruments that measure outcomes of comprehensive medical rehabilitation at the level of impairment are plentiful. Many of the measures are physiologically oriented, involve technologically sophisticated instrumentation, and are usually highly reliable and well validated. They yield information that is used by physicians and others both for initial assessments and for monitoring the effectiveness of treatments. An example is the measurement of vital capacity to assess lung function in connection with a variety of conditions, including asthma, pneumonia, or chronic obstructive pulmonary disease.

Some impairment measures like vital capacity are used across many diagnostic categories; others are used to assess impairment associated with a particular diagnosis. A few examples of specialized scales are given below.

Glasgow Coma Scale (GCS) This scale was designed by neurosurgeons in response to clinical and research needs for a common terminology characterizing the duration and degree of coma following traumatic head injury (Teasdale & Jennett, 1974). The GCS is valuable because it is easily administered and understood and because changes in levels of consciousness can be followed over time. Additional discussion of the scale is provided by Diller and Ben-Yishay (Chapter 16).

Standards for Neurological Classification of Spinal Cord Injury Patients As discussed by Whiteneck (Chapter 17), the American Spinal Injury Association (ASIA, 1982) has developed a standardized procedure for assessing the functioning of persons with spinal injury. Motor and sensory scores are computed for both sides of the body to determine the levels of complete or incomplete spinal cord injury. A Total Motor Index Score also can be computed to document improvement or deterioration of motor functioning for outcome assessment.

Disability The most frequently used scales in outcome studies concern disability. By definition, these scales measure "any restriction or lack of ability to perform an everyday activity in a manner or within the range considered normal for a person of the same age, culture and education" (WHO, 1980). Most instruments designated in the literature as functional assessment measures are directed at assessing disability. Many of the instruments are described in texts by Halpern and Fuhrer (1984) and Granger and Gresham (1984), and analytical reviews have been published by Brown et al. (1983) and Granger (1982).

In comprehensive medical rehabilitation, functional assessment is largely concerned with evaluating the degree of assistance the patient requires in performing ADL skills. The emphasis on ADL skills has at least two reasons. First, activities such as dressing and personal hygiene are of self-evident importance in daily life. Second, minimizing patients' dependency on assistance by others is one of rehabilitation's most cherished goals. In addition to ADL, many functional assessment scales are concerned with the individual's mobility (e.g., the Expanded Disability Status Scale, Kurtzke, 1983; LaRocca, Chapter 11), communication (e.g., the Level of Rehabilitation Scale [LORS], Carey & Posavac, 1978), and interpersonal skills (e.g., the Patient Evaluation Conference System [PECS], Harvey & Jellinek, 1981).

The most widely used functional assessment scales in medical rehabilitation outcomes research are the PULSES (Moskowitz & McCann, 1957) and the Barthel Index (Mahoney & Barthel, 1965). These scales were both originally designed for use by rehabilitation professionals in a hospital setting. The patient's ability to perform various activities is observed and a numerical score is yielded that indicates the individual's overall functional status.

Disability and Handicap There are several instruments that predominantly assess disability, but that include some items dealing with handicap. In addition to ADL, the LORS assesses mobility in the community and participation in social activities (Carey & Posavac, 1978). The Disability Rating Scale (DRS), which is used primarily with traumatic brain injury, assesses disability in terms of cognitive ability required for self-care, and handicap in terms of the client being an employee, homemaker, or student (Rappaport, Hall, Hopkins, Belleza, & Cope, 1982). The DRS was specifically designed to track patients' progress after discharge from inpatient rehabilitation.

Increasing attention to outcomes at the level of handicap reflects in part the influence of the independent living movement on medical rehabilitation. In a study of outcomes of persons with spinal cord injury, DeJong and Hughes (1982) proposed that two outcome measures are of prime relevance: 1) the degree to which the individual lives in a less restrictive living situation, and 2) the degree to which the individual is productive as a member of society. They stated, "society, as represented through various funding sources, will want to know whether medical rehabilitation's efforts ultimately contributed—with all due considerations of other intervening variables—to a person's ability to live independently" (p. 73).

Intended Users

It is axiomatic that rating scales and other measures must be designed with intended users in mind. In this respect, instruments with applications in comprehensive medical rehabilitation differ substantially depending on whether they were developed for a single facility's use or for general use.

Single Facility User A number of comprehensive medical rehabilitation facilities have developed their own ADL scales for the clinical purpose of documenting patient progress. There are several advantages to using these scales for assessing program outcomes in those facilities. Staff members already know how to use the instrument, and they are committed to recording the data consistently because they find it clinically useful. A disadvantage is that because of the idiosyncratic features of the scales, results based on them cannot be readily compared with data yielded by other instruments used in other settings. Their uniqueness also makes it difficult to communicate resulting data to sponsors and referrers.

Multiple Facility Users A number of measures are available that are for general use. Some of these scales were designed originally to meet a particular facility's needs, but they were then developed further until they became appropriate for general use. That was the history, for example, of the PECS (Harvey & Jellinek, 1981) and the LORS (Carey & Posavac, 1978). Other scales intended for general use from inception include the DRS (Rappaport et al., 1982), the Self-Observation and Report Technique (SORT; Rintala et al., 1984), Rehabilitation Indicators (RI; Brown, Gordon & Diller, 1984), and the Functional Independence Measure being developed in connection with the Uniform National Data System for Medical Rehabilitation (Hamilton, Granger, Sherwin, Zielezny, & Tashman, Chapter 10).

Scales for general use af_____ tages. Detailed information / regarding the scale's reliabi_____ regarding standardized methods __ istration. Published data may also be available about outcomes for patients in other facilities so that comparisons can be made. A frequent disadvantage is that scale items are included only if they are thought to reflect the program aims of most potential user facilities. A particular facility often must add items to obtain a complete assessment of outcomes congruent with its particular program aims.

Intended Target Group

Outcome measures in comprehensive medical rehabilitation are designed for use with a single, specific diagnosis or with multiple diagnoses. This difference strongly influences the content and applications of any particular measure.

Single Diagnosis–Oriented Measures
Examples of instruments designed for a single diagnostic group are the DRS (Rappaport et al., 1982) and the Glasgow Outcome Scale (Jennett & Bond, 1975), both used in traumatic brain injury. Consistent with the clinically recognized effects of such injury, these scales measure outcomes in a variety of cognitive and physical areas. In a different domain, the National Spinal Cord Injury Database (NSCIDB) contains no item dealing with cognitive functioning, but it contains many concerned with pathophysiology and disability associated with spinal cord injury (Young, Burns, Bowen, & McCutchen, 1982). An advantage of the single diagnosis outcome measure is that only information relevant to that condition need be collected. A disadvantage is that professionals who work with patients with several diagnoses must become familiar with multiple measures. Another disadvantage is that if a facility treats several diagnostic groups and assesses each with a different measure, it may not be possible to compare outcomes across groups. For example, the NSCIDB documents an individual's vocational status in terms of items dealing with employment at follow-up compared with employment preinjury. The DRS does not assess if patients are employed, but rather if they are employable in a restricted, competitive, or

_neltered setting. A sponsor would have difficulty determining if the facility did as well in meeting the vocational needs of persons with spinal cord injury as it did persons with traumatic brain injury.

Multiple Diagnoses–Oriented Measures Many available instruments were designed for use with a variety of diagnostic groups. The RI (Brown et al., 1984), the LORS (Carey & Posavac, 1978), and the PECS (Harvey & Jellinek, 1981), for example, were designed for use with the kinds of diagnoses typically treated in comprehensive medical rehabilitation facilities. An advantage of this type of instrument is that, once staff members learn how it is used, they can use it for many patient groups and results can be compared across diagnostic categories. A disadvantage is that outcome variables relevant only to a particular diagnosis tend to be omitted.

Kinds of Behavior Recorded

One of the principle aims of comprehensive medical rehabilitation is to provide the services necessary for patients to achieve maximum independence in performing tasks of daily living. Outcome assessments, therefore, must provide information on how fully that aim is achieved. Either of two approaches to assessing performance is possible: in terms of capability or in terms of typical performance. Associated with these different approaches are marked differences in types of measures and methods of data collection.

Capability On capability measures, the rater records whether the patient can perform a task in a defined manner. In the Barthel Index (Mahoney & Barthel, 1965), for example, the rater records whether the patient can independently or dependently walk up a flight of stairs. The assessment is focused on the ability to perform the act in a controlled situation.

This approach to outcome assessment is especially useful when services are concerned with teaching skills or competencies. Service effectiveness can be monitored by documenting changes in functional capabilities from admission to discharge and at follow-up. Individual life-style or environmental variances do not confound outcome results based on measuring

capability. However, capability often gives a distorted view of the outcome picture. An individual who is capable of driving but who has no vehicle continues to have a transportation handicap. Some persons may be capable of eating independently but, because of the time involved, may choose to hire an attendant to assist them.

Typical Performance Some measures have been designed to assess how a person typically performs an activity. The SORT (Rintala et al., 1984) and the RI (Brown et al., 1984) document how the patient actually accomplishes various daily activities. In the SORT, information is obtained by a 15–45-minute interview that quantifies a person's activities during a 24-hour period. In the sections of the RI that document a person's typical performance, the data are collected through written self-report.

An advantage of basing outcomes on typical performance is that this directly reflects the success of the rehabilitation program in achieving the widely expressed goal of assessing the disabled person's ability to live in the community independently and without restrictions. Another advantage is the opportunity to assess the meaningfulness of skills being taught during rehabilitation. An individual may be trained to use a piece of equipment to enable grasp, but then discard it after discharge because another solution was found. If this happens frequently, a review of the equipment training effort may be warranted. In addition, by portraying disabilities and handicaps that remain for the individual, the treatment plan can be realigned with actual needs.

Because of the multiplicity of influences that shape an individual's typical performance, it is often difficult to know whether observed changes are related to the treatment or to situational or individual preferences. Another problem is that normative data are frequently unavailable for the population at large to interpret findings for a disabled group.

ISSUES IN COMPREHENSIVE MEDICAL REHABILITATION

Several other issues are discussed below that warrant attention in planning outcome studies of comprehensive medical rehabilitation.

Assessing Services
Aimed at Family Members

Two different rationales exist for providing services to members of the disabled individual's family. Each has distinctive implications for outcome analysis. The prevailing reason is that services for nondisabled family members will maximize chances of a successful rehabilitation outcome for the disabled individual. This justification rests on the understanding that family members who have accepted the individual's disability will be better equipped to provide the emotional and practical support that the disabled individual requires. The success of those services are therefore evaluated in terms of the disabled family member's rehabilitation outcome.

There is advocacy from professionals and from representatives of disabled persons to provide services to nondisabled family members on the grounds that the family unit per se is the appropriate focal point of rehabilitation services. The need to consider the family unit as a recipient of services is particularly emphasized in pediatric interventions (Allen, Chapter 14) and in traumatic brain injury (Diller and Ben-Yishay, Chapter 16). From this vantage, the dysfunction created by severe impairment is viewed as extending beyond the disabled individual to include some or all family members. It is argued in such cases that providing services for nondisabled family members is not less justified than for the disabled individual. For services provided according to this rationale, outcome assessment should focus on the behavior of each family member for whom they were provided.

In the current practice of comprehensive medical rehabilitation, services focus overwhelmingly on patients themselves. When family members are included, the interventions are justified for the most part in terms of benefits that the patient will derive. This state of affairs largely reflects the fact that sponsorship is seldom available to serve nondisabled family members, not that medical rehabilitation professionals devalue the importance of the family unit.

Impact of Aging on
Longitudinal Outcome Analysis

The aging process must be considered in designing many outcome studies and in interpreting their results. This is especially true if the changes being documented occur over a relatively long time span. Both ends of the age continuum are potentially of concern. Children's physical and behavioral functioning can be expected to improve with time in relation to the developmental process. Difficulties in discerning which changes are due to development and which are due to interventions are discussed by Miner, Fletcher, and Ewing-Cobbs (1986). Elderly patients manifest changes that are generally associated with advancing age. Included are changes in living situations as a result of retirement, altered finances, or a spouse's death. Failure to document such changes may result in unaccounted for variability in outcome results pertaining, for example, to service recipients' kinds and degree of social participation.

Spontaneous Recovery or Deterioration

Many of the underlying pathologies treated during comprehensive medical rehabilitation have an evolving natural history that may be associated with progressive changes at the levels of impairment, disability, or handicap. For example, cerebral edema (swelling) associated with some forms of stroke can resolve with the passage of time. Those changes enable improved neural functioning that, in turn, enable improved cognitive and interpersonal functioning. Such improved functioning may be viewed as an instance of "spontaneous recovery." Other diseases such as multiple sclerosis are associated with progressively deteriorating physical states that may be reflected in progressive dysfunction at the psychological, behavioral, and interpersonal levels (LaRocca, Chapter 11). Many aspects of a condition's natural history may affect measures chosen to document outcomes. Consequently, changes on these measures may be attributed mistakenly to the intervention, although they actually reflect the natural history of the underlying condition. Because of this possibility, many authors recommend obtaining data from matched control groups (e.g., Carey & Posavac, 1978; Forer & Miller, 1980; Watson & Kendall, 1983). Other designs that allow effects of natural history to be distinguished from effects of intervention are discussed by Rintala (Chapter 7).

Timing of Outcome Analysis

The plan of a typical outcome study calls for acquiring data at some point after the completion of services. The criteria for judging whether or not services were completed can be surprisingly problematic. In too many outcome studies, discharge from the inpatient rehabilitation program is accepted uncritically as the criterion for program completion. That is a mistake, because discharge is an ambiguous indicator of program completion. There are other reasons for discharge, but they may not be readily discernable, especially in retrospective studies that depend on conventional medical records. Some discharges occur, for example, because inpatient sponsorship dwindles and the patient must be released before maximum benefit has been achieved. Other discharges occur in connection with a treatment plan that consists of a period of inpatient rehabilitation followed by discharge to the community, and then by one or more planned, relatively brief readmissions for inpatient services. In such plans, opportunities to leave the hospital are justified in many ways, for instance, to allow time at home to practice ADL and mobility skills before readmission for advanced training.

Regardless of whether it reflects sponsorship constraints, the overall treatment plan, or other considerations, discharge per se need not signify completion of the rehabilitation program. The common practice of basing outcome results on all discharged patients ignores this fact and is likely to produce a diluted picture of a program's effectiveness. Additionally, the opportunity is lost to assess the effectiveness of different intensities of service by grouping patients according to the reasons for discharge.

After deciding what constitutes the completion of services, the interval(s) at which outcome analysis is to be done must be chosen. The Commission on the Accreditation of Rehabilitation Facilities (1979, p. 19) recommends that the evaluation should occur long enough after the intervention that an accurate assessment of outcomes can be obtained, but soon enough that one can infer a causal relationship. Identifying a point in time that fulfills the CARF recommendation is difficult at best. A patient's comprehensive medical rehabilitation program entails numerous services objectives that are specified in very different time domains. For example, the objective of a patient education program on skin care may be to minimize the number of pressure sores acquired by patients with paraplegia. Attainment of such an objective is evaluated most appropriately at an interval relatively long after discharge from services. On the other hand, the desired outcome of a treatment to teach patients how to transfer from a bed to a wheelchair without assistance is appropriately evaluated at discharge or before. The point is that limiting outcome assessment to a single point in time will be decidedly suboptimal for fulfilling the CARF recommendation for at least some variables studied. Repeated outcome assessments designed to collect data at several points in time following the completion of services are the preferred alternative. An additional benefit of multiple follow-up intervals is the ability to track changes in the durability of outcomes over time.

Norms

Meaningful interpretation of rehabilitation outcome data often presupposes availability of norms for the population at large. For example, a study may report on the percentage of service recipients who, following comprehensive medical rehabilitation services, participate weekly in leisure activities out of the home. Interpreting the reported percentage depends to some extent on knowing the percentage of nondisabled persons in the general population of similar age, gender, and socioeconomic class who pursue leisure activities out of the home. Unfortunately, such data are seldom available. Where normative data are available, they need to be cited more frequently in published outcome studies (Wagner, 1986). For example, according to the 1980 census (U.S. Department of Commerce, 1983), the divorce rate in Houston, Texas was 8.4/1,000 population. That fact could be important, for example, in comparing comprehensive medical rehabilitation results in Houston with results for a program in San Diego, where the divorce rate was 5.5/1,000 population.

Normative data are also important for interpreting results of a given program's performance over time. Assuming that the probability of acquiring a job is related to the number of jobs available, interpreting year-to-year outcomes of rehabilitation programs in Houston should be tempered by knowing that the annual unemployment rates in 1980, 1981, 1982, and 1983 were 4.2, 4.1, 7, and 9.3, respectively. If a Houston rehabilitation program were to show equal percentages of employed patients over the 4 years, it might well be viewed as becoming increasingly successful.

SUMMARY

In the past comprehensive medical rehabilitation emphasized the inpatient care process. The major focus of outcome analysis was on medical concerns such as complications and on patient functional gains. Results of functional assessments were used for managing individual patients and for demonstrating to other professionals that the services were effective. How a person would function in society following discharge was of secondary importance.

As rehabilitation services broadened, the literature reflected a trend toward assessing psychosocial outcomes in addition to medical outcomes. In a study by Gerhards, Florin, and Knapp (1984), for example, rehabilitation outcomes for patients with amputation was regarded as a "multifacet phenomenon comprising medical, social, vocational, and psychological aspects." Cummings, Kener, Arones, and Steinbock (1985) reported on outcomes of rehabilitation services provided by a day hospital program. They assessed impacts on patients' psychological adjustment and on their families as well as changes in ADL, mobility, and the number of medical problems. In discussing outcomes for patients with arthritis, Fries, Spitz, Kraines, and Holman (1980) stated, "Outcome measures must be appropriate to the disease condition being evaluated . . . and in chronic disease must be defined in terms that include patients' social, physical and mental functioning" (p. 137). This view of arthritis rehabilitation outcomes is shared by Wegener, Brunner, and Stabenow (Chapter 12). Psychosocial outcomes are similarly prominent in the study of burn rehabilitation patients by Questad, Boltwood, Alquist, and deLateur (Chapter 13).

In the future, researchers will be challenged to design evaluation studies in keeping with the changing nature of comprehensive medical rehabilitation programs. At least three changes can be envisioned: 1) increasing alternatives to extended inpatient care, 2) greater emphasis on networking the rehabilitation program with other services, and 3) even more stress on cost containment.

Emerging alternatives to extended patient care include alternating periods of inpatient and outpatient care as well as replacing inpatient care with day care services. These arrangements permit more influences to shape program outcomes than if interventions consisted only of inpatient care. One of these influences, for example, is the patient's compliance with outpatient plans. Special attention will be required to design outcome analysis that separates such influences from impacts of the rehabilitation program itself.

To ensure the continuity of services that patients need, networking must occur among programs that care for patients before rehabilitation is appropriate and that serve them after rehabilitation is complete. However, networking poses difficulties in interpreting results of long-term outcome studies. Foremost is the problem that outcomes cannot be attributed unequivocally to the rehabilitation program itself. This is likely to lead to greater emphasis on proximate measures of rehabilitation outcomes.

Pressure on comprehensive medical rehabilitation programs to produce outcome data will continue in connection with the mounting emphasis on reducing health care costs. The challenge is to design outcome analyses that demonstrate the cost-effectiveness of services in permitting persons with disabilities to function as contributing members of the community.

REFERENCES

American Spinal Injury Association. (1982). *Standards for neurological classification of spinal injury patients*. Chicago: Author.

Brown, M., Gordon, W. A., & Diller, L. (1983). Functional assessment and outcome measurement: An integrative review. In E. L. Pan, T. E. Backer, & C. L. Vask (Eds.),

Annual review of rehabilitation (Vol. 3). New York: Springer-Verlag.

Brown, M., Gordon, W. A., & Diller, L. (1984). Rehabilitation indicators. In A. S. Halpern & M. J. Fuhrer (Eds.), *Functional assessment in rehabilitation* (pp. 187–203). Baltimore: Paul H. Brookes Publishing Co.

Carey, R. G., & Posavac, E. J. (1978). Program evaluation of a physical medicine and rehabilitation unit: A new approach. *Archives of Physical Medicine and Rehabilitation, 59*, 330–337.

Commission on Accreditation of Rehabilitation Facilities. (1979). *Program evaluation in inpatient medical rehabilitation facilities.* Tucson: Author.

Cummings, V., Kener, J. F., Arones, S., & Steinbock, C. (1985). Day hospital service in rehabilitation medicine: An evaluation. *Archives of Physical Medicine and Rehabilitation, 66*, 86–91.

DeJong, G., & Hughes, J. (1982). Independent living methodology for measuring long-term outcomes. *Archives of Physical Medicine and Rehabilitation, 63*, 68–73.

DeLoach, C. P., Wilkins, R. D., & Walker, G. W. (1983). *Independent living.* Baltimore: University Park Press.

Forer, S. K., & Miller, L. S. (1980). Rehabilitation outcome: Comparative analyses of different patient types. *Archives of Physical Medicine and Rehabilitation, 61*, 359–365.

Frankel, H. L. (1969). The value of postural reduction in the initial management of closed injuries of the spine with paraplegia and tetraplegia. *Paraplegia, 7*, 179–192.

Fries, J., Spitz, P., Kraines, R. G., & Holman, H. R. (1980). Measurement of patient outcome in arthritis. *Arthritis and Rheumatism, 23*, 137–145.

Gerhards, F., Florin, I., & Knapp, T. (1984). The impact of medical reeducational and psychological variables on rehabilitation outcome in amputees. *International Journal of Rehabilitation Research, 7*, 379–388.

Granger, C. V. (1982). Health accounting—functional assessment of the long-term patient. In F. J. Kottke, G. K. Stillwell, & J. F. Lehmann (Eds.), *Krusen's handbook of physical medicine and rehabilitation* (3rd ed.), pp. 252–274). Philadelphia: W. B. Saunders.

Granger, C. V., & Gresham, G. E. (1984). *Functional assessment in rehabilitation medicine.* Baltimore: Williams & Wilkins.

Halpern, A. S., & Fuhrer, M. J. (Eds.). (1984). *Functional assessment in rehabilitation.* Baltimore: Paul H. Brookes Publishing Co.

Harvey, R. F., & Jellinek, H. M. (1981). Functional performance assessment: A program approach. *Archives of Physical Medicine and Rehabilitation, 62*, 456–461.

Jennett, B., & Bond, B. (1975). Assessment of outcome after severe brain damage. *Lancet, 1*, 480.

Kurtzke, J. F. (1983). Rating neurological impairment in multiple sclerosis: An expanded disability status scale. *Neurology, 33*, 1444–1452.

Luker, K. A. (1981). An overview of evaluation research in nursing. *Journal of Advanced Nursing, 6*, 87–93.

Mahoney, F. T., & Barthel, D. W. (1965). Functional evaluation: The Barthel Index. *Maryland State Medical Journal, 14*, 61–65.

Miner, M. E., Fletcher, J. M., & Ewing-Cobbs, L. (1986). Recovery versus outcome after head injury in children. In M. E. Miner & K. A. Wagner (Eds.), *Neurotrauma: Treatment, rehabilitation and related issues* (pp. 233–241). Boston: Butterworths.

Moskowitz, E., & McCann, C. B. (1957). Classification of disability in the chronically ill and aging. *Journal of Chronic Disease, 5*, 342–346.

Rappaport, M., Hall, K. M., Hopkins, K., Belleza, T., & Cope, D. N. (1982). Disability rating scale for severe head trauma: Coma to community. *Archives of Physical Medicine and Rehabilitation, 63*, 118–123.

Rintala, D., Uttermohlen, D., Buck, E. L., Hanover, D., Alexander, J., Norris-Baker, C., Stephens, M. A. P., Willems, E. R., & Halstead, L. S. (1984). Self-observation and report technique (SORT): Description and clinical applications. In A. S. Halpern & M. J. Fuhrer (Eds.), *Functional assessment in rehabilitation* (pp. 205–221). Baltimore: Paul H. Brookes Publishing Co.

Teasdale, G., & Jennett, B. (1974). Assessment of coma and impaired consciousness: A practical scale. *Lancet, 2*, 81–84.

U.S. Department of Commerce, Bureau of the Census. (1983). *County and City Data Book* (10th ed.). Washington, DC: U.S. Department of Commerce.

Wagner, K. A. (1986). Sociological parameters affecting comparison of long-term outcome. In M. E. Miner & K. A. Wagner (Eds.), *Neurotrauma: Treatment, rehabilitation and related issues* (pp. 213–222). Boston: Butterworths.

Watson, D., & Kendall, P. C. (1983). Methodological issues in research on coping with chronic disease. In *Coping with chronic disease* (pp. 39–81). New York: Academic Press.

World Health Organization. (1980). *International classification of impairments, disabilities, and handicaps.* Geneva: Author.

Young, J. S., Burns, P. E., Bowen, A. M., & McCutchen, R. (1982). *Spinal cord injury statistics.* Phoenix, AZ: National Spinal Cord Injury Data Research Center.

Chapter 3

Outcome Analysis for Persons with Mental Retardation

Andrew S. Halpern

In many ways, the measurement practices that have emerged within the field of mental retardation are inextricably bound to the concept of mental retardation, since the definition of this condition is essentially psychometric. Because of this close tie of the definition to assessment, measurement issues have always been present and at times predominant throughout the development of this field.

These issues originally focused primarily on diagnosis and classification of people with mental retardation. During the past two decades, however, there has been a strong shift in emphasis toward examining the relevance of assessment for decision making within the service delivery process, as a supplement to the more traditional concerns about incidence, prevalence, and prevention of mental retardation. As this shift in emphasis occurred, assessment issues began to emerge concerning the planning and evaluation of services. This includes, of course, a major concern with the measurement of service outcomes.

Because the label "mental retardation" covers an extremely broad range of human behavior, from the most severe disability imaginable to only a slight deviation from expected social norms, the stipulation and measurement of outcomes in this field is a very complex endeavor. Equally complex is the range of services required to respond appropriately to the diverse needs of this population.

To explore outcome analysis issues within such a broad and complex contextual framework, this chapter has been organized to include the following major components: 1) assessment issues that emerge from the definition of mental retardation, 2) an overview of relevant outcomes, 3) an overview of relevant services, 4) a description of assessment issues that emerge from an analysis of service delivery models, and 5) a description of measurement issues that are particularly relevant to assessment activities involving people with mental retardation. An attempt is made both to document the current state of the art and to articulate major problems and issues that still remain unresolved.

MENTAL RETARDATION AS A PSYCHOMETRIC CONCEPT

Many definitions of mental retardation have emerged over the years from all corners of the world. Because the term refers to a rather broad set of behaviors rather than a specific disease, the definition and diagnosis of mental retardation have always been intrinsically tied to the parameters of psychometric assessment. Furthermore, achieving an accurate diagnosis has often been difficult because discriminating between mild retardation and normal behavior is frequently difficult.

This difficulty emerges from an inherent ambiguity in the concept of social competence, which is a central component of nearly all definitions of mental retardation. In essence, people with mental retardation are viewed as having a limited repertoire of available social skills and minimal insight into the causes and consequences of their behavior. During recent years, the term "adaptive behavior" has replaced "social competence" as a label for this defining characteristic of mental retardation.

Intelligence is the second major concept found in most current definitions of mental retardation. Following the invention of intelligence testing during the early 20th century, a low IQ score became the primary defining characteristic of mental retardation. This happened because an IQ score gives the appearance of objectivity, whereas limited social competence or adaptive behavior has always been difficult to measure operationally.

These two criteria—limited adaptive behavior and subaverage intelligence—are the major components of the most widely acknowledged definition of mental retardation in the United States, which was first offered by the American Association on Mental Deficiency (AAMD) in 1959 and revised in 1983:

> Mental retardation refers to significantly subaverage general intellectual functioning existing concurrently with deficits in adaptive behavior and manifested during the developmental period. (Grossman, 1983, p. 1)

The third component of this definition—manifestation during the developmental period—is generally interpreted to mean that the initial diagnosis occurs before the age of 18.

From the perspective of outcome assessment, the measurement of intelligence has little value, whereas the measurement of adaptive behavior has a major potential for impact. The intelligence component of the diagnosis serves only the purpose of documenting an impairment, because the raising of intelligence is not normally a reasonable goal of the habilitation process. Adaptive behavior, on the other hand, is frequently involved in the goals of habilitation, either as an attempt to reduce disability (i.e., improve skills) or as an attempt to reduce handicap (i.e., provide opportunities to enjoy socially valued roles). In this sense, adaptive behavior is both an integral component of the definition of mental retardation and an appropriate target for outcome assessment. Since adaptive behavior will manifest itself differently in different environments, measures of outcome must be concerned with both client assessment and environmental assessment.

RELEVANT OUTCOMES

Many attempts have been made to develop a taxonomy of relevant outcomes. When dealing with disability, such outcomes are usually described as a set of client skills that can be construed as the desired outcomes of instruction. Brolin (1983) offered a system that identifies 22 broad competencies and more that 100 subcompetencies. Halpern, Lehmann, Irvin, and Heiry (1982) described a similar system consisting of 15 domains and 51 subdomains, each associated with one or more standardized assessment instruments. Both taxonomies (and others like them) cover a broad range of academic, vocational, independent living, and social skills that are frequently the targets of instructional programs for people with mental retardation.

Skill attainment, however, is only one step along the road toward reducing handicap. The achievement of satisfactory community adjustment depends not only upon client skills but also upon opportunities and characteristics of the environment. In other words, skills are a necessary but insufficient condition for surviving, and perhaps even thriving, in one's community.

To reduce handicap as a goal of service delivery and a target of outcome assessment, one must identify and develop a multidimensional taxonomy of community adjustment that reflects both skill attainment and environmental demands or opportunities. Such a taxonomy should include at a minimum the following four components: 1) occupation and financial security, 2) residential adjustment, 3) social support networks and safety, and 4) client satisfaction (Halpern, Close, & Nelson, 1986). The first three dimensions represent societal values, irrespective of the personal preferences of the client. The fourth dimension takes into account the client's own perspective concerning adjustment. This distinction between client and societal perspectives is discussed again later in this chapter.

Occupational and financial security clearly represent a cornerstone of community adjustment within American society. Whenever possible, this includes securing and maintaining a good job with decent wages. The employment histories for people with mental retardation, however, are not very rosy, with most follow-up studies indicating unemployment and/or underemployment rates between 30% and 70% (Edgar, 1985; Halpern et al., 1986; Hasazi, Gordon, & Roe, 1985; Will, 1984a). For some of this group (but clearly not all), other options to employment must be considered, including a regular routine of nonvocational day activities and income subsidies to provide financial security.

Residential adjustment for people with mental retardation has passed through many stages of development. A quarter century ago, the primary alternative to remaining with one's family was placement in a large residential institution, usually far removed from other community resources and basically custodial in nature. The indignities of this approach have been documented poignantly by Blatt (1981). During the 1970s, a national policy on deinstitutionalization led to the proliferation of community residential facilities, offering skill training in more homelike settings in addition to around the clock supervision (Bruininks, Meyers, Sigford, & Lakin, 1981; O'Connor, 1976). The newest alternative in the array of residential options emerged primarily in the 1980s, with several major improvements over the options of the past. Instead of locating clients in "group homes," this program places clients in ordinary homes and apartments in the community. Supervision and training are provided only as needed by the client, often at a level of only 10 or 15 hours per month. Even though this type of program is relatively new, a recent thorough examination has clearly demonstrated its effectiveness (Halpern et al., 1986).

The development of, and participation in, social support networks, accompanied by personal safety, is considered by many people to be the most important dimension of all for adults with mental retardation (Landesman-Dwyer & Berkson, 1984; O'Connor, 1983). This includes friendship, leisure activities, family relationships, intimate relationships, and experience in either avoiding or dealing effectively with major and minor abuse. Although success in this area has clearly been shown to be possible (Halpern et al., 1986), there are times when success occurs only with the assistance of a "benefactor" (Edgerton, 1967, 1984). A benefactor is someone who provides assistance, without remuneration, to a person with mental retardation in many ways, including money management, personal advice, and crisis intervention.

These three societal dimensions of community adjustment—occupation, residence, and social networks—along with the personal dimension of client satisfaction, provide a structure for identifying the ultimate targets of outcome analysis for adults with mental retardation. Skill attainment, as the goal of instruction, provides intermediate targets that pave the way for achievement of the ultimate goals. Such achievement will also often require environmental modification and assessment to improve the match between client skills and instructional demands or between client behavioral performance and the environmental requirements or opportunities of the subculture in which the client lives. The proposed model for representing all of these components is presented in Table 1.

RELEVANT SERVICES

As Table 1 illustrates, outcome analysis can be understood best within the context of a broader

Table 1. An assessment model for adolescents and adults with mental retardation

	Purpose of assessment		
	Eligibility determination	Service delivery	Outcome evaluation
Focus of measurement	Intelligence	Learner Skills	Client Performance
	Adaptive Behavior	Academic	Occupation
		Vocational	Residential adjustment
		Independent living	Social networks/safety
		Social/interpersonal	Satisfaction
		Instructional requirements	Environmental requirements

model that also represents eligibility determination and service delivery as entities influencing the attainment of outcomes. Before exploring the nature of these influences, those services provided most frequently to adolescents and adults with mental retardation are described. Five types of particularly relevant services have been identified: educational services, vocational services, residential services, transfer payments, and case management.

Educational services refer to any attempt to provide systematic instruction, whether in a high school or a postsecondary environment such as a community college or a rehabilitation facility. These services normally focus upon the skill-building component of the model presented in Table 1. The focus of instruction can usually be described as falling into one or more of the following areas: remedial academic skills, vocational skills, independent living skills, and/or social/interpersonal skills (Brolin, 1983; Halpern et al., 1982).

Vocational services are also provided frequently in both high school and postsecondary environments. Helping clients seek and secure a job is the most critical service in this area, although training clients for specific jobs is obviously quite important. Many workers with mental retardation also need special assistance in developing good social relationships on the job. Over the years, this problem has often been found to be the primary reason why people with mental retardation lose their jobs (Foss & Bostwick, 1981). In other instances, modifying a job or providing special ongoing supervision may also be necessary to maintain a worker successfully in competitive employment. This type of service, called "supported employment," has received a substantial amount of attention during recent years (Kiernan & Stark, 1986; Wehman, 1981; Will, 1984b).

Residential services have followed the trends mentioned above from placement in large isolated institutions to community-based group homes to semi-independent living opportunities in ordinary homes or apartments. The services associated with these placements have also shifted dramatically from custodial to training and supervision. Evidence suggests that, as this shift has occurred, the qualifications of service providers have improved substantially (Gollay, Freedman, Wyngaarden, & Kurtz, 1978; Landesman-Dwyer, Sackett, & Kleinman, 1980), although this unfortunately has not been accompanied by an appropriate improvement in salaries (Halpern et al., 1986).

Assistance in the securing of transfer payments is a fourth type of service that is often needed by adults with mental retardation. This may include, in varying combinations, income maintenance, medical care, food stamps, and housing subsidies. Despite the wide array of such programs that are theoretically available, it is discouraging to discover that a large proportion of adults with mental retardation are still living at or below the national poverty level (Halpern et al., 1986).

Case management has evolved as a specific service program that is often needed by adults with mental retardation. Typically administered at the local level (city or county), this service emerged in response to the acknowledged service needs and program jurisdictions that must be somehow brought together in the development of a good service plan. Services provided under the rubric of case management include placement in an appropriate agency program, coordination of services among agencies that are working simultaneously with the same client, supervision of clients, and crisis intervention. Although the concept of case management looks good on paper, its implementation has often been compromised by the existence of excessively large case loads. When this occurs, the job of case manager becomes primarily one of managing paper rather than people.

CONTEXTUAL ISSUES AFFECTING ASSESSMENT

Basic descriptions have now been provided of the major services that have an impact on community adjustment outcomes for adults with mental retardation. As Table 1 illustrates, however, there are several points in an integrated model of assessment where issues may emerge that have a direct impact on any attempt to measure and evaluate outcomes. Accordingly, some of the issues that emerge during eligibility determination, service delivery, and outcome specification are examined here as a precursor to describing some of the assessment practices and problems that are particularly relevant for people with mental retardation.

Eligibility

Problems with assessment in the field of mental retardation clearly begin at the stage of eligibility determination. These problems are perhaps exacerbated by the fact that the term "mental retardation" refers to such a wide range of human behavior. The issue emerges under two rubrics: disability labels and level of disability.

Problems of Labeling Disability labels are legally required in order to justify expenditures for most publicly sponsored programs in special education and adult service agencies. The validity of these labels, however, can often be challenged at two levels: their definitional adequacy and their programmatic relevance.

Inadequate definitions are extremely troublesome because they undercut the validity of both service planning and service evaluation. In essence, when definitions are inadequate, we cannot know how well or consistently they have been operationalized in the placement of clients or the selection of samples for evaluation projects.

An example may suffice to illustrate this problem. As mentioned above, intelligence, as measured primarily by IQ, is one of the two major defining characteristics of the condition we call mental retardation. The validity of this measure, however, was challenged both legally and conceptually when it was discoverd that a disproportionate number of blacks and Hispanics have been labeled as mildly mentally retarded and placed in special education classes (Mercer, 1973). As an outcome of litigation, it is now illegal to even use IQ as a diagnostic criterion for special class placement in some states (Galagan, 1985). This example raises the specter of misdiagnosis and misclassification as a problem that could affect adversely any attempts to interpret the findings of outcome analysis.

Programmatic relevance is a second issue that has emerged from the literature on diagnostic labeling. At one level, there is no issue. We need labels in order to document expenditures under the current methods of funding. At another level, a substantial body of research literature suggests that there is little predictive validity for many labels. For example, the evidence is overwhelming that IQ scores are not particularly useful for predicting level of community adjustment (Charles, 1953; Kennedy, 1966; McCarver & Craig, 1974). On the other hand, a "functional" approach to assessment is highly predictive of such outcomes, when appropriate interventions are provided in response to the functional assessment (Halpern, 1984).

Level of Disability A growing awareness of the desirability of functional assessment has resulted in a movement within special education toward "noncategorical" models of service delivery. This means that services are organized around levels of disability (e.g., mild versus severe) rather than type (e.g., mental retardation versus psychiatric impairment) of disability. A counterargument has also emerged asserting that noncategorical approaches tend to disregard the unique aspects of specific impairments that are instructionally relevant. Since there is probably some truth to both positions, the field is left with an unresolved issue having a clear potential for impact on the selection of outcomes to be pursued.

Another "eligibility" issue associated with the severity of disability concerns the placement of a student with mental retardation within a "regular" or "alternative" school program. This decision typically results in the student either receiving or not receiving a regular diploma upon graduation. For students with mild disabilities and their families, this decision is often difficult, frustrating, and painful, since it affects greatly the selection of desired outcomes, and predictive guidelines are fairly poor concerning who will and will not succeed in the more difficult (regular) program.

Eligibility for adult services presents a different kind of problem than eligibility for school, since only the latter is construed as a constitutional right for all people. In the vocational rehabilitation program, eligibility depends in part on the counselor's judgment as to whether or not the potential client's rehabilitation goal is "feasible," meaning that the disability is not so severe as to preclude a successful outcome, yet is severe enough to warrant the provision of services. Severity of disability is clearly a requirement for some other services, such as income maintenance, medical care, certain residential programs, and ongoing case management. The issue that emerges concerning all of these eligibility decisions is the ambiguity that surrounds both the definition and documentation of "severe." Different applications of this criterion will, of course, affect the potential outcomes of any services that are provided. In the field of mental retardation, there is a tendency to underestimate client potential and therefore underestimate the targeted outcomes for service delivery (Halpern et al., 1986; Kiernan & Stark, 1986).

Service Delivery

Once eligibility decisions have been reached, a myriad of service delivery issues emerge as programs are adopted in pursuit of educational and rehabilitation goals. These issues have been organized into four categories: 1) design of instruction, 2) classroom organization, 3) program coordination, and 4) program documentation. The resolution of these issues will have direct implications for the evaluation of service outcomes. As studies are designed to provide such evaluations, controlling these "independent variables" carefully will become crucial to take full advantage of other efforts aimed primarily at controlling measurement error.

Design of Instruction   Assuming that appropriate content has been identified for the instructional programs provided to adolescents or adults with mental retardation, certain important issues still arise with respect to instructional design. These issues involve the contrast between a functional versus a developmental approach, an inductive versus a deductive approach, a scripted versus a flexible approach, and a learning strategies versus a tutorial approach.

The developmental approach in curriculum organizes instruction around the attainment of learner skills, which are presumed then to function as basic tools for subsequent problem solving by the learner. The student's potential for learn-

ing such skills is also viewed as "developmental," with the acquisition of certain skills serving as a foundation for subsequent acquisition of other skills. One's ability to solve problems is viewed as a function of the level of developmental skill attainment. Looking at problem solving from a "functional" approach instead, curriculum developers of this persuasion regard the articulation of specific problems as the starting point of instructional design. Once these problems have been identified, instructional procedures are developed and, if necessary, modified until the problem has been solved. The onus is placed on the teacher to find "some way" of helping the student achieve the desired outcome, rather than on the student "preparing" for problem solving encounters that may occur at some later point in time.

The maintenance and generalization of newly acquired knowledge and skills is another major concern in the area of instructional design for people with mental retardation. The question being addressed here is whether or not students will be able to apply what they have learned during instruction in other settings and at other times. This question becomes particularly relevant when the skills being taught are used mostly or even exclusively in a nonschool environment (e.g., banking, home management, public transportation). From the perspective of outcome analysis, the question becomes whether or not the outcomes of instruction are satisfactory "predictors" of outcome performance in a natural environment.

Both inductive and deductive instructional methods have been developed for enhancing maintenance and generalization. The inductive approach presents many examples, from representative environments, of opportunities to perform an instructionally targeted skill. If these examples are well chosen to represent the universe of opportunities, it is assumed that the student will eventually be able to perform the skill in situations that have not previously been experienced. The deductive approach is more cognitive in style, teaching a rule for behavior on the assumption that knowing *why* is as or more important than knowing *how,* when the goal of instruction is maintenance and generalization. Students with severe disabilities seem to respond well only to inductive approaches, whereas students with mild disabilities can respond well to either approach, and there is no clear evidence yet concerning which approach works best (Stokes & Baer, 1977).

A third curriculum issue is the contrast between a scripted and a flexible approach to the delivery of instruction. In a scripted approach, the sequence and the content of instruction are tightly designed, including the very words that are spoken by a teacher as instruction is delivered and student errors are corrected. The assumption behind this position is that learning occurs best under very tightly controlled conditions of instruction. The more flexible approach, on the other hand, presumes that many learning opportunities cannot be engineered in advance, and that the teacher must be able to recognize such opportunities and respond appropriately. In a sense, the issue becomes one of allocating control over the direction of instruction between the teacher and the student. This decision will, of course, also affect the stipulated outcomes of instruction.

The contrast between a learning strategies and a tutorial approach to instruction involves primarily the opportunities that are made available to students whose disability is at the mild end of the continuum. In particular, this issue pertains to the subset of these students for whom "mainstreaming" into the regular academic curriculum is appropriate. For many years, the main instructional approach provided to such students has been tutorial assistance in specific content area courses. This meant, of course, that the special education teacher had to be a jack of all trades, teaching language arts one period and math the next. An alternative approach, called "learning strategies" instruction, changes the focus of instruction to teaching students "learning" and "study" skills that might generalize across different content areas (Alley & Deshler, 1979).

Classroom Organization In addition to issues of instructional design, some related issues concerning classroom organization have an impact on high school programs for students with mental retardation. These issues pertain to the location(s) in which instruction is provided.

The classic issue in this area concerns the contrast between special class, resource room, and mainstream classes, all viable alternatives for students with mental retardation. The choice among these alternatives depends largely, of course, on the goals and methods of instruction that have been adopted. As a rule of thumb, special classes should be used only for group instruction in those aspects of the curriculum that are completely unique for students with disabilities, whereas the other options should be used to provide individualized instruction to and to facilitate integration of students with disabilities into the regular high school curriculum. One must ascertain whether or not there is a proper match for any given student between classroom organization and the goals and methods of instruction. Any mismatch will adversely affect both the selection and achievement of outcomes.

A more recent issue concerning classroom organization is the delivery of instruction in a school building versus some other appropriate location in the community. This issue emerges most clearly when the content of the curriculum focuses on vocational training or skills in independent living. In such situations, a strong argument can be mustered for "moving the classroom into the community," even though this presents many logistical and administrative difficulties that must be solved. The validity of this approach is still open for evaluation (Falvey, 1986).

Collaboration The successful preparation of high school students with mental retardation for transition into the community requires extensive collaboration both within departments of a school program and between the school and several adult service agencies. Within the school system, the primary departments are special education, vocational education, and regular academic education, compounded by the use of support services such as counseling and speech therapy. The adult service agencies that become involved most frequently are vocational rehabilitation, mental retardation case management agencies, vocational training facilities, residential programs, and income maintenance programs. The problems and issues pertaining to collaboration affect the selection, monitoring, and evaluating of service outcomes.

With all this complexity encountered, it is not surprising that coordination has emerged as a major problem to be solved, both within school programs and between school programs and adult service agencies (Halpern & Benz, in press). In essence, no one has typically been assigned responsibility for crossing divisional and/or agency boundaries to coordinate services that are or might be provided to a given student. As a consequence of this lack of coordination, any given student may experience both duplication of services and lack of a needed service. From the service provider's perspective, lack of coordination tends to produce inefficiency at best and chaos at worst when attempts at collaboration are made.

Certain attitudinal barriers have also been a historical deterrent to collaboration. Within school programs, vocational education instructors have frequently been unmotivated to work with students who have disabilities. Such instructors were more concerned with dispelling the reputation of vocational education as a "dumping ground" for students who could not succeed in the regular academic curriculum. These instructors also believed that encouraging the participation of students with disabilities would enhance the negative reputation of vocational education. Another example of an attitudinal barrier is the perception of some special education teachers that vocational rehabilitation is basically a "paper shuffling" agency, with no truly useful services to provide. Other examples could be cited, but the underlying theme is the same: a lack of desire to collaborate.

Heavy work loads present another reality that can interfere with the possibilities for collaboration. For example, teachers in the regular vocational and academic programs of high schools are often responsible for between 150 and 200 students in five or more daily classes. Preparations, paper grading, and teaching time to fulfill these responsibilities create more than a full-time job. How can we ask these people to provide additional time and effort to address the needs of students with disabilities? So long as collaboration requires "adding on" responsibilities, it will be difficult to entice participation from those whose burdens would grow heavier.

Even when a desire to collaborate is present, administrative problems and issues tend to interfere. These include deficiencies in information sharing, ambiguity concerning supervisory roles, and some problems that have come to be known as "similar benefits" regulations, whereby services that are available from one agency are not allowed to be provided by another.

Lack of information sharing has often been identified as a barrier to effective collaboration (Edgar, 1985; Halpern & Benz, in press). For example, public schools rarely inform adult service agencies of the number of students with disabilities who will be leaving school and possibly requiring postschool assistance. Young adults with disabilities may have to apply separately to each adult service agency they need, providing the same application information over and over again. The underlying problem is a lack of effective and appropriate procedures for sharing relevant information.

When collaboration has been negotiated between separate agencies, the question of supervision has often emerged. Who is really responsible for developing and implementing a service plan? If this responsibility is shared between professionals from different agencies, who supervises whom? What happens to the student/client as this responsibility is passed around? Difficulties in answering such questions have led to the demise of some collaborative programs, such as the popular work/study program of the 1960s and 1970s, which involved negotiated agreements between public schools and vocational rehabilitation agencies (Halpern, 1974).

A final potential deterrent to collaboration has emerged from the "similar benefits" requirements of many service programs. Briefly, this requirement states that funds shall not be expended on a given service if that service is available from some other source. The idea is to avoid duplication of services and also preserve agency funds for those mandates that are uniquely its own. Unfortunately, it is sometimes unclear whether one agency has more or less responsibility than another for providing a given service. When this occurs, a client can sometimes fall between the cracks of agency fiscal responsibility.

Program Documentation The final service delivery area that has potential impact on outcomes is the documentation that is required as people with disabilities receive services both in school and from adult service agencies. Documentation refers both to planning requirements prior to service delivery and to closure practices and requirements as people exit from their programs.

The planning documentation requirements that affect outcome evaluation are derived from major pieces of federal legislation that govern most school and adult service programs for people with disabilities. A common feature of this legislation is the requirement for producing "individualized program plans" as a precondition for service delivery. These plans must include several components, among which are documentation of need for services, long-range goals and short-term objectives (i.e., outcomes), specification of services to be delivered, and timelines for implementation of the plan. All affected parties must participate in the development of the plan, including service providers, service recipients, and family members when appropriate. The planning process must also be repeated and updated periodically.

The outcome of this process is the development of a formal document, such as the individualized education program (IEP) in special education and the individualized written rehabilitation program (IWRP) in vocational rehabilitation. These documents serve several purposes, including the structuring of a data base that can be used for outcome evaluation. The issue that emerges is the validity of this data base. Because the information is produced in order to comply with various laws (and thereby to receive federal funds), there is a tendency for people to fill out the forms in a "boiler plate" manner, complying with the letter of the law but not necessarily its spirit. This is not always the case, but sorting out the good data from the bad can become difficult.

The "closure" documents that accompany the termination of services can also present some problems for outcome evaluation. In education, the issue is whether the person leaving school will receive a diploma or a "certificate of completion." The distinction between these two is not always clear and uniform across school districts, and the problem will surely become worse as the current movement toward "excellence in education" accelerates and graduation requirements become more and more stringent. From the perspective of evaluation, the problem becomes one of attaching meaning to the attainment of a diploma as an outcome criterion.

A somewhat similar problem exists within the rehabilitation agency, where closure status is simply documented with a code number indicating overall success or failure in attaining the rehabilitation goal(s) expressed in the IWRP. Since these goals can vary greatly in their complexity and qualitative merit, a dichotomous, "on/off" scoring system will minimize the interpretative power of evaluation efforts that use such scores.

Service Outcome

Even though eligibility and service delivery issues are obviously relevant to the planning and evaluation of service outcomes, there are several issues to be considered simply from the perspective of the outcomes themselves. These issues can be characterized as 1) multilevel definition of outcomes, 2) multidimensional definition of outcomes, and 3) societal versus client perspectives.

Multilevel Definition of Outcomes Differences in severity of disability are likely to have a major impact on the outcomes of service programs. For example, people with the most severe levels of mental retardation are likely to pursue outcome goals that are substantially different from those goals that are sought by people with mild mental retardation. The main outcome concern is whether or not eventual adult adjustment will require ongoing support from other people.

Two current examples of this issue can be cited, one from employment and the other from independent living. A major outcome goal for most people with disabilities is to achieve the maximum level of employment possible, given any constraints imposed by the consequences of impairment. For many people, this will mean regular competitive employment in the community. For others, however, competitive employment may only be achievable if accompanied by ongoing support from a person whose job is to troubleshoot problems or provide the employee with assistance in avoiding problems (Kiernan & Stark, 1986; Will, 1984b). Similar residential programs, called "semi-independent living" programs, provide clients with the minimum amount of training and supervision necessary to maintain their homes in the community (Halpern et al., 1986).

The existence of different outcome "levels," although clearly appropriate for many service programs, also presents a problem in outcome evaluation. When evaluating the impact of programs, we must attempt to neither over- nor underestimate the "potential" of a given student when outcome goals are selected. If easy (but inappropriate) goals are selected, programs may appear to perform more effectively than they really do. If difficult goals are unnecessarily avoided, clients may be inappropriately denied opportunities to enhance their level of adjustment. Evaluations must be designed very carefully in order to avoid (or at least account for) this source of potential bias.

Multidimensional Definition of Outcome Community adjustment has been presented in Table 1 as a multidimensional set of outcomes, including residential environment and social networks in addition to employment. There is a need both to define these dimensions operationally and to examine whatever relationships may exist between the defined dimensions.

Outcome dimensions are not easy to define because they represent a wide array of social values. Is it more important to earn a lot of money or to do work that is interesting? Is it more important to have many friends or to nurture a few deep relationships? Many models of community adjustment have been suggested, and the adoption of a particular model will have obvious implications for how the components of outcome dimensions are operationalized and measured. For example, the outcome components of the model presented in Table 1 have been operationalized in one study by 12 discrete variables (Halpern, Nave, Close, & Nelson, in press), with the model playing a major role in identifying these variables.

Assuming that a multidimensional model of community adjustment is eventually adopted as the appropriate goal of service programs, a new issue will emerge concerning the degree of independence between different dimensions of the model. If the dimensions are highly related to one another, programs geared to address only one dimension may have "spillover" effects onto the others. On the other hand, if the dimensions are largely independent of one another, then programs will need to attend specifically to each desired dimension. Otherwise, success in one area, such as employment, may be offset by failure in another, such as the quality of social networks. Recent evidence strongly suggests that outcome dimensions for adults with mental retardation are, in fact, largely independent of one another (Halpern et al., in press).

Societal versus Client Perspective Even with the adoption of a multidimensional model of outcomes, one further issue must be resolved. Most proposed models of adjustment focus on societal values for their articulation. This includes employment, independent living, and the development of social networks. The valuing of specific elements within such dimensions, however, can vary greatly from individual to individual, to the point where a personal definition might vary substantially from a societal definition. It would, therefore, be prudent for any outcome model adopted to represent both client and societal perspectives. Research evidence has shown that obtaining reliable and valid self-reports from people with mental retardation is possible, as long as appropriate precautions are observed during the data collection process to ensure that interviewees understand the questions and interviewers understand the answers (Sigelman et al., 1981).

SPECIFIC MEASUREMENT ISSUES

The above discussion has focused primarily on issues and problems of design that must be identified and controlled to evaluate properly the array of programs and services for people with mental retardation. There are also both conceptual and methodological issues in measurement that have a potential impact on the evaluation of outcomes. The conceptual issues include the contrasts between functional and structural assessment, student and environmental assessment, and process and product assessment. Methodological issues include format limitations on assessment tools imposed by impairment, and the level of examinee involvement in the assessment process.

Conceptual Issues

Structural versus Functional The distinction between structural and functional assessment has already been introduced as a diagnostic issue, where it was argued that functional assessment is more relevant than structural assessment for determining eligibility. A very similar argument can be stated forcefully for the measurement of outcomes. In essence, functional assessment deals with behaviors that are relatively molecular, such as budgeting or home management skills, whereas structural assessment concerns molar constructs that are inferred from assessment performance, such as intelligence or adaptive behavior. Since outcomes are usually most interpretable as goals when they are articulated at the molecular level, functional assessment becomes the desirable approach for measurement of outcomes. Many instruments have been identified that are appropriate for providing functional assessments of adolescents and adults with mental retardation (Halpern, 1984; Halpern et al., 1982).

Student versus Environmental The role of environmental assessment is very closely related to the role of functional assessment within the service delivery process in that both are required to facilitate good decision making. The outcome of a functional assessment is a profile of personal strengths and weaknesses along one or more dimensions of behavior that are relevant to the educational or community adjustment objective. To make an appropriate decision about service delivery, however, one must also document the environmental demands and resources that are available to solve a given problem. Once this "environmental assessment" has been completed, an attempt can be made to match student needs with environmental opportunities (Wallace & Larsen, 1978). Given the importance of en-

vironmental assessment within a functional approach to decision making, it is unfortunate to observe that very little work has been done in the field of mental retardation toward the development of procedures and instruments that focus on environmental assessment (Halpern, 1984).

Product versus Process Approach A third conceptual issue in the area of assessment is the distinction between a product and a process approach to assessment. In the former approach, which is also the most ubiquitous, assessment is concerned only with the products of past learning, and it is assumed that the examinee's prior opportunities to learn have been adequate. Assessment is geared toward measuring what an examinee can do at the present time *without assistance,* rather than investigating what might be required in the process of instruction to enhance the likelihood of future success. It is possible, however, to focus on the process of instruction as an object rather than an assumption of assessment. This transforms the salient assessment question from "How well does a person perform?" to "What resources are required to attain a given level of performance?" Although this approach is relatively new, a technology of process assessment is available for answering certain questions more appropriately than through the use of more familiar product approaches to assessment (Browning & Irvin, 1981; Feuerstein, 1979; Halpern, 1984).

Methodological Issues

Certain impairment-related characteristics must be considered when selecting an assessment instrument (Halpern et al., 1982). For example, if a norm-referenced instrument is selected for addressing a particular problem, one must ascertain whether or not people with impairments similar to the person being evaluated have been included in the standardization sample. Testing format can also present problems, as illustrated by the use of instruments requiring high reading levels with students who have mental retardation. Unless the skill being evaluated *itself* requires reading, such an instrument will confound reading ability with whatever skill is actually of concern, leading to a spuriously low interpretation.

A focus on functional assessment leads to another methodological issue concerning the extent of student involvement in the assessment process. This approach to assessment works best when the examinee is thoroughly involved in all stages of the assessment process, including interpretation and ultimate decision making (Vash, 1984). Questions have been raised, however, about the extent of involvement possible when the person being evaluated has limited abilities and/or certain behavioral problems. This issue surfaces in studies that attempt to evaluate the impact of examinee involvement on the outcomes of assessment.

CONCLUSION

When outcome evaluation is placed in the broader context of a complete service delivery model, it quickly becomes apparent that issues of evaluation design and outcome measurement are inextricably intertwined with one another. An attempt has been made in this chapter to identify these issues and elucidate their relationships. If the lessons to be learned are followed, it is both possible and rewarding to incorporate good outcome evaluation in the management of educational and habilitation programs for people with mental retardation.

REFERENCES

Alley, G., & Deshler, D. (1979). *Teaching the learning disabled adolescent: Strategies and methods*. Denver: Love Publishing Co.

Blatt, B. (1981). *In and out of mental retardation: Essays on educability, disability, and human policy*. Baltimore: University Park Press.

Brolin, D. (1983). *Life centered career education: A competency based approach* (rev. ed.). Reston, VA: The Council for Exceptional Children.

Browning, P., & Irvin, L. (1981). Vocational evaluation, training and placement of retarded persons. *Rehabilitation Counseling Bulletin, 24,* 374–408.

Bruininks, R., Meyers, C., Sigford, B., & Lakin, K. (Eds.). (1981). Deinstitutionalization and community adjustment of mentally retarded people. Washington, DC: *American Association on Mental Deficiency Monographs,* No. 4.

Charles, D. (1953). Ability and accomplishments of persons earlier judged as mentally retarded. *Genetics Psychology Monograph, 47,* 3–71.

Edgar, E. (1985). How do special education students fare after they leave school: A response to Hasazi, Gordon, and Roe. *Exceptional Children, 51,* 470–473.

Edgerton, R. (1967). *The cloak of competence: Stigma in the lives of the mentally retarded*. Berkeley: University of California Press.

Edgerton, R. (Ed.). (1984). Lives in process: Mildly retarded adults in a large city. Washington, DC: *American Association on Mental Deficiency Monographs,* No. 6.

Falvey, M. (1986). *Community-based curriculum: Instructional strategies for students with severe handicaps*. Baltimore: Paul H. Brookes Publishing Co.

Feuerstein, R. (1979). *The dynamic assessment of retarded performers*. Baltimore: University Park Press.

Foss, G., & Bostwick, D. (1981). Problems of mentally retarded adults: A study of rehabilitation service consumers and providers. *Rehabilitation Counseling Bulletin, 25,* 66–73.

Galagan, J. (1985). Psychoeducational testing: Turn out the lights, the party's over. *Exceptional Children, 52,* 288–299.

Gollay, E., Freedman, R., Wyngaarden, M., & Kurtz, N. (1978). *Coming back*. Cambridge, MA: Abt Books.

Grossman, H. J. (1983). *Classification in mental retardation*. Washington, DC: American Association on Mental Deficiency.

Halpern, A. (1974). Work-study programs for the mentally retarded: An overview. In P. Browning (Ed.), *Mental retardation: Rehabilitation and counseling*. Springfield, IL: Charles C Thomas.

Halpern, A. (1984). Functional assessment and mental retardation. In A. Halpern & M. Fuhrer (Eds.), *Functional assessment in rehabilitation*. Baltimore: Paul H. Brookes Publishing Co.

Halpern, A., & Benz, M. (in press). A statewide examination of secondary special education students with mild disabilities: Implications for the high school curriculum. *Exceptional Children*.

Halpern, A., Close, D., & Nelson, D. (1986). *On my own: The impact of semi-independent living programs for adults with mental retardation*. Baltimore: Paul H. Brookes Publishing Co.

Halpern, A., Lehmann, J., Irvin, L., & Heiry, T. (1982). *Contemporary assessment for mentally retarded adolescents and adults*. Baltimore: University Park Press.

Halpern, A., Nave, G., Close, D., & Nelson, D. (in press). An empirical analysis of the dimensions of community adjustment for adults with mental retardation and borderline intelligence. *Australia and New Zealand Journal of Developmental Disabilities*.

Hasazi, S., Gordon, L., & Roe, C. (1985). Factors associated with the employment status of handicapped youth exiting high school from 1979 to 1983. *Exceptional Children, 51,* 455–469.

Kennedy, R. (1966). *A Connecticut community revisited: A study of the social adjustment of a group of mentally deficient adults in 1948 and 1960*. Hartford, CT: Connecticut State Department of Health, Office of Mental Retardation.

Kiernan, W., & Stark, J. (1986). *Pathways to employment for adults with developmental disabilities*. Baltimore: Paul H. Brookes Publishing Co.

Landesman-Dwyer, S., & Berkson, G. (1984). Friendship and social behavior. In J. W. Wortis (Ed.), *Mental retardation and developmental disabilities: Annual review* (Vol. 13). New York: Plenum Press.

Landesman-Dwyer, S., Sackett, G., & Kleinman, J. (1980). Relationship of size to resident and staff behavior in small community residences. *American Journal of Mental Deficiency, 85,* 6–17.

McCarver, R., & Craig, E. (1974). Placement of the retarded in the community: Prognosis and outcome. In N. R. Ellis (Ed.), *International review of research in mental retardation* (Vol. 7). New York: Academic Press.

Mercer, J. (1973). *Labeling the mentally retarded.* Berkeley: University of California Press.

O'Connor, G. (1976). Home is a good place: A national perspective of community residential facilities for developmentally disabled persons. Washington, DC: *American Association on Mental Deficiency Monographs,* No. 2.

O'Connor, G. (1983). Social support of mentally retarded persons (1983 presidential address to the American Association on Mental Deficiency, Dallas). *Mental Retardation, 21,* 187–196.

Sigelman, C., Schoenrock, C., Winer, J., Spanhel, C., Hromas, S., Martin, P., Budd, E., & Bensberg, G. (1981). Issues in interviewing mentally retarded persons: An empirical study. In R. Bruininks, C. Meyers, B. Sigford, & K. Lakin (Eds.), Deinstitutionalization and community adjustment of mentally retarded people. Washington, DC: *American Association on Mental Deficiency Monographs,* No. 4.

Stokes, T., & Baer, D. (1977). An implicit technology of generalization. *Journal of Applied Behavior Analysis, 10,* 349–367.

Vash, C. (1984). Evaluation from the client's point of view. In A. Halpern & M. Fuhrer (Eds.), *Functional assessment in rehabilitation.* Baltimore: Paul H. Brookes Publishing Co.

Wallace, G., & Larsen, S. (1978). *Educational assessment of learning problems: Testing for teaching* (Chapter 4). Boston: Allyn and Bacon.

Wehman, P. (1981). *Competitive employment: New horizons for severely disabled individuals.* Baltimore: Paul H. Brookes Publishing Co.

Will, M. (1984a). *OSERS programming for the transition of youth with disabilities: Bridges from school to working life.* Washington, DC: Office of Special Education and Rehabilitative Services.

Will, M. (1984b). *Supported employment for adults with severe disabilities: An OSERS program initiative.* Washington, DC: Office of Special Education and Rehabilitative Services.

Chapter 4

Outcome Analysis
in Psychiatric Rehabilitation

Marianne Farkas and William A. Anthony

Outcome studies in psychiatric rehabilitation have been complicated by the varied definitions of rehabilitation and the resultant differences in what was considered appropriate outcome. Historically, the psychiatric population has been treated in terms of the diagnostic categorization of the patient or client sample. Studies focused on the treatment of schizophrenia or the treatment of the borderline personality. The *International Classification of Impairments, Disabilities, and Handicaps* (World Health Organization, 1980) has helped to differentiate the focus of *treatment* for the psychiatric population and *rehabilitation* for the psychiatric population. The classification essentially implies that "treatment-oriented" techniques be used for the impairment related to the disorder. In other words, clinical treatment focuses on reducing the symptoms of pathology. Symptom reduction is thus an appropriate outcome measure for clinical treatment. Rehabilitation, on the other hand, focuses on the disability, that is, the decreased ability to perform certain skills and activities as well as the societal handicaps that accompany such disabilities (Anthony, Cohen, & Danley, in press). Changes in functioning or in living, learning, or working status become appropriate outcome measures for studies related to rehabilitation.

Over the last two decades, a number of studies have assessed the efficacy of rehabilitation programs for persons with severe psychiatric disabilities (Anthony, Buell, Sharrett, & Althoff, 1972; Anthony, Cohen, & Vitalo, 1978; Bachrach, 1976; Erickson, 1975). In addition to these general overviews, there have been reviews of outcome in specific psychiatric rehabilitation and community support settings—for example, community residential facilities (Carpenter, 1978; Goldmier, 1977), halfway houses (Cometa, Morrison, & Zishoren 1979), and day hospitals (Moscowitz, 1980). Still other reviews have assessed the effectiveness of various skill-training approaches (Anthony, 1979; Anthony & Margules, 1974; Hersen & Bellack, 1977; Morrison & Bellack, 1984; Wallace et al., 1980); drug therapy, alone or in combination with psychosocial rehabilitation (Davis, Schaffer, Killian, Kinard, & Chan, 1980; Engelhardt & Rosen, 1976; Gardos & Cole, 1976; Goldberg, Schooler, Hogarty, & Roper, 1977; Schooler & Severe, 1984; Tobias & MacDonald, 1974); and the major community support intervention approaches (Test, 1984; Test & Stein, 1978).

The research of the last several decades has focused on three major contributors to client rehabilitation outcome variance:

1. Skill training interventions, which teach skills necessary for success in a particular environment.
2. Drug therapy interventions, which reduce symptomatology and prevent relapse.
3. Community support interventions, which enhance the client's ability to function in specific community settings.

These three interventions are the treatment modalities that a psychiatrically disabled client will most typically experience (excluding custodial care).

Two other interventions, psychotherapy and family treatment, have been used and researched less often. Psychotherapy research with severely disabled clients was on the wane during the 1970s (Mosher & Keith, 1979), whereas family treatment, albeit with a less dynamic and more supportive-educational approach than formerly, attracted renewed research interest (Anderson, Hogarty, & Reiss, 1980; Falloon, Boyd, McGill, Strang, & Moss, 1981).

Although the focus of a research study may be on one particular intervention strategy, a researcher must control for the fact that a client is often concurrently receiving one or both of the other interventions. All three types of intervention are known to contribute to some of the same measures of rehabilitation outcome (Anthony, 1979).

Early studies of psychiatric rehabilitation relied almost exclusively on recidivism, relapse, and, to a lesser extent, employment data as outcome criteria (Anthony et al., 1972; Mosher & Keith, 1979), all measures of changes in the psychiatric handicap. Although these measures have undeniable advantages—they are easily objectified and readily understood by lay people, imply tangible economic benefits, and make it possible to compare studies using similar outcome measures—the importance of using a broader range of outcome measures has been stressed repeatedly (Anthony et al., 1972, 1978; Bachrach, 1976; Erickson, 1975; Mosher & Keith, 1979).

Most recent studies of psychiatric rehabilitation have investigated the outcomes of a psychiatric rehabilitation intervention for severely psychiatrically disabled persons by measuring: 1) client behavioral change, or measures related to changes in the disability, or 2) client and society benefits (Anthony, 1984; Anthony & Farkas, 1982). Measures of client behavioral change indicate whether the clients are able to do anything differently as a result of their involvement in a psychiatric rehabilitation intervention—that is, what skills (e.g., conversing with parents) or activities (e.g., joining a club) are they now performing, either in the rehabilitation setting (e.g., completing work tasks on time at the sheltered workshop) or in a nonrehabilitation environment (e.g., conversing with parents at the dinner table). Measures of client and society benefits indicate what the client and/or society re-

ceives because of the psychiatric rehabilitation intervention. Simple measures of recidivism and days spent in the hospital or community may be used as rough estimates of client and society benefits. Other types of benefit measures are estimates of the clients' satisfaction with their life situation and measures of living, learning, and working status, such as level of employment, degree of independent living, and educational achievement.

In this chapter, the nature of psychiatric rehabilitation and its target population are described first. Available information is then summarized regarding recidivism and the residential, educational, and vocational status of psychiatrically disabled persons. The following section overviews the current practice of outcome analysis in psychiatric rehabilitation, with a review of the types of studies typically conducted. Problems and unresolved issues in the analysis of psychiatric rehabilitation outcome are discussed in the next chapter section. The final section describes one study as an example of how some of these issues can be addressed.

THE INTERVENTION AND THE TARGET GROUP

The field of psychiatric rehabilitation is increasing in popularity. More and more mental health professionals have come to recognize the need for a rehabilitation intervention to complement existing treatment approaches (Anthony et al., 1972; Anthony, Cohen, & Farkas, 1986). The term *rehabilitation* is used increasingly in our professional jargon and program descriptions. Inpatient as well as community programs are described as having a rehabilitation orientation (Allen & Velasco, 1980; Fairweather, 1978; Furman & Lund, 1979).

The psychiatric rehabilitation approach has progressed to the stage where its mission and philosophy can be articulated, the characteristics of its intended recipients described, its outcomes specified and measured, and its major interventions described and monitored. In essence, the overall mission of psychiatric rehabilitation is to ensure that the person with a psychiatric disability can perform those physical, emotional, and intellectual skills needed to live, learn, and work in his or her own particular community, given the least amount of intervention necessary from agents of the helping professions (Anthony, 1979). The major clinical interventions by which this mission is accomplished involve either developing the specific skills clients need to function effectively in their lives and/or developing the community supports needed to accommodate or strengthen the client's present level of functioning (Anthony, 1979; Anthony & Margules, 1974; Liberman & Foy, 1983).

The *target population* of psychiatric rehabilitation is those persons who have become disabled as a result of psychiatric illness. Several definitions of severe psychiatric disability characterize this target population. The definition used for this review is consistent with the definition currently used by the National Institute of Mental Health's Community Support Program (CSP), the Rehabilitation Services Administration's (RSA) definition of severe disability, and Goldman's (Goldman, Galtozzi, & Taube, 1981) definition of the "chronically mentally ill." Each of these definitions (CSP, RSA, Goldman) shares common elements: a diagnosis of mental illness, of prolonged duration, with resulting functional or role incapacity. It has ben estimated that between 1.7 and 2.4 million persons in the United States are severely psychiatrically disabled (Goldman et al., 1981). The appendix to this chapter lists the components of the CSP definition (Stroul, 1984), which at the present time appears to be the most accepted definition.

Implications for Outcome Assessment

The field of psychiatric rehabilitation has progressed from a singular emphasis on vocational functioning to the clients' functioning in all areas of their lives. Simple reliance on a working/not working outcome dichotomy, or a recidivist/non-recidivist distinction, is being replaced. Consistent with the current practice of psychiatric rehabilitation, more complex outcome measures remain to be developed for the various living, learning, and working environments in which clients function. Also important is having a sense of

what the base rate of functioning is in each of these areas. The available information is summarized below.

Historically, the *living* status of persons who are psychiatrically disabled has usually been assessed in two ways: recidivism rates and place of residence. Although the use of hospital recidivism figures has been repeatedly critiqued because of its susceptibility to a variety of influences other than persons' adjustment to their living situation (Anthony et al., 1972, 1978; Bachrach, 1976), it continues to be a measure that is routinely collected. Comprehensive reviews of the literature indicate a gradually increasing rate of recidivism as the follow-up period lengthens. The recidivism rate at 6 months is approximately 30%–40%; at 12 months, 35%–50%; and at 5 years, 67%–75% (Anthony et al., 1972, 1978).

Not many data about the psychiatrically disabled person's residence are comparable across studies. Thus, no accurate estimates exist of the typical degree of independent living status of severely psychiatrically disabled persons. A multistate sample of clients attending community support programs indicates that 40% were living in a private home or apartment, 12% in board and care settings, and 10% in family foster care placements; other residential categories had less than 10% each (Tessler & Goldman, 1982). The National Plan for the Chronically Mentally Ill (U.S. Department of Health and Human Services, 1980) estimated that, of those persons residing in the community, 38%–50% were in board and care settings and 19%–21% lived with families. A nationwide survey of family members of severely psychiatrically disabled persons, who were also members of the National Alliance for the Mentally Ill (NAMI), reported that approximately 30% lived at home with family, 15% in a community residence, and 18% in a hospital (Spaniol, Zipple, & Fitzgerald, 1984). It is clear from these studies that the type of definition of residential categories varies from study to study, thus precluding, for the time being, national estimates of independent living status.

Data about the *educational* status of severely psychiatrically disabled persons have received scant attention in the literature. However, the available data serve as a reminder of the advanced educational status of many severely psychiatrically disabled persons. It appears, depending on the particular sample taken, that 52%–92% of severely psychiatrically disabled persons are high school graduates, and that 15%–60% of these high school graduates have attended college (Fountain House, 1985; Goering, Wasylenki, Farkas, Lancee, & Ballantyne, 1986; Spaniol et al., 1984; Tessler & Goldman, 1982).

Studies containing data on the competitive employment rates of persons discharged from psychiatric hospitals have been periodically surveyed by Anthony and associates (Anthony et al., 1972, 1978; Anthony, Howell, & Danley, 1984). The data have been fairly consistent, suggesting a full-time competitive employment figure of 20%–25% for all persons discharged from psychiatric hospitals. However, if just severely psychiatrically disabled persons are studied, the full- and part-time competitive employment figure drops to approximately 15% and below. For example, the NAMI survey data of well-educated, severely psychiatrically disabled persons from middle to upper income families reported a full-time employment rate of only 6% (Spaniol et al., 1984). Farkas, Rogers, and Thurer (1986) followed up 54 long-term state hospital inpatients who had been targeted for deinstitutionalization in 1979. Over a 5-year period, none obtained competitive employment. Tessler and Goldman (1982) reported an 11% full- and part-time competitive employment rate for Community Support Program clients. Wasylenki, Goering, Lancee, Ballantyne, and Farkas (1985) reported that 11% of their hospitalized sample were competitively employed prior to admission. When Dion (1985) followed up patients hospitalized with bipolar disorder, he found evidence of the impact of severity on vocational outcome. At 6 months' follow-up, 64% of first-admission patients were employed at some level of competitive employment, versus 33% of persons with one or more hospitalizations. Interestingly, only 20% of the total sample were functioning at their expected level of employment, that is, at the occupational level expected given previous work history and education.

CURRENT PRACTICE OF OUTCOME ANALYSIS

Types of Outcomes

In a comprehensive review of outcome measures used in psychiatric rehabilitation, Anthony and Farkas (1982) concluded that:

1. Change on a single measure of client outcome does not indicate that seemingly related measures of change have been affected.
2. A positive effect on one client outcome measure may have an associated negative effect on the other.

Thus, it behooves researchers to study the impact of their intervention with a wider range of outcomes and to make no assumptions about the intervention's impact on outcomes not specifically studied. In general, the recent research literature seems compatible with these guidelines.

The types of outcomes used in the studies reviewed indicate the manner in which outcome measures have been refined. Simple yes/no measures of employment status have been complemented by measures of types of employment, for example, vocational, transitional, part-time, full-time (Fountain House, 1985); earnings (e.g., Bond, 1984); satisfaction with work (Rehabilitation Research Brief, 1980); productivity (Hoffman, 1980); and instrumental role functioning (Goering, Farkas, Wasylenki, Lancee, & Ballantyne, 1986).

Regarding living status, simple recidivism measures have been all but replaced by measures of total days in the community (e.g., Cannady, 1982), social adjustment (e.g., Linn, Caffey, Klett, Hogarty, & Lamb, 1979), number of friends and activities (Rehabilitation Research Brief, 1980; Vitalo, 1979), degree of independent living (e.g., Mosher & Menn, 1978), satisfaction with community adjustment (e.g., Katz-Garris, McCue, Garris, & Herrign, 1983), and social skills (e.g., Aveni & Upper, 1977).

Educational status has been the subject of very few studies. Yet many academically capable young adults have had their educational progress interrupted by a psychiatric disability (Spaniol et al., 1984; Unger & Anthony, 1983). The outcome of rehabilitation interventions designed to improve educational functioning could be assessed by using such outcome measures as degree programs entered or completed, courses completed, professional/educational certificate programs completed, academic skills learned, course grades, and achievement test scores.

Typical Outcome Studies

A variety of settings have served as the location of psychiatric rehabilitation studies, the most common being psychosocial rehabilitation centers and hospitals. Community mental health centers and offices of state divisions of vocational rehabilitation have also been used. A number of studies have investigated the delivery of psychiatric rehabilitation–type interventions by the collaborative efforts of more than one setting or agency. These studies include hospital/community linkages (Paul & Lentz, 1977; Wasylenki et al., 1985) and mental health and vocational rehabilitation programming (Dellario, 1984; Rogers, Spaniol, Dellario, & Danley, 1984). Even many of the settings that appear autonomous, such as psychosocial rehabilitation centers, actually involve places outside the center's physical setting, such as employment sites (Fountain House, 1985). The fact that the rehabilitation intervention often occurs in more than one place illustrates the need for a thorough understanding by researchers of the comprehensive nature of the psychiatric rehabilitation intervention.

As expected, a good deal of the psychiatric rehabilitation outcome literature focuses on the vocational environment. In part, this appears to be due to the original emergence of the term *rehabilitation* in a vocational context, that is, the vocational rehabilitation of the physically disabled. Within the mental health field, however, the rehabilitation concept has included a concern with the person's adjustment to his or her living situation as well, a fact reflected in the early and routine collection of recidivism data. The research investigations reviewed are characteristic of the field's interest in working and living environments.

In contrast, as evidenced by the types of outcome measures used, investigations related to

improving the person's educational status have rarely been forthcoming. However, an ongoing research project investigating a university-based rehabilitation program for young adults indicates the need for such programming (Unger & Anthony, 1983). The announcement of this program to a selected group of mental health agencies in the Boston area has generated over 75 completed applications for the first 26 available spots.

There are several obvious limitations in the manner in which the interventions have been studied. First, many of the interventions are not described in sufficient detail to permit replication, either in future research studies or in clinical practice. Simply knowing the setting in which the intervention occurred provides little information about the specific intervention. Although limitations imposed by journal space no doubt account for some of this brevity, the references accompanying most articles do not indicate the existence of any manuals and videotapes that might facilitate replication. Some exceptions are the interventions modeled after the psychiatric rehabilitation intervention developed by Anthony and his colleagues (e.g., Goering, Farkas et al., 1986; Rehabilitation Research Brief, 1980; Vitalo, 1979; Wasylenki et al., 1985); the Fountain House transitional employment approach (e.g., Fountain House, 1985); Paul's social learning approach (e.g., Paul & Lentz, 1977); and Azrin's job-seeking skills program (see H. E. Jacobs, Kardashian, Kreinbring, Ponder, & Simpson, 1984).

Another problem is the difficulty in differentiating the unique contributions to rehabilitation outcome of skill development from supportive interventions. Support typically occurs by means of programs that shelter or otherwise accommodate psychiatrically disabled persons who do not have the skills to consistently meet the demands of the environment. Rehabilitation support is also provided by people in these programs who offer personal support, companionship, advocacy, and practical assistance. Most of these supportive programs and people also provide opportunities for persons with severe psychiatric disabilities to learn skills. Some may promote the skill-learning process by providing an environment that facilitates learning, whereas others provide a relatively more structured, formalized skill-learning program. Still others, of course, fall somewhere in between.

From a research perspective, skill development and supports have been inextricable. Investigations have lacked either the technology or the intent to study the relative merits of the two types of interventions. At the present time, the research suggests that interventions that give the client the opportunity to both learn and receive support remain the preferred rehabilitation interventions.

Results of Outcome Studies

Anthony and Dion (1986) have conducted the most recent review of psychiatric rehabilitation outcome studies. Particularly significant are the studies that reported improved outcome through joint programming between two different settings or agencies. These coordinated efforts included cooperative hospital and community programming (Paul & Lentz, 1977; Wasylenki et al., 1985) and collaborative mental health and vocational rehabilitation efforts (Dellario, 1984; Rogers et al., 1984).

The ability of collaborative interventions initiated from a hospital base to produce rehabilitation outcome in the community is particularly noteworthy. Dellario and Anthony (1981), Kileser (1982), and Test and Stein (1978) concluded that hospital care and community-based care should not be compared to one another, but rather to the stated mission of the agency, no matter what its location. This, of course, presumes a statement of mission that articulates exactly the intended outcomes for each facility—an apparently nonexistent condition for many settings (Farkas, Cohen, & Nemec, 1986). Nevertheless, hospital and community rehabilitation efforts can be successful if properly coordinated and if committed jointly to the provision of rehabilitation programming without arbitrary time limits.

The positive vocational outcomes associated with collaborative mental health and vocational rehabilitation interventions confirm the benefits of better coordination between services that are already available. In an era of cost containment, such data give impetus to efforts at increasing the

effectiveness of those service components already in place. More efficient service delivery need not sacrifice improved client outcome; indeed, it may improve it.

With the continued nationwide development of psychosocial rehabilitation centers, research conducted at these centers takes on increasing importance. Several of the interventions carried out at psychosocial rehabilitation centers were studies of Transitional Employment Programming (TEP), a vocational training innovation currently used in many psychosocial rehabilitation agencies around the country (Fountain House, 1985). In a TEP, a client of the psychosocial rehabilitation agency is placed in an entry-level job in a normal place of business. All placements are temporary (3–9 months), typically half-time, and supervised by the psychosocial agency (Beard, Propst, & Malamud, 1982). A TEP is designed to develop the self-confidence, job references, and work habits necessary to secure employment.

Until recently, there has been little research studying the effectiveness of TEPs. Typically, studies have examined the vocational outcomes of persons served by a psychosocial rehabilitation agency, whose services included a TEP. In a very early study, Beard, Pitt, Fischer, & Goertzel (1963) reported no significant differences in employment between experimental and comparison subjects. In a randomized control group design, Dincin and Witheridge (1982) found no differences in employment at 9 months' follow-up.

A major follow-up of Fountain House members who spent at least 1 day in a TEP has just been completed (Fountain House, 1985). The results from 527 individuals who received a TEP indicated the employment outcome increased as a function of the time since the initial TEP. For those whose initial TEP was at least 42 months ago, 36% were competitively employed. At 12 months and 24 months, the employment rates were 11% and 19%, respectively.

Also just completed was a study of Thresholds' psychosocial rehabilitation center of two different types of TEPs, an accelerated and a traditional one. At 15 months' follow-up, the 20% and 7% employment rates in the accelerated and traditional TEP conditions approximated Fountain House's employment figure for the same time period (Bond & Dincin, 1986).

The results of current TEP research to date suggest the TEPs have a significant impact on employment as the follow-up period increases. The recent research out of Thresholds suggest that for a person with prior work experience, the entrance into a TEP could be accelerated and the time needed to obtain employment shortened.

Psychiatric rehabilitation outcome studies are somewhat unique in the mental health field in that many of the intended outcomes are specific, observable, understandable, and valued by the general public. Various methods of skill development and/or support development interventions have been found to impact such seemingly straightforward outcome criteria as days in the community (Cannady, 1982; Paul & Lentz, 1977), earnings (Bond, 1984), reduction in disability pensions (Jensen, Spangaard, Juel-Neilsen, & Voag, 1978), and employment (Turkat & Buzzell, 1983). Other outcomes produced, although somewhat more complex in terms of measurement, have meaning to the lay person, for example, independent living (Bond, 1984; Mosher & Menn, 1978), productivity (Ryan & Bell, 1985), work satisfaction (Rehabilitation Research Brief, 1980), increased friendships and activities (Vitalo, 1979), role performance (Goering, Farkas et al., 1986; Goering, Wasylenki et al., 1986; M. K. Jacobs & Trick, 1974), and increased skills (LaPaglia, 1981; Vitalo, 1979). The intended outcome goals of psychiatric rehabilitation interventions are typically very specific. As outcome measurements in psychiatric rehabilitation studies have become more refined by measuring degrees of improvement over time rather than at one time, the findings of psychiatric rehabilitation interventions have become more positive. For example, studies that have not shown the expected change on measures of recidivism did report results on measures of community tenure (Beard, Malamud, & Rossman, 1978) and role functioning (Goering, Farkas, Wasylenki, Lancee, & Ballantyne, 1986).

In several studies, the longer the follow-up period the more dramatic the findings. For example, differences in instrumental role functioning and social adjustment increased from 6 months'

to 2 years' follow-up (Goering, Farkas, Wasylenki, Lancee, & Ballantyne, 1986; Goering, Wasylenki, Farkas, Lancee, & Ballantyne, 1986), differences in employment that were not apparent at 9 months appeared at 15 months (Bond & Dincin, 1986), and the longer the transitional employment placement the greater the vocational outcome (Fountain House, 1985).

UNRESOLVED PROBLEMS IN ASSESSMENT

Rehabilitation researchers tend to think of their interventions as having an impact only on the outcome goals of immediate interest to them. Concern with measuring expected outcomes often obscures the importance of investigating other potential outcomes. For example, Vitalo (1971, 1979) reported that his experimental group surpassed the control group in targeted interpersonal skills but was also rated as more anxious. Thus, researchers must examine a range of outcomes, assessing both intended and unintended effects.

One of the most difficult problems in assessing psychiatric rehabilitation outcome is effectively measuring changes in clients' level of skills. Many measures, particularly those adapted from the social skill training literature, reflect molecular behavior. Moving from such measures as frequency counts of the number of eye contacts made in 3 minutes of conversation to the more complex assessment of social behavior involves a loss of clarity and specificity. Two common responses to the problem of vagueness have been either to further refine the assessment of molecular behavior (Wallace et al., 1980) or to develop idiosyncratic measures for each new set of research problems. Because of journal space limitations, instruments often are not described in sufficient detail. Consequently, replicating the study is as difficult as replicating the rehabilitation interventions, which are also incompletely described. Many studies do not even reference the instruments that were used, making it more difficult to identify the potential standardized measures.

Another problem is that reliability and validity measures are often not reported (Ciminero, Calhoun, & Adams, 1977). Reliability tends to be more frequently reported than validity—perhaps reflecting the problems that arise in establishing convergent or concurrent validity for a vaguely defined set of complex behaviors (Alevizos & Callahan, 1977). Indeed, the question of the validity of behavioral measures has rarely been considered (Wallace et al., 1980).

For community adjustment measures, however, even formal tests of reliability are seldom documented (Waskow & Parloff, 1975). Many instruments used in outcome research were developed on acute inpatients or outpatients and then applied to the chronic population, for lack of a population-specific instrument. When the researcher moves beyond direct measurements of change (e.g., number of days attending a workshop) and applies assessment techniques standardized on other populations, problems with reliability and validity arise.

Researchers are unanimous in calling for more measures designed to assess the generalization of skill acquisition. Hersen and Bellack (1977, p. 510) stated that the "importance of generalization in most behavioral research has been acknowledged more in print than in actual practice." There is an acknowledged lack of a systematic framework in which to produce generalization techniques or measures that are ethical and naturalistic (Curran, 1980; Hersen & Bellack, 1977). Only 40% of studies targeting the skills behaviors of the chronically disabled addressed some aspect of the problem of skill application (Wallace et al., 1980). In those studies that have addressed generalization, frequency counts of behaviors and unstructured or structured questionnaires have typically been the assessment format used (Hollingsworth & Foreyt, 1975; Patterson & Teigen, 1973; Tracey, Briddell, & Wilson, 1974).

In addition to assessing whether the skills learned in training are applied in the targeted environment, there is a pressing need for the development of skill acquisition measures that positively correlate with concrete measures of client benefits. Skill outcome measures developed by Paul and Lentz (1977) and by Griffiths (1973) are models in this regard. Predictive validity based on measures of inpatient be-

haviors has been reported by Power (1979) and Redfield (1979) using the Clinical Frequencies Recording System and the Time Sample Behavioral Checklist, respectively. Both these instruments were developed and standardized in the decade-long investigation conducted by Paul and his associates. Predischarge scores on these instruments can significantly predict the discharged patient's functioning in the community (Paul, 1984).

Designed to measure vocational skills of psychiatrically disabled clients, the Standardized Assessment of Work Behavior (Griffiths, 1973, 1974; Watts, 1978) assesses a broad range of skills (e.g., uses tools/equipment, communicates spontaneously, grasps instructions quickly). Items are rated on a continuum from skill strength (e.g., looks for more work) to skill deficit (e.g., waits to be given work). Both reliability and productive validity data are available for this scale.

Recently, interest has increased in outcome measures of overall level of functioning, compatible with the increased use of functional assessment in psychiatric rehabilitation practice (Cohen & Anthony, 1984). Many states have developed forms for measuring the functional levels of their Community Support Programs clients. These forms often include ratings of client skills. The CSS-100 (New York State Office of Mental Health, 1979) is used by many community support systems. Separate scales measure adjustment to environment (e.g., using public transportation, managing funds, dressing self) and behavioral problems or symptoms (e.g., hospitalization, employment-related services, community living programs, socialization activities). Similarly, the Multi-Function Needs Assessment (Angelini, Potthof, & Goldblatt, 1980) used in Rhode Island and Connecticut includes assessment of functioning self-maintenance, environmental interactions, psychiatric symptoms, and current use of services. Other forms, developed along the same lines, are in use in New Jersey (New Jersey Division of Mental Health and Hospitals, 1979) and Michigan (Cornhill Associates, 1980). These scales have shown promise in outcome studies using a large number of subjects (e.g., all patients in the hospital, all mentally ill clients served by the state).

In addition to the shortcomings of most measurement tools, there are deficiencies in the research design of most outcome studies. However, outcome studies do exist, and in increasing frequency, that have randomly assigned subjects to experimental and control groups (Bond, 1984; Bond & Dincin, 1986; Dincin & Witheridge, 1982; Paul & Lentz, 1977; Ryan & Bell, 1985; Wolkon, Karmen, & Tanaka, 1971) or matched experimental and control groups (Beard et al., 1982; Goering, Wasylenki et al., 1986; Hoffman, 1980; Matthews, 1979; Mosher & Menn, 1978; Vitalo, 1979; Wasylenki et al., 1985). The positive outcomes of these studies seem in no way different from the outcomes generated by quasi-experimental designs.

Unfortunately, the design deficiencies in the psychiatric rehabilitation field are still readily apparent. First, there is a gross lack of studies employing designs that permit reasonable causal inferences to be made. Second, many designs are plagued by inadequate sample size, heterogeneity of population, nonrandom assignment, lack of specificity and replicability of treatment approach, brief follow-up periods, and lack of reliable, valid outcome measures appropriate to the interventions used. Third, the vast majority of studies used one-group, posttest only designs.

Despite the fact that the field's data base rests on a number of nonexperimental studies, these studies still do have value. They have provided the empirical and conceptual foundation for the experimental studies that have begun to appear. Current researchers have seized the data that were available from these studies to fashion more specific interventions that can now be researched experimentally. Much of this previous research can be considered exploratory, examining the practical significance of interventions prior to the experimental test so that new outcome strategies and methodologies could be developed.

OVERCOMING SOME OF THE PROBLEMS OF PSYCHIATRIC REHABILITATION OUTCOME RESEARCH: A CURRENT EXAMPLE

A recent study conducted by the Center for Psychiatric Rehabilitation of Boston University in conjunction with the Clarke Institute of Psychiatry of Toronto attempted to address some of the outcome research issues outlined: sample size, heterogeneity of population, random assignment, specificity of intervention, relevant outcome variables, instrumentation, and length of follow-up. The study focused on chronically psychiatrically disabled patients managed by community-based practitioners trained in psychiatric rehabilitation compared with patients whose discharge planning was arranged by inpatient staff members (Wasylenki et al., 1985).

Sample Size

A multisite strategy provided the research project with a large pool of subjects. In each of the four hospital settings, consecutively admitted patients were screened for chronicity, poor employment history, social isolation, and residential instability. These criteria predicted poor outcome 6 months and 2 years postdischarge in a previous descriptive study (Goering, Wasylenki, Lancee, & Freeman, 1984). Ninety-two matched control patients were identified from the pool of 505 subjects interviewed in the original aftercare study. The two groups were matched for diagnoses, number of previous admissions, employment prior to admission, and hospital setting. Fortunately, there were no differences between the two groups in demographic or treatment characteristics.

Heterogeneity of the Population

Global variables, such as age, sex, marital status, education and diagnostic categories, number of previous admissions, and employment prior to admission were used to match the group in the comparative study with the historical controls. Employing statistical controls allowed the researchers to use the population they had at hand without reducing the sample size.

Random Assignment

The screened patients were randomly selected to participate in the rehabilitation case management program. Those not selected for the rehabilitation program were given the discharge plans usual for the hospital in which they were patients. The random assignment did not pose the usual ethical

problems encountered in the field, since most of
the hospital staffs were quite pleased with their
discharge methodology and did not believe that
their patients were being deprived of treatment.
This was one instance in which reticence on the
part of the setting being researched in fact helped
the research design.

Specificity of the Intervention

One of the ongoing problems in rehabilitation research has always been the lack of specificity of
the intervention, which impedes the ability of
other researchers to replicate the study. The skills
of Community Service Coordination (in which
the case managers were trained) have been detailed (Cohen, Vitalo, Anthony, & Pierce, 1980)
and a written curriculum has been used to train
Master's students as well as practitioners in the
field. The curriculum breaks each skill down into
component parts and presents didactic, modeling, and experiential material to help practitioners learn the standardized sets of skills needed.
This training has been successfully replicated for
case managers in regular training offered by the
Center for Psychiatric Rehabilitation.

Outcome Variables

Given that the rehabilitation program being evaluated was designed to link patients from inpatient settings to services that met their identified
needs, the outcome variables were: percentage of
identified needs for which referrals were made,
use of aftercare services for which links were
made, satisfaction with services, symptomatology and social functioning, and recidivism.

Case management is designed to provide support for effective linking of the patient with the
aftercare service, rather than any direct service.
The variables of symptomatology, social functioning, and recidivism thus were included more
because of the interest in the field in these variables than because they represented any intended
outcome of the rehabilitation case management
program. These outcome variables became measures of the unintended effects of the case management program.

Instrumentation

The study used five standardized instruments—
Brief Follow Up Scale (Soskis, 1970); Housing

Scale (Clare & Cairns, 1978); Social Functioning
Scale (Remington & Tyrer, 1979); Brief Psychiatric Rating Scale (Overall & Gorham, 1962);
and General Health Questionnaire (Goldberg &
Hiller, 1979). It also included a questionnaire designed to evaluate the patients' satisfaction with
their services and their degree of involvement in
the process (Farkas, 1982). This questionnaire
had been reliably used in many other studies conducted by the Center for Psychiatric Rehabilitation. The interviewers were trained to use all of
the instruments, and a reliability check was carried out. The interviewers also contacted by
phone or in person all agencies and individuals
that had provided aftercare to at least five or more
of the subjects. They also contacted a random
sample of those treating fewer subjects. Information from aftercare service providers was comparable to that obtained from subjects about their
use of services during the 6 months postdischarge.

Length of Follow-Up

Because psychiatrically disabled persons are
often hard to find once they have left confined
facilities such as hospitals, many outcome studies have a very brief follow-up period (3–6
months). Often, however, changes do not occur
until much later in the process (Harding, Brooks,
Ashikaya, & Strauss, 1982). The case management study conducted a 6-month follow-up
(Goering, Farkas, Wasylenki, Lancee, & Ballantyne, 1986) and a 2-year follow-up (Goering,
Wasylenki, Farkas, Lancee, & Ballantyne,
1986). Of the original 92 subjects, only 10 were
lost to follow-up. The single interviewer used for
the 2-year follow-up study was the same person
who conducted the 6-month follow-up study. The
advantage of this strategy was that she knew the
patients well enough to be able to find them when
they had left no forwarding address or did not
show up at their homes for a lengthy period of
time. Furthermore, when she did find them, they
knew her and were comfortable enough to talk to
her again, thus lowering the rate of refusal to be
interviewed.

Preliminary Results

The 82 subjects remaining at 2 years' follow-up
were matched with historical controls from the

original descriptive aftercare study (Goering et al., 1984) for hospital setting, number of previous admissions, diagnosis, and employment status. There were no significant differences in the demographic or clinical characteristics of the experimental and control groups in instrumental role functioning (unintended outcome), changes in occupational and housing status, and social isolation. There was no difference in recidivism rates or total number of readmissions. If these outcomes had been the only ones used, it would have appeared as though the intervention had no effect.

SUMMARY

The study described above is one example of attempting to overcome the traditional problems of conducting rehabilitation research with the chronically psychiatrically disabled population. The experiences of the researchers in this study indicate that paying attention to the details of planning and the human factors involved, and a great deal of persistence, do result in data that can be a valid and reliable contribution to the field.

The field of outcome research in psychiatric rehabilitation is in its infancy. Current research has had to begin to identify research designs, instrumentation, and methods of collecting data as well as methods of analyzing the "in vivo" results that are meaningful and valid. Although, as pointed out in this chapter, some of these efforts are beginning to bear fruit, there is much room for the enterprising researcher to contribute new methods to what promises to be an exciting and productive field of inquiry.

APPENDIX: NIMH OPERATIONAL DEFINITION OF THE CSP POPULATION[1]

Based on the first 3 years of the pilot CSP initiative, in 1980 the National Institute of Mental Health (NIMH) developed an operational defini-

tion for use in identifying CSP clients, planning service system improvements, and evaluating national CSP efforts. All NIMH-supported CSP activity must focus on persons who meet the following criteria:

1. **Severe disability resulting from mental illness**
   A CSP client typically meets at least *one* of the following criteria:
   - Has undergone psychiatric treatment more intensive than outpatient care more than once (e.g., emergency services, alternative home care, partial hospitalization, or inpatient hospitalization)
   - Has experienced a single episode of continuous, structured supportive residential care other than hospitalization for a duration of at least 2 months

2. **Impaired role functioning**
   In addition, such an individual typically meets at least *two* of the following criteria, on a continuing or intermittent basis for at least 2 years:
   - Is unemployed, is employed in a sheltered setting, or has markedly limited skills and a poor work history
   - Requires public financial assistance for out-of-hospital maintenance and may be unable to procure such assistance without help
   - Shows severe inability to establish or maintain a personal social support system
   - Requires help in basic living skills
   - Exhibits inappropriate social behavior which results in demand for intervention by the mental health and/or judicial system

People who meet these program criteria and who do not *appropriately* require long-term, full-time, skilled, or semiskilled care in a medical or nursing facility should be conceptually included regardless of where they may be residing at a particular time.

[1]Portions of this appendix have been reprinted with minor modifications from Stroul, B. A. (1984, June). *Toward community support systems for the mentally disabled: The NIMH community support program.* Boston: Center for Rehabilitation Research and Training in Mental Health, Boston University.

REFERENCES

Alevizos, P., & Callahan, E. (1977). The assessment of psychotic behavior. In A. Ciminero, K. Calhoun & H. Adams (Eds.), *Handbook of behavioral assessment* (pp. 683–721). New York: John Wiley & Sons.

Allen, R. E., & Velasco, R. D. (1980). An inpatient setting: The contributions of a rehabilitation approach. *Rehabilitation Counseling Bulletin, 24,* 108–117.

Anderson, C. M., Hogarty, G. E., & Reiss, D. J. (1980). Family treatment of adult schizophrenic patients: A psycho-educational approach. *Schizophrenia Bulletin, 6,* 490–505.

Angelini, D., Potthof, P., & Goldblatt, R. (1980). *Multi-Functional Assessment Instrument.* Unpublished manuscript, Rhode Island Division of Mental Health, Cranston, RI.

Anthony, W. A. (Ed.). (1979). *The principles of psychiatric rehabilitation.* Baltimore: University Park Press.

Anthony, W. A. (1984). The one-two-three of client evaluation in psychiatric rehabilitation settings. *Psychosocial Rehabilitation Journal, 8,* 83–95.

Anthony, W. A., Buell, G. J., Sharrett, S., & Althoff, M. F. (1972). The efficacy of psychiatric rehabilitation. *Psychological Bulletin, 78,* 447–456.

Anthony, W. A., Cohen, M. R., & Danley, K. S. (in press). The psychiatric rehabilitation model as applied to vocational rehabilitation. In M. Bell and J. Ciardiello (Eds.), *Vocational rehabilitation of persons with prolonged disorders.* Baltimore: Johns Hopkins University Press.

Anthony, W. A., Cohen, M. R., & Farkas, M. (1986). Training and technical assistance in psychiatric rehabilitation. In A. Meherson (Ed.), *Psychiatric disability: Clinical, administrative and legal aspects.* Washington, DC: American Psychiatric Association Press.

Anthony, W. A., Cohen, M. P., & Vitalo, R. (1978). The measurement of rehabilitation outcome. *Schizophrenia Bulletin, 4,* 365–383.

Anthony, W. A., & Dion, G. (1986). *Psychiatric rehabilitation: Rehabilitation research review.* Washington, DC: Catholic University Press.

Anthony, W. A. & Farkas, M. (1982). A client outcome planning model for assessing psychiatric rehabilitation interventions. *Schizophrenia Bulletin, 8,* 13–38.

Anthony, W. A., Howell, J., & Danley, K. (1984). The vocational rehabilitation of the psychiatrically disabled. In M. Mirabi (Ed.), *The chronically mentally ill: Research and services.* New York: SP Medical and Scientific Books.

Anthony, W. A., & Margules, A. (1974). Towards improving the efficacy of psychiatric rehabilitation: A skills training approach. *Rehabilitation Psychology, 21,* 101–105.

Aveni, C. A., & Upper, D. (1976). *Training psychiatric patients for community living.* Paper presented at Midwestern Association of Behavior Analysis meeting, Chicago, IL.

Bachrach, L. L. (1976). A note on some recent studies of released mental hospital patients in the community. *American Journal of Psychiatry, 133,* 73–75.

Beard, J. H., Pitt, R. B., Fisher, S. H., & Goertzel, V. (1963). Evaluating the effectiveness of a psychiatric rehabilitation program. *American Journal of Orthopsychiatry, 33,* 701–712.

Beard, J. H., Malamud, T. J., & Rossman, E. (1978). Psychiatric rehabilitation and long-term rehospitalization rates: The findings of two research studies. *Schizophrenia Bulletin, 4,* 622–635.

Beard, J. H., Propst, R. N., & Malamud, T. J. (1982). The Fountain House model of psychiatric rehabilitation. *Psychosocial Rehabilitation Journal, 5,* 47–52.

Bond, G. R. (1984). An economic analysis of psychosocial rehabilitation. *Hospital and Community Psychiatry, 35(4),* 356–362.

Bond, G. R., & Dincin, J. (1986). Accelerating entry into transitional employment in a psychosocial rehabilitation agency. *Rehabilitation Psychology, 31(3).*

Cannady, D. (1982). Chronics and cleaning ladies. *Psychological Rehabilitation Journal, 5,* 13–16.

Carpenter, M. D. (1978). Residential placement for the chronic psychiatric patient: A review and evaluation of the literature. *Schizophrenia Bulletin, 4,* 384–398.

Ciminero, A., Calhoun, K., & Adams, H. (1977). *Handbook of behavioral assessment.* New York: John Wiley & Sons.

Clare, A., & Cairns, V. E. (1978). Design, development and use of a standardized interview to assess social maladjustment and dysfunction in community studies. *Psychological Medicine, 8,* 589–604.

Cohen, B., & Anthony, W. A. (1984). Functional assessment in psychiatric rehabilitation. In A. Halpern & M. Fuhrer (Eds.), *Functional assessment in rehabilitation.* Baltimore: Paul H. Brookes Publishing Co.

Cohen, M., Vitalo, R., Anthony, W., & Pierce, R. (1980). *The skills of community service coordination* (Psychiatric Rehabilitation Practice Series, Book 6). Baltimore: University Park Press.

Cometa, M. S., Morrison, J. K., & Zishoren, M. (1979). Halfway to where? A critique of research on psychiatric halfway houses. *Journal of Community Psychology, 7,* 23–27.

Cornhill Associates. (1980). *Needs Assessment Instrument.* Unpublished manuscript, Newton, MA.

Curran, T. (1980). A procedure for the assessment of social skills: The simulated social interaction test. In T. Curran & P. Monti (Eds.), *Social skills training: A practical handbook for assessment and treatment.* New York: Guilford Press.

Davis, J. M., Schaffer, C. B., Killian, G.A., Kinard, C., & Chan, C. (1980). Important issues in the drug treatment of schizophrenia. *Schizophrenia Bulletin, 6,* 70–87.

Dellario, D. (1984, March). The relationship between MH/VR interagency functioning and vocational rehabilitation outcome in the psychiatrically disabled. *Rehabilitation Counseling Bulletin,* pp. 167–170.

Dellario, D., & Anthony, W. A. (1981). On the relative effectiveness of institutional and alternative placement for the psychiatrically disabled. *Journal of Social Issues, 37,* 21–33.

Dincin, J., & Witheridge, T. F. (1982). Psychiatric rehabilitation as a deterrent to recidivism. *Hospital and Community Psychiatry, 33,* 645–650.

Dion, G. L. (1985). *Parameters and predictors of functional outcome in bipolar patients hospitalized for a manic episode: Results of two and six month follow-up.* Unpublished doctoral dissertation, Boston University.

Engelhardt, D. M., & Rosen, B. (1976). Implications of drug treatment for the social rehabilitation of schizophrenic patients. *Schizophrenia Bulletin, 2,* 454–462.

Erickson, R. (1975). Outcome studies in mental hospitals: A

review. *Psychological Bulletin, 82,* 519–540.

Fairweather, G. (1978). The development, evaluation and diffusion of rehabilitative programs: A social change process. In L. Stein & M. Test (Eds.), *Alternatives to mental hospital treatment.* New York: Plenum Press.

Falloon, I. R., Boyd, J. L, McGill, C. W., Strang, J. S., & Moss, H. B. (1981). Family management training in the community care of schizophrenia. In M. Goldstein (Ed.), *New directions for mental health services: New developments in interventions with families of schizophrenics* (pp. 61–67). San Francisco: Jossey-Bass.

Farkas, M. (1982). *Client satisfaction questionnaire.* Boston: Center for Psychiatric Rehabilitation, Boston University.

Farkas, M., Cohen, M., & Nemec, P. (1986). *Psychiatric rehabilitation programs: Putting concepts into practice?* Boston: Center for Psychiatric Rehabilitation, Boston University.

Farkas, M., Rogers, S., & Thurer, S. (1986). *Rehabilitation outcome for the recently deinstitutionalized client: The ones left behind.* Boston: Center for Psychiatric Rehabilitation, Boston University.

Fountain House. (1985). *Evaluation of clubhouse model community based psychiatric rehabilitation.* Final report. (Contract No. 300-84-0124). Washington, DC: National Institute of Handicapped Research.

Furman, W. M., & Lund, D. A. (1979). The assessment of patient needs: Description of the level of care survey. *Journal of Psychiatric Treatment and Evaluation, 1,* 51–56.

Gardos, G., & Cole, J. O. (1976). Maintenance antipsychotic therapy. Is the cure worse than the disease? *American Journal of Psychiatry, 133*(11), 32–36.

Goering, P. N., Farkas, M., Wasylenki, D., Lancee, W. J., and Ballantyne, R. (1986). *Improved functioning for clients of a rehabilitation case management program.* Manuscript submitted for publication.

Goering, P. N., Wasylenki, D., Farkas, M., Lancee, W., & Ballantyne, R. (1986). *Two year follow-up of a rehabilitation case management program. What happens to the chronically disabled psychiatric clients?* Manuscript submitted for publication.

Goering, P. N., Wasylenki, D., Lancee, W., & Freeman, S. (1984). From hospital to community: Six-month and two-year outcomes for 505 patients. *Journal of Nervous and Mental Disease, 172,* 667–673.

Goldberg, D. P., & Hiller, V. E. (1979). A scaled version of the general health questionnaire. *Psychological Medicine, 9,* 139–145.

Goldberg, S. C., Schooler, N. R., Hogarty, G. E., & Roper, M. (1977). Prediction of relapse in schizophrenia outpatients treated by drug and sociotherapy. *Archives of General Psychiatry, 34,* 171–184.

Goldman, H. H., Galtozzi, A. A., & Taube, C. A. (1981). Defining and counting the chronically mentally ill. *Hospital and Community Psychiatry, 32,* 21–27.

Goldmier, J. (1977). Community residential facilities for former mental patients: A review. *Psychosocial Rehabilitation Journal, 1*(4), 1–46.

Griffiths, R. (1973). A standardized assessment of the work behavior of psychiatric patients. *British Journal of Psychiatry, 123,* 403–408.

Griffiths, R. (1974). Rehabilitation of chronic psychotic patients. *Psychological Medicine, 4,* 316–325.

Harding, C. M., Brooks, G., Ashikaya, T., & Strauss, J. (1982, June). *Social functioning in chronic patients 21–58 years after admission.* Paper presented at the Conference on Schizophrenia, Paranoia and Schizophreniform Disorders in Later Life, Center for Studies of Mental Health on the Aging and Schizophrenia, NIMH, Bethesda, MD.

Hersen, M., & Bellack, A. (1977). The assessment of social skills. In A. Ciminero, K. Calhoun, & H. Adams (Eds.), *Handbook of behavioral assessment* (pp. 509–554). New York: John Wiley & Sons.

Hoffman, D. A. (1980). *The differential effects of self-monitoring, self-reinforcement, and performance standards on the production output, job satisfaction and attendance of vocational rehabilitation clients.* Doctoral dissertation, Catholic University of America. (University Microfilms ABG80-18439)

Hollingsworth, R., & Foreyt, J. (1975). Community adjustment of released token economy patients. *Journal of Behavior Therapy and Experimental Psychiatry, 6,* 271–274.

Jacobs, H. E., Kardashian, S., Kreinbring, R. K., Ponder, R., & Simpson, A. R. (1984). A skills oriented model for facilitating employment among psychiatrically disabled persons. *Rehabilitation Counseling Bulletin, 28,* 87–96.

Jacobs, M. K., & Trick, O. L. (1974). Successful psychiatric rehabilitation using an inpatient teaching laboratory—one-year follow-up study. *American Journal of Psychiatry, 131,* 145–148.

Jensen, K., Spangaard, P., Juel-Neilsen, N., & Voag, V. H. (1978). Experimental psychiatric rehabilitation unit. *International Journal of Social Psychiatry, 24,* 53–57.

Katz-Garris, L., McCue, M., Garris, R. P., & Herrign, J. (1983). Psychiatric rehabilitation: An outcome study. *Rehabilitation Counseling, 26,* 329–335.

Kiesler, C. A. (1982). Mental hospitals and alternative care. *American Psychologist, 37,* 349–360.

Lapaglia, J. E. (1981). *The use of role-play strategies to teach vocationally related social skills to mentally handicapped persons: Three studies of training and generalization.* Doctoral dissertation, Vanderbilt University. (University Microfilms ABG81-21551)

Liberman, R. P., & Foy, D. W. (1983). Psychiatric rehabilitation for chronic mental patients. *Psychiatric Annals, 13,* 539–545.

Linn, M. W., Caffey, E. M., Klett, J., Hogarty, G. E., & Lamb, R. (1979). Day treatment and psychotropic drugs in the aftercare of schizophrenic patients. *Archives of General Psychiatry, 36,* 1055–1066.

Matthews, W. C.(1979). Effects of a work activity program on the self-concept of chronic schizophrenics. *Dissertation Abstracts International, 41*(1), 358B. (Ann Arbor, University Microfilms No. 8816281, 98)

Morrison, R. L., & Bellack, A. S. (1984). Social skills training. In A. S. Bellack (Ed.). *Schizophrenia: Treatment, management and rehabilitation* (pp.274–279). Orlando, FL: Grune & Stratton.

Moscowitz, I. (1980). The effectiveness of day hospital treatment: A review. *Journal of Community Psychology, 8,* 155–164.

Mosher, L. R., & Keith, S. J. (1979). Research on the psychosocial treatment of schizophrenia: A summary report. *American Journal of Psychiatry, 136,* 623–631.

Mosher, L. R., & Menn, A. Z. (1978). Community residential treatment for schizophrenia: Two-year follow-up. *Hospital and Community Psychiatry, 29,* 715–723.

New Jersey Division of Mental Health and Hospitals. (1979). *General level of functioning scale.* Princeton, NJ: Office of Evaluation.

New York State Office of Mental Health. (1979). *CSS-100. Community support systems, NIMH client assessment.* Unpublished manuscript, Albany, NY.

Overall, J. E., & Gorham, D. R. (1962). The brief psychiatric rating scale. *Psychological Reports, 10,* 799–819.

Patterson, R., & Teigen, J. (1973). Conditional and post-hospital generalization of non-delusional responses in chronic psychotic patients. *Journal of Applied Behavior Analysis, 6,* 65–70.

Paul, G. (1984). Residential treatment programs and aftercare for the chronically institutionalized. In M. Mirabi, (Ed.), *The chronically mentally ill: Research and services* (p. 239). New York: Spectrum Publications.

Paul, G. L., & Lentz, R. J. (1977). *Psychosocial treatment of chronic mental patients: Milieu vs. social-learning programs.* Cambridge, MA: Harvard University Press.

Power, C. (1979). The time-sample behavior checklist: Observational assessment of patient functioning. *Journal of Behavior Assessment, 1(3),* 199–210.

Redfield, J. (1979). Clinical frequencies recording systems: Standardizing staff observations by event recording. *Journal of Behavior Assessment, 1,* 199–210.

Rehabilitation Research Brief. (1980). *A skills training approach in psychiatric rehabilitation.* Washington, DC: National Institute of Handicapped Research.

Remington, M., & Tyrer, P. (1979). The social functioning schedule: A brief semi-structured interview. *Social Psychiatry, 14,* 151–157.

Rogers, E. S., Spaniol, L., Dellario, D., & Danley, K. (1984). *The development, implementation, and evaluation of an integrated service delivery system within a rural setting. Project R-12.* In Center for Rehabilitation Research and Training in Mental Health Final Report (Grant no. GOO8005486). Washington, DC: National Institute of Handicapped Research.

Ryan, E. R., & Bell, M. D. (1985). *Rehabilitation of chronic psychiatric patients: A randomized clinical study.* Paper presented at the meeting of the American Psychiatric Association, Los Angeles.

Schooler, N. R., & Severe, J. B. (1984). Efficacy of drug treatment for chronic schizophrenic patients. In M. Mirabi (Ed.), *The chronically mentally ill: Research and services* (pp. 125–142). New York: Spectrum Publications.

Soskis, D. (1970). A brief follow-up scale. *Comprehensive Psychiatry, II,* 445–449.

Spaniol, L., Zipple, A. M., & Fitzgerald, S. (1984). How professionals can share power with families: A new approach to working with families of the mentally ill. *Psychosocial Rehabilitation Journal, 18,* 77–84.

Stroul, B. A. (1984, June). *Toward community support systems for the mentally disabled: The NIMH community support program.* Boston: Center for Rehabilitation Research and Training in Mental Health, Boston University.

Tessler, R. C., & Goldman, H. H. (1982). *The chronically mentally ill: Assessing community support systems.* Cambridge, MA: Ballinger Press.

Test, M. A. (1984). Community support programs. In A. S. Bellack (Ed.), *Schizophrenia: Treatment, management and rehabilitation* (pp. 347–373). Orlando, FL: Grune & Stratton.

Test, M. A., & Stein, L. I. (1978). Community treatment of the chronic patient: Research overview. *Schizophrenia Bulletin, 4,* 350–364.

Tobias, L. L., & MacDonald, M. L. (1974). Withdrawal of maintenance drugs with long-term hospitalized mental patients: A critical review. *Psychological Bulletin, 81,* 107–125.

Tracey, D., Briddell, D., & Wilson, G. (1974). Generalization of verbal conditioning to verbal and non-verbal behavior: Group therapy with chronic psychiatric patients. *Journal of Applied Behavior Analysis, 7,* 391–402.

Turkat, D., & Buzzell, U. M. (1983). Are families satisfied with services to young adult chronic patients? A recent survey and a proposed alternative. In B. Pepper & H. Ryglewicz (Eds.), *New directions for mental health services sourcebook.* San Francisco: Jossey-Bass.

Unger, K., & Anthony, W. (1983). Are families satisfied with services to young adult chronic patients? A recent survey and a proposed alternative. In B. Pepper & H. Ryglewicz (Eds.), *New Directions for Mental Health Services Sourcebook* (pp. 91–98). San Francisco: Jossey-Bass.

U.S. Department of Health and Human Services. (1980). *Toward a national plan for the chronically mentally ill.* Report to the Secretary by the Department of Health and Human Services Steering Committee of the Chronically Mentally Ill. Washington, DC: Author.

Vitalo, R. (1971). Teaching improved interpersonal functioning as a preferred mode of treatment. *Journal of Clinical Psychology, 27,* 166–171.

Vitalo, R. (1979). An application in an aftercare setting. In W. A. Anthony (Ed.), *Principles of psychiatric rehabilitation.* Baltimore: University Park Press.

Wallace, C., Nelson, C., Liberman, R., Aitchinson, R., Lukoff, D., Eider, J., & Ferris, C. (1980). A review and critique of social skills training with schizophrenic patients. *Schizophrenia Bulletin, 6,* 42–63.

Waskow, I., & Parloff, M. (Eds.). (1975). *Psychotherapy change measures* (AIM 74-120). Rockville, MD: National Institute of Mental Health.

Wasylenki, D. A., Goering, P. N., Lancee, W. J., Ballantyne, R., & Farkas, M. (1985). Impact of a case manager program on psychiatric aftercare. *The Journal of Nervous and Mental Disease, 173,* 303–308.

Watts, R. (1978). A study of work behavior in a psychiatric rehabilitation unit. *British Journal of Clinical Psychology, 17,* 85–92.

Wolkon, G. H., Karmen, M., & Tanaka, H. T. (1971). Evaluation of a social rehabilitation program for recently released psychiatric patients. *Community Mental Health Journal, 7,* 312–322.

World Health Organization. (1980). *International classification of impairments, disabilities, and handicaps.* Geneva: Author.

Chapter 5

Outcome Analysis
in Vocational Rehabilitation

Brian Bolton

Since the inception of the state/federal vocational rehabilitation (VR) program two thirds of a century ago, the goal of service provision has been to return persons with disabilities to the competitive labor market. Consequently, the criteria by which the VR program traditionally has been judged and justified have been *economic* measures, that is, placement in employment, salary earned, and discontinuation or reduction of public financial support. The emphasis on "hard" economic indicators of success continues to this day because the state/federal VR program is justified legislatively as an excellent investment of taxpayers' money. Estimates of benefit-to-cost ratios exceed 10 for some categories of disabled former clients, that is, $10 is returned to the economy for every $1 expended for rehabilitation services.

Needless to say, continued reliance on economic measures of success has been severely criticized by many rehabilitationists as too narrow in focus. It is not true, of course, that vocational rehabilitation programs have entirely neglected the humanitarian argument. Efforts directed at employers to encourage them to "hire the handicapped" stress both economic benefits and civic responsibility. Still, the substantial burden on VR administrators is to demonstrate the economic viability of the program. And the most stringently applied of the three eligibility criteria for state/federal VR services is the requirement that the applicant be "feasible," that there exist a reasonable probability that the individual will be

employable after the provision of needed services. What all of this means is that outcome analysis is almost synonymous with economic justification in publicly supported VR programs.

This chapter is concerned primarily with assessment of clients' outcomes in the state/federal VR program and in facilities that contract with state programs to provide intensive vocational evaluation, adjustment, and related preparatory services. However, much of the discussion also applies to outcome analysis in the private, for-profit rehabilitation sector. This chapter does not deal with the translation of outcome measures into economic indices, or what is generally called benefit–cost analysis, because that topic is addressed in Chapter 8. Overlap with Chapter 16 is also minimized by focusing on problems, issues, and techniques in VR outcome analysis, rather than on VR outcome analysis systems.

Although this chapter is of necessity eclectic in composition because there is no systematized body of knowledge on outcome analysis in VR, one perspective is relied upon to provide an overall theoretical framework. The Minnesota Theory of Work Adjustment (MTWA) has been researched continuously and refined for the past 30 years. Begun in 1957 with the support of the Vocational Rehabilitation Administration (VRA) as the Work Adjustment Project at the University of Minnesota, the MTWA evolved into a psychological conceptualization of the VR process. Especially relevant for this chapter is the MTWA's delineation of vocational outcomes and the de-

Preparation of this chapter was supported by Research and Training Center grant G0083C0010/03 from the National Institute of Handicapped Research.

velopment of instruments for measuring these outcomes. Readers desiring an axiomatic presentation of the MTWA are referred to the volume by Dawis and Lofquist (1984); a succinct overview of the MTWA is available in the recent chapter by Dawis (1986).

The remainder of the chapter consists of seven sections:

1. Descriptions of the state/federal VR service program and the population served
2. Delineation of the scope of VR outcome analysis
3. Reviews of milestone studies in VR outcome analysis
4. Summaries of four VR outcome studies that illustrate the variety of client variables that can be assessed
5. Overviews of four conceptual/statistical issues in VR outcome analysis
6. Descriptions of eight VR outcome analysis instruments
7. Discussions of instrument applications in analyzing VR outcomes and needed research in VR outcome analysis

VR SERVICE INTERVENTIONS AND TARGET GROUPS

The state/federal VR program serves more than a half million persons with disabilities every year. The primary agent of service delivery is the field counselor, who manages the case from the point of application for services through case closure. With the exception of general vocational counseling, most client services are purchased from registered vendors. Services typically include medical and psychological examinations, appropriate restorative services, and specialized work adjustment and vocational training programs. In some cases, psychosocial adjustment preparation, independent living training, family counseling, or individual psychotherapy may be provided.

State/federal VR services are *not* available to all disabled persons. To qualify for VR services, an applicant must be judged eligible to receive services. Eligibility includes three requirements, all of which must be satisfied:

1. Presence of a diagnosable condition of medical, psychiatric, or intellectual disablement

2. Determination that the disabling condition constitutes a handicap to employment, broadly defined
3. Reasonable expectation that the provision of necessary services will render the individual employable

The state/federal VR program serves persons with all types and degrees of disabling conditions, subject only to the eligibility requirements stated above.

The implications of the eligibility requirements for the analysis of VR program outcomes are twofold. First, outcome measures must bear directly on vocational functioning generally and employment particularly, or a strong case must be made that any outcome measures are at least vocationally relevant. Second, the heterogeneity of the target group served, which encompasses persons with all types of disabilities, and the wide range of services that may be provided necessitate an equally broad-ranging and comprehensive approach to VR outcome analysis.

Walls and Tseng (1986) outlined the VR process as an input–intervention–output model and reviewed client statuses in the VR service program. Assessments of VR clients' characteristics and outcomes are appropriately completed at three points in time: 1) acceptance for services (at status 10); 2) case closure (in statuses 26, 28, or 30); and 3) follow-up 1 year after case closure. Instruments administered before acceptance for services can serve both a diagnostic function (see Bolton, 1986a, 1986d) and as a baseline for assessing clients' change as a result of VR service provision. Measures of severity of disability administered at status 10 can be used to evaluate the suitability of clients' outcomes at closure and follow-up. It should be stressed that a 1-year follow-up assessment of former VR clients is *not* legally mandated; clients closed successfully (status 26) must have been suitably employed for 60 days, however.

SCOPE OF VR OUTCOME ANALYSIS

A system for comprehensively measuring client outcomes of the VR process is not currently available. This is not because substantial effort has not been expended, but rather is a reflection of the complexity of the problem. This section defines some terms, and the two sections that immediately follow summarize selected studies from the short history of VR outcome analysis research. Then four critical conceptual/statistical issues are briefly outlined.

As stated above, measures of successful outcome in VR have traditionally been economic. Nobody disagrees with the claim that placement in permanent employment is the ultimate goal of VR services, but there are certainly degrees of success within this broad outcome category. Some employees are more satisfied with their jobs than are others, and, conversely, employers are usually more satisfied with some employees than with others. Employment tenure is only a minimal (although highly meaningful) indicator of vocational adjustment. Salary earned is also a very important measure of vocational success, of course. However, it is the thesis of this chapter that many other factors must also be considered in assessing VR outcomes.

Although distinctions could be drawn among terms such as *work*, *occupation*, *employment*, *vocation*, and *job*, they are considered synonymous and interchangeable here. Using the structural approach of the MTWA, vocational adjustment is defined as purposive engagement in some type of economic or work-related activity. This activity is usually paid employment, but not necessarily so. Vocational adjustment is indicated by the individual's *satisfaction* with the work activity and by the *satisfactoriness* of the individual's performance. The MTWA postulates that tenure, or continuation in the particular work activity, is a function of both satisfaction and satisfactoriness.

Many authorities in VR believe that restriction to measures that are primarily work related, although not strictly economic indicators, still neglects an important aspect of vocational adjustment. They argue that vocational adjustment is inseparable from the individual's adjustment in nonwork spheres. For severely disabled persons, who are often restricted to sheltered or supported work environments, nonvocational benefits are often the most important consequence of return

to employment, especially when productivity is extremely limited and work serves a substantially therapeutic function. I personally find this argument compelling and thus pay considerable attention to measurement of psychosocial adjustment as a legitimate facet of VR outcome analysis.

This raises the inevitable question about how severity of disablement can best be considered when analyzing VR outcomes. The direct approach to this issue is to quantify severity in terms of functional limitations, both at initiation of services and again at the time when VR clients are judged to be ready for placement in some form of employment. Assessment of functional limitations has received considerable attention in medical rehabilitation, originally in conjunction with assessment of activities of daily living (ADL), and more recently in attempts to measure broader categories of skills and capabilities that individuals retain or regain following disablement. The reader is referred to the chapter by Crewe (1986) for an overview of measurement in this area.

MILESTONE STUDIES IN VR OUTCOME ANALYSIS

It was not until the 1950s that professionals in VR began to think seriously about the "criterion problem" in analyzing client outcomes. This is not to suggest that rehabilitation counselors and administrators had not realized previously that simple economic measures do not tell the whole story. However, with the initiation of advanced graduate training in vocational rehabilitation in the late 1940s, persons with academic skills in psychology and statistics began entering the field. Within a decade, the state/federal VR program had shifted from a medical restoration and job placement service to an identifiable profession for which specialized training of practitioners was required.

Despite recognition more than 25 years ago of the critical need to resolve the criterion problem in conceptualizing and measuring work adjustment (Scott, Dawis, England, & Lofquist, 1960), and numerous research projects that have been carried out since then, the problem has not been solved as of this writing, although many of the elements of a solution are currently available, including a variety of suitable assessment techniques. The criterion problem is: How can VR program outcomes be properly quantified? More specifically this means: How can outcomes be measured in such a way as to fully reflect the benefits conferred by providing appropriate VR services to disabled clients? Desirable (if not essential) characteristics of the solution include comprehensiveness, parsimony, and practicality. Comprehensiveness refers to appropriate measurement of economic, vocational, and psychosocial variables; parsimony requires that a minimum number of key measures be identified; and practicality means that outcome assessment procedures should be suitable for implementation in state VR agency operations.

With this modest explication of the criterion problem in mind, it is easy to appreciate the relevance of the next milestone research project in VR outcome analysis. Eber (1966) factor analyzed data for a large sample of clients of a state rehabilitation agency. Two outcome factors were identified, vocational adequacy at case closure and vocational adequacy at follow-up. Vocational adequacy at closure was defined by four variables: work status at closure, occupational level of job, weekly earnings, and closure code. Examination of the variables reveals that this dimension is a pure economic composite. Vocational adequacy at follow-up was also defined by four variables: employment status at follow-up, work status improvement from closure, job satisfaction, and the counselor's estimate of success. Although still emphasizing economic indices, the follow-up dimension also includes two judgmental variables, the client's reported job satisfaction and the counselor's global assessment of case success. As a general rule, follow-up studies of VR outcomes encompass a much broader range of measures.

The advances in VR outcome analysis provided by the results of Eber's (1966) statistical investigation were in parsimony and practicality. Instead of viewing discrete variables such as work status, salary, and job satisfaction as separate indicators, Eber's findings demonstrated that

just two underlying factors could explain most of the variance in clients' vocational outcomes (at least with the fairly restricted set of variables used in his study). Because the variables he analyzed were for the most part routinely collected by the agency, the application of appropriate weighting formulas to generate scores on the two vocational dimensions was a simple, practical matter. It is also worth noting that clients' vocational outcomes were substantially predictable from their demographic characteristics and case service information. The obvious weakness of Eber's results is in comprehensiveness—the two vocational success composites are primarily composed of economic indices.

It is in the area of comprehensiveness that the Rehabilitation Gain Scale developed by Reagles, Wright, and Butler (1970) made the next important contribution to VR outcome analysis. In addition to standard economic items (e.g., work status, salary, and primary source of income) and noneconomic vocational items (e.g., difficulty locating a job and optimism about finding a job), the Rehabilitation Gain Scale includes a variety of items reflecting clients' personal and social adjustment (e.g., assessments of physical and mental health, extent of participation in community activities, and membership in organizations). Responses to the 20 items composing the scale are summed to a total score, on the very questionable assumption that economic, vocational, and psychosocial variables all reflect a single, underlying dimension of rehabilitation status. Considerable evidence suggests that VR outcome is a multidimensional construct (see Bolton, 1979, chap. 5).

During the 1970s, considerable progress was made in refining the outcome analysis strategy known generically as case weighting methods. Because case weighting procedures have been used principally to evaluate the efficacy of service delivery units, rather than to quantify individual client benefits, the topic is only indirectly related to the central concern of this chapter. Cooper and Harper (1979) defined a case weighting system as any procedure designed to give differential value to the work done by agency service units with clients having different characteristics, service needs, or outcomes. Readers interested in an overview of case weighting systems in vocational rehabilitation are referred to the chapter by Cooper and Harper (1979).

Numerous instruments have been developed for analyzing rehabilitation outcomes during the past 20 years. For capsule reviews of a wide variety of VR measures, see Bolton (1985), Roessler and Bolton (1983), and Walls and Tseng (1986). From this population of instruments, I have selected eight that are especially appropriate for outcome analysis in state/federal VR programs. The criteria of appropriateness are the three desirable characteristics mentioned above: comprehensiveness, parsimony, and practicality. Because brief descriptions are given later in this chapter, this unreferenced list is provided only to complete the historical review: Functional Assessment Inventory, Human Service Scale, Minnesota Satisfaction Questionnaire, Minnesota Satisfactoriness Scales, Minnesota Survey of Employment Experiences, Service Outcome Measurement Form, Sixteen Personality Factor Questionnaire (Form E), and Work Personality Profile.

SELECTED VR OUTCOME STUDIES

Literally hundreds of studies of VR clients' rehabilitation outcomes have been reported in the literature during the past 35 years. These investigations have typically been restricted to an examination of relationships between standard client biographical variables, (e.g., age, marital status, education, IQ, and disability) and a few indices of employment status at case closure. Some studies have included variables that quantified type and intensity of VR services provided, and some have encompassed a wider range of service outcome measures. Walls and Tseng (1986) presented a selective review of recent vocational rehabilitation outcome studies. In general, it has been longitudinal follow-up research efforts that have attempted to comprehensively analyze VR outcomes. This makes sense because only when a substantial interval of time has elapsed can client outcome criteria "mature"; client outcomes are in actuality a lifelong process rather than an event or occurrence.

In this section, four VR outcome studies reported during the last decade are summarized. Reflecting the characterization of criterion maturation given above, all four studies are follow-up investigations of various samples of former VR clients. What distinguishes these studies from the "historical milestones" described previously is the focus on technology of outcome analysis in the former, whereas follow-up research projects are concerned with evaluation of VR services as indicated by the long-term benefits conferred on former clients. To accomplish the goal of comprehensive evaluation, investigations in the latter group have assessed the full range of client outcome: economic, vocational, and psychosocial variables. The brief descriptions below indicate the range of client outcomes that may be analyzed in VR.

Tseng (1975) collected information from 65 former clients who had been closed successfully after provision of VR services and were employed at follow-up. Information was also obtained from the employers of the former clients. In addition to standard demographic items (e.g., marital status, number of dependents, and recent vocational training) and information about employment (e.g., occupation, salary, and hours worked per week), former clients responded to questions about their job satisfaction, attitudes toward work, work behavior, self-acceptance, and family harmony. Employers rated former clients on work personality variables (e.g., punctuality, cooperativeness, and motivation) and work proficiency variables (e.g., job knowledge, job skill, and safety practices), in addition to providing basic information about clients' employment and an overall judgment of work performance.

Floor and Rosen (1976) investigated the effects of specialized services on 113 adults with cerebral palsy, almost all of whom had previously been VR clients. In individual interviews conducted prior to provision of specialized services and again 1 year later, extensive information about clients' personal and vocational adjustment was obtained. This information included disability condition, living situation, financial dependency, employment history, use of transportation, social activities, emotional problems, and other aspects of clients' adjustment. Interviewers rated clients' degree of physical handicap, employment potential, self-care skills, and daily living skills using standardized scales. A battery of psychological tests, including intelligence, perceptual-motor, and academic achievement measures, was administered before services were rendered. In addition to routine statistical analyses, narrative case reports were written for each client to provide a better understanding of how various facets of rehabilitation outcome combine and interact in the individual situation.

Bolton (1983) obtained follow-up data for 211 former VR clients 2 years after case closure. In addition to standard demographic information collected at intake, the Wechsler Adult Intelligence Scale and Sixteen Personality Factor Questionnaire–Form E were administered before VR services were initiated. The five-page follow-up questionnaire consisted of a variety of multiple-choice and short-answer items covering current employment status, sources of income and financial status, health and psychosocial adjustment, family support, and time spent in various types of nonwork activities. For respondents who were not employed at follow-up, questions about difficulties locating work and perceived prospects for employment were asked. The last page of the questionnaire contained the short form of the Minnesota Satisfaction Questionnaire and was completed by currently employed respondents only.

Roessler and Bolton (1984) performed an intensive follow-up investigation of 57 former VR clients with substantial deficits in employability skills. Personal interviews were conducted with each former client using a standard interview guide. Questions were asked about current and previous employment (e.g., occupation, hours worked, and salary), problems on the job (e.g., production, supervision, and co-workers), job satisfaction, adequacy of vocational preparation, barriers to employment (e.g., inadequate skills, disability problems, and lack of transportation), health status, support from family and friends, perceived employer attitudes toward handicapped persons, and time spent in nonwork activities (e.g., hobbies, watching TV, and social

participation). Employers completed the Minnesota Satisfactoriness Scales for former clients who had worked during the follow-up period.

These four studies illustrate the range and variety of measures that can be used to assess VR outcomes, encompassing numerous economic, vocational, and psychosocial variables. The fundamental principle that is manifested in VR follow-up research is that clients' adjustment is a continuing process, rather than an event that can be assessed at a single point in time, such as at case closure. Follow-up studies also enable deriving more stable indices of adjustment by averaging behavior over time periods (e.g., proportion of time employed during a given interval), as well as calculating change scores. Many researchers and administrators think that a formal follow-up assessment 1 year after case closure should be required in the state/federal VR system. A review and integrated summary of the results of VR follow-up studies is available in an earlier article in which I advocated implementation of a lifelong follow-up system in vocational rehabilitation (Bolton, 1981).

ISSUES IN VR OUTCOME ANALYSIS

Four conceptual statistical issues are central to progress on, and ultimately resolution of, the criterion problem in VR outcome analysis. Because I have previously reviewed these issues in outcome analysis in some detail (see Bolton, 1979, chap. 5), only short summaries are given here.

Economic versus Noneconomic Indices

This issue, already mentioned above, concerns the conceptual range or scope of VR outcome analysis. Economic indices are clearly relevant to vocational success. Equally obvious to most VR practitioners is that noneconomic vocational measures are very important. Although there is less agreement on inclusion of nonvocational or psychosocial indicators of VR success, in my opinion it would be a serious error to exclude this segment of clients' adjustment from the legitimate domain of VR outcomes. Hence, this chapter assumes that comprehensive VR outcome analysis includes psychosocial measures, as well as economic and vocational indices of clients' adjustment.

Agency versus Client Perspectives

The issue of measurement perspectives refers to the source of data or information. Even responses to items such as salary or employment status may be subject to interpretation, contingent on the informant's point of view. Historically, the VR service program (and other social service programs as well) has relied upon agency data for the evaluation of client outcomes, usually referring to such recorded information as "objective data." The implication of this practice, of course, is that clients' opinions, and often counselors' judgments as well, are "subjective" and therefore untrustworthy or useless. Most outcome measures are completed by the VR counselor (representing the agency) or by the client using self-report instruments of psychosocial adjustment or job satisfaction; however, family members and employers are also valuable data sources.

Unidimensional versus Multidimensional Outcome

This issue, known as dimensionality of outcome, has been partially resolved. There is no logical or psychometric justification for summing disparate and distinct aspects of VR outcome into a single composite score to represent overall client "success." In other words, vocational outcome is *not* unidimensional; however, the number of primary dimensions necessary to adequately represent variability in client outcomes has not been determined. The little evidence that exists suggests that there are probably at least four classes (or second-order factors) of VR program outcomes: purely economic indices (e.g., salary and productivity), noneconomic-vocational measures (e.g., job search efforts and job satisfaction), psychosocial adjustment measures (e.g., increased socialization and reduced anxiety), and psychopathology measures (i.e., reduction of psychiatric symptomatology). However, the primary factors of VR outcome and their interrelationships are not known.

Status versus Change Measures

The basic issue here is whether or not it is necessary or desirable to measure relevant variables two or more times in order to quantify individual benefits of VR services. The general answer to the implied question is that, for most aspects of rehabilitation outcome, preservice and postservice assessments are desirable. In some areas, such as job satisfaction, only postservice assessment is realistic. Obviously, job satisfaction measurement presumes placement in some type of sustained work activity. However, for most VR outcome areas, some type of preservice assessment is feasible. The assessment of functional limitations is a more general type of preservice assessment that attempts to quantify "severity of disablement" as a basis for adjusting or interpreting various postservice assessments. Problems with, and techniques for, analyzing pre- and post-data are discussed in Chapter 7.

VR OUTCOME ANALYSIS INSTRUMENTS

In my opinion, adequate instrumentation for analyzing outcomes in VR is currently available. The eight instruments listed previously provide comprehensive coverage of the VR outcome domain. The standard data form used in the state/federal VR program (called the Statistical Reporting Form R-300) already includes client demographic data (e.g., age, education, work history, and occupational skills), VR services provided (e.g., medical treatment, vocational training, and family counseling), and vocational outcome information (e.g., work status, occupation, salary, and public assistance received). The capsule descriptions that follow indicate the variables measured by the selected instruments and summarize their technical characteristics. The most suitable applications of the instruments in VR outcome analysis are outlined in the final section of this chapter.

Functional Assessment Inventory (FAI)

The FAI (Crewe & Athelstan, 1984) is a counselor rating instrument designed to assess VR clients' employment-relevant capacities. It consists of 30 items that specify functional limitations and 10 special strength items. The 30 behaviorally anchored items each describe four levels of clients' capabilities, beginning with "no significant impairment" and progressing through three degrees of increasing limitations that approximate mild, moderate, and severe conditions. The descriptors emphasize vocationally pertinent skills and behaviors. The 10 special strength items require only a check to identify clients' exceptional assets that may act to neutralize the impact of disablement on employment. The FAI can be scored on seven factor scales—adaptive behavior, motor functioning, cognition, physical condition, communication, vocational qualifications, and vision—as well as a total functional limitations (FL) score. The strength items can be summed to a total strength score. Interrater agreement and internal consistency reliability of the FAI items, subscales, and total score are generally high.

Several studies support the validity of the FAI as a measure of vocational potential. Concurrent judgments of "severity of disability" and "employability" correlated in the .50s with the total FL score in several samples of VR clients. Predictive validity coefficients for total FL against work status and earnings at closure were both .50, which is a relatively high level of predictive accuracy for VR clients. Although the authors expressed reasonable reservations about using the FAI on a pre–post basis to assess clients' change as a result of VR services, this should not deter assessors from applying the FAI to "adjust" other vocational measures, enabling consideration of clients' permanent functional limitations in vocational capacities. The FAI has been translated into a self-report inventory, the Personal Capacities Questionnaire (PCQ; Crewe & Athelstan, 1984), which was designed to be completed by clients. The PCQ enables clients to give their own perspectives on their self-perceived limitations.

Human Service Scale (HSS)

The HSS (Kravetz, Florian, & Wright, 1985) was designed to assess clients' rehabilitation needs as a basis for providing appropriate services, and to measure (by retest) the extent to which services were successful in satisfying the rehabilitation needs. Eighty items that require either biographical information or self-ratings are scored on seven-factor analytically derived subscales that are closely related to Maslow's basic need categories: physiological, emotional security, economic security, family, social, economic self-esteem, and vocational self-actualization. The internal consistency reliability coefficients for the HSS subscales range from 0.69 to 0.97, with a median of 0.86.

Several investigations have provided evidence supporting the validity of the HSS: successfully closed VR clients reported greater gains on five of seven subscales than did unsuccessful clients or clients still receiving services, three HSS scales (physiological, family, and economic self-esteem) correlated significantly with independent ratings of similar attributes by VR counselors, and five of seven scales (physiological and emotional security excepted) were independent of psychopathology as measured by the Minnesota Multiphasic Personality Inventory (MMPI). Instructions for HSS administration and normative tables for 10 disability groups are available in mimeographed form, technical information about HSS development is presented in Kravetz et al. (1985), and suggestions for the use of the HSS are given by Reagles and Butler (1976). Unfortunately, no manual for the HSS has been published even though the instrument has been available for use for more than a decade.

Minnesota Satisfaction Questionnaire (MSQ)

The MSQ (Weiss, Dawis, England, & Lofquist, 1967) was designed to measure an individual's satisfaction with 20 different aspects of the work environment, such as ability utilization, achievement, advancement, co-workers, independence, responsibility, variety, and work conditions. The long-form MSQ consists of 100 items that are scored on 20 scales or classes of job reinforcers. The short-form MSQ consists of 20 items, one selected from each of the 20 categories of job reinforcers, that are scored on intrinsic, extrinsic, and general satisfaction scales. For the long-form MSQ, 25 occupational norm groups are available, including professional, clerical, service, benchwork, and unskilled occupations. Seven occupational norm groups ranging from engineers to janitors are provided for the short-form MSQ.

Median internal consistency reliabilities for the long-form MSQ scales range from .78 to .93, with a median of .86. Retest reliabilities with a 1-week interval for a heterogeneous sample of employees ranged from .66 to .91, with a median of .83. Retest stability coefficients with a 1-year interval ranged from .35 to .71, with a median of .61. Median internal consistency reliabilities for the short-form MSQ were .86, .80, and .90 for intrinsic, extrinsic, and general satisfaction, respectively. One-week retest reliability and 1-year stability coefficients for general satisfaction were .89 and .70, respectively.

Concurrent validity of the MSQ was supported by differences among occupational groups in average job satisfaction. For both long-form and short-form MSQs, professional groups reported the highest job satisfaction and unskilled groups reported the least satisfaction, a finding consistent with the existing literature on job satisfaction. Construct validity evidence for the MSQ derives from a variety of investigations of theoretical propositions concerning the antecedents and consequences of job satisfaction (see Bolton, 1986c, for details).

Minnesota Satisfactoriness Scales (MSS)

The MSS (Gibson, Weiss, Dawis, & Lofquist, 1970) is an observer rating instrument that summarizes an employee's level of job performance as judged by the employer. The instrument consists of 28 multiple-choice items that can be completed by an employee's supervisor in about 5 minutes. Scores are calculated on four subscales: 1) performance—how well employees handle their work tasks; 2) conformance—refers to employees' cooperation with supervisors and co-workers; 3) personal adjustment—concerns employees' mental health and personal behavior on the job; and 4) dependability—reflects employees' disciplinary problems and work habits. Raw scores for each of the subscales and a total score, general satisfactoriness, can be converted to percentiles using normative tables for four occupational groups and a workers-in-general group that is representative of the entire U.S. labor force.

Internal consistency reliabilities for the MSS are .90 for performance, .85 for conformance, .74 for personal adjustment, .95 for dependability, and .94 for general satisfactoriness. Retest stability coefficients with a 2-year interval between administrations were .59, .50, .49, .45, and .59, respectively. Research indicates that the MSS is a valid measure of employees' satisfactoriness; satisfactory workers are less likely to leave their jobs than unsatisfactory workers. The MSS has been used in several studies of handicapped employees, with the general finding that former VR clients are typically judged to be only slightly less satisfactory than their nonhandicapped co-workers. For details about the MSS, readers are referred to Bolton (1986b).

Minnesota Survey of Employment Experiences (MSEE)

The MSEE (Tinsley, Warnken, Weiss, Dawis, & Lofquist, 1969) is a follow-up questionnaire designed to be completed without professional assistance by former VR clients. This feature enables agencies to conduct inexpensive follow-up surveys by mailing the MSEE to former clients. Twenty-two questions are presented on four pages that are carefully formatted to minimize confusion and errors. Some items are simple yes/no questions, but the majority require choices from several options or ask the respondent to list activities, such as jobs held, with dates of employment and salary earned. Four types of information are obtained: 1) work experience prior to VR services, 2) work experience from case closure to follow-up contact, 3) details about current employment situation, and 4) related vocational information, such as influence of handicap and job search problems. The last page of the MSEE contains the short form of the Minnesota Satisfaction Questionnaire (MSQ) described above.

The MSEE has been modified for use in a variety of follow-up studies of former VR clients. All indications are that it is a practical, efficient data-collecting device. The only statistics that bear on its "reliability," or perhaps utility, are that, of 5,000 MSEEs returned in a large-scale follow-up project, only 4,000 (80%) were judged to contain "usable information" (Tinsley et al., 1969, p. 4). It is reasonable to assume, however, that there were a multiplicity of reasons why a returned questionnaire was declared unusable. Still, this is an area that should concern outcome analysts; of course, the more fundamental problem of accuracy (or validity) of self-reports should not be neglected.

Service Outcome
Measurement Form (SOMF)

The SOMF (Westerheide, Lenhart, & Miller, 1975) is a counselor rating instrument developed to reflect the employment orientation of the state/federal VR service program. Six subscales or areas of functioning are measured: difficulty, education, economic-vocational status, physical functioning, adjustment to disability, and social competency. Education requires only information about years of schooling; 23 rating items, each with five alternatives, indicate clients' levels of functioning in the other five areas. The anchors emphasize clients' capabilities in relationship to their employment potential. The SOMF can be completed by VR field counselors using routinely available case information in less than 10 minutes.

Interrater reliabilities for the SOMF subscales (except education) for a sample of VR counselors were .69, .95, .75, .79, and .89, respectively (Westerheide & Lenhart, 1973, p. 21). Clients may be evaluated at acceptance for services and again at case closure, with acceptance ratings indicating initial status (or difficulty), closure ratings indicating VR outcome status, and difference scores reflecting benefits due to rehabilitation service (see Westerheide et al., 1975). The SOMF is accompanied by an instruction manual (Westerheide, Lenhart, & Miller, 1974, pp. B12–B46), which include directions for each item and case examples for practice.

Sixteen Personality Factor
Questionnaire–Form E (16 PF-E)

The 16 PF-E (Institute for Personality and Ability Testing [IPAT], (1985) is a self-report personality inventory, designed for use with persons of limited educational and cultural background. It has been used with a variety of rehabilitation populations, including mentally retarded adults, schizophrenic patients, and general caseload VR cli-

ents. The 16 PF-E measures 16 primary dimensions of normal personality functioning, such as warmth, dominance, sensitivity, imagination, insecurity, and self-sufficiency, and five second-order factors: extraversion, adjustment, tough-mindedness, independence, and discipline.

Parallel-form reliabilities for the primary scales are almost all in the .50s and .60s and range from .69 to .86 for the five secondary scales. Eleven primary scales and all five secondary scales had stability coefficients above .40 over a 6-year interval for a sample of VR clients; extraversion (.67) and tough-mindedness (.75) were highly stable, whereas adjustment (.40) and its primary components were much more susceptible to modification as a result of rehabilitation services. Norm tables based on a heterogeneous sample of 992 general VR clients are included in the 16 PF-E manual (IPAT, 1985, pp. 22–26).

Work Personality Profile (WPP)

The WPP (Roessler & Bolton, 1985) is an observer rating instrument designed to be used in conjunction with situational assessments of VR clients' work performance. The WPP consists of 58 items that specify behaviors critical to job maintenance. Each item or work performance characteristic is evaluated using a four-point rating format, with anchors ranging from "employment strength" to "definite problem." The WPP is usually completed by vocational evaluators, but it may be used by employers to identify work problems on the job. The 58 items are scored on 11 work performance scales (acceptance of work role, ability to profit from instruction, work persistence, work tolerance, amount of supervision required, extent trainee seeks assistance, degree of comfort or anxiety with supervisor, appropriateness of personal relations with supervisor, teamwork, ability to socialize with co-workers, and social communication skills) and on five second-order factor scales (task performance, social skills, work motivation, conformance, and personal presentation).

Internal consistency reliabilities for the work performance primary scales range from .71 to .92, with a median of .84, and range from .83 to .91 for the five factor scales, with a median of .89. Retest ratings after 1 week by the same raters are uniformly reliable for all scales, typically in the .70s and .80s. However, interrater agreement is generally much lower, with most coefficients in the .40s, .50s, and .60s. This is not unusual for ratings of observed work behavior and suggests that independent evaluations by two or more raters should be averaged into composite scale scores, a realistic procedure considering the simplicity and brevity of the WPP.

Many other excellent instruments are available for analyzing VR outcomes. Omission from this chapter does not imply that instruments are defective in some way, or even that they are necessarily second choices. The eight instruments described here were selected to encompass the VR outcome domain as efficiently, and yet as comprehensively, as possible. The evaluation below could be applied just as well as to any other set of VR outcome analysis instruments.

APPLICATIONS AND NEEDED RESEARCH

In Table 1, the characteristics of the eight outcome analysis instruments that I selected to be most suitable for use by VR agencies are evaluated according to four conceptual/statistical measurement issues. This brief synopsis provides a

handy reference for use by VR program evaluators who desire to develop a comprehensive outcome analysis system. However, the "issues" of dimensions and time periods in Table 1 are not identical to the measurement issues discussed previously. "Dimensions" in Table 1 refers to intrainstrument dimensionality and scoring procedures, whereas the unidimensional versus multidimensional issue in VR outcome analysis concerns interrelationships among scales across several instruments. "Time periods" in Table 1 denotes three primary assessment points in the VR service/follow-along sequence; measurement of client change is obviously feasible only when an instrument is administered at two or more time periods.

A reasonable conclusion drawn from the discussion thus far is that a comprehensive outcome analysis scheme for VR should measure all three classes of variables (economic, vocational, and psychosocial) from two primary perspectives (agency and client) at three time periods (pretest, closure, and follow-up). Of course, it would be highly desirable to have an assessment by employers at the follow-up period. Careful examination of Table 1 suggests that a number of different combinations of instruments meet the requirements of a comprehensive outcome analysis system. Because the various instruments measure

Table 1. Evaluation of instruments according to measurement issues

Instruments	Variables[a]			Perspectives[b]			Dimensions[c]			Periods[d]		
	E	V	P	A	C	E	P	S	T	P	C	F
FAI		X	X	X	X[e]		X		X	X	X	
HSS	X	X	X		X		X			X	X	X
MSQ		X			X		X[f]	X	X			X[h]
MSS	X	X				X	X		X			X[h]
MSEE	X	X			X							X
SOMF	X	X	X	X			X		X	X	X	
16 PF-E		X			X		X	X		X	X	X
WPP		X		X		X	X	X	X	X[g]		X[h]

[a]Three classes of variables are coded: economic (E), vocational (V), and psychosocial (P).

[b]Three perspectives are coded: agency (A), client (C), and employer (E).

[c]Three levels of dimensions are coded: primary scales (P), second-order factors (S), and total score (T).

[d]Three time periods for assessment are coded: pretest before service initiation (P), case closure (C), and follow-up (F).

[e]The Personal Capacities Questionnaire (PCQ) provides a client-reported assessment of functional limitations.

[f]The long-form MSQ measures satisfaction with 20 primary classes of job reinforcers; the short-form MSQ measures two second-order factors, intrinsic and extrinsic satisfaction.

[g]The WPP requires an extended period to observe clients' work behavior.

[h]The MSQ, MSS, and WPP presume that clients are either employed at follow-up or engaged in some other type of vocational activity.

clients' characteristics and attributes in slightly different ways, considerable flexibility in conceptualizing and analyzing VR outcomes is available to program evaluators and administrators.

By far the single greatest research need in VR outcome analysis is large-scale investigations of instrument interrelationships and dimensionality of comprehensive systems for outcome measures, as defined in the preceding paragraph. The primary goal of this research should be the delineation and specification of a set of major VR outcome dimensions, operationalized in a series of linear equations applicable to various combinations of scores obtained at the three assessment time periods. Such equations would allow psychometrically meaningful, standardized assessment of client outcomes throughout the state/federal VR program.

The organization of occupational aptitudes, normal personality, work values, and many other psychological and vocational domains is hierarchical in structure, with 3 to 5 higher order factors and 12 to 15 primary dimensions. Preliminary evidence supports a similar arrangement of VR outcomes. Once the structure of VR client outcomes is ascertained and standardized scoring equations are developed and published, outcome analysis research can move to another plane of activity. The objective of the second stage of outcome research should be to identify relationships between client characteristics, services provided, and VR outcomes achieved. Such studies would clarify the nature of the constructs represented by the standardized outcome equations, as well as enhance understanding of the VR service system. The ultimate goal of outcome analysis research, then, should be to establish a scientific basis for the improvement of VR services for persons with disabilities.

REFERENCES

Bolton, B. (1979). *Rehabilitation counseling research* (Rev. ed.). Austin, TX: Pro-Ed.

Bolton, B. (1981). Follow-up studies in vocational rehabilitation. *Annual Review of Rehabilitation, 2*, 58–82.

Bolton, B. (1983). Psychosocial factors affecting the employment of former vocational rehabilitation clients. *Rehabilitation Psychology, 28*, 35–44.

Bolton, B. (1985). Measurement in rehabilitation. *Annual Review of Rehabilitation, 4*, 115–144.

Bolton, B. (1986a). Clinical diagnosis and psychotherapeutic monitoring. In R. B. Cattell & R. Johnson (Eds.), *Functional psychological testing*, (pp. 348–376) New York: Brunner/Mazel.

Bolton, B. (1986b). Minnesota Satisfactoriness Scales. In D. J. Keyser & R. C. Sweetland (Eds.), *Test critiques: Vol. 4*, (pp. 434–439) Kansas City, MO: Test Corporation of America.

Bolton, (1986c). Minnesota Satisfaction Questionnaire. In D. J. Keyser & R. C. Sweetland (Eds.), *Test critiques: Vol. 5* (pp. 255–265). Kansas City, MO: Test Corporation of America.

Bolton, B. (1986d). Vocational assessment of psychiatrically disabled persons. In J. A. Ciardiello & M. D. Bell (Eds.), *Vocational rehabilitation of persons with prolonged mental illness*. Baltimore, MD: Johns Hopkins University Press.

Bolton, B., & Roessler, R. (1986). *Manual for the work personality profile*. Fayetteville, AR: Arkansas Research and Training Center in Vocational Rehabilitation.

Cooper, P. G., & Harper, J. N. (1979). Case weighting systems. In B. Bolton, *Rehabilitation counseling research* (pp. 213–228). Austin, TX: Pro-Ed.

Crewe, N. M. (1987). Assessment of physical functioning. In B. Bolton (Ed.), *Handbook of measurement and evaluation in rehabilitation* (2nd ed., pp. 235–247). Baltimore: Paul H. Brookes Publishing Co.

Crewe, N. M., & Athelstan, G. T. (1984). *Functional Assessment Inventory manual*. Menomonie: Materials Development Center, University of Wisconsin–Stout.

Dawis, R. V. (1987). The Minnesota Theory of Work Adjustment. In B. Bolton (Ed.), *Handbook of measurement and evaluation in rehabilitation* (2nd ed., pp. 203–217). Baltimore: Paul H. Brookes Publishing Co.

Dawis, R. V., & Lofquist, L. H. (1984). *A psychological theory of work adjustment*. Minneapolis: University of Minnesota Press.

Eber, H. W. (1966). Multivariate analysis of a vocational rehabilitation system. *Multivariate Behavioral Research*, Monograph No. 66-1.

Floor, L., & Rosen, M. (1976). New criteria of adjustment for the cerebral palsied. *Rehabilitation Literature, 37*, 268–274.

Gibson, D. L., Weiss, D. J., Dawis, R. V., & Lofquist, L. H. (1970). *Manual for the Minnesota Satisfactoriness Scales* (Minnesota Studies in Vocational Rehabilitation: 27). Minneapolis: Vocational Psychology Research, University of Minnesota.

Institute for Personality and Ability Testing. (1985). *Manual for Form E of the 16 PF*. Champaign, IL: Author.

Kravetz, S., Florian, V., & Wright, G. N. (1985). The development of a multifaceted measure of rehabilitation effectiveness: Theoretical rationale and scale construction. *Rehabilitation Psychology, 30*, 195–208.

Reagles, K. W., & Butler, A. J. (1976). The Human Service Scale: A new measure for evaluation. *Journal of Rehabilitation, 42*, 34–38.

Reagles, K. W., Wright, G. N., & Butler, A. J. (1970). *A scale of rehabilitation gain for clients of an expanded vocational rehabilitation program*. (Wisconsin Studies in Vocational Rehabilitation: 13). Madison: Regional Rehabilitation Research Institute, University of Wisconsin.

Roessler, R., & Bolton, B. (1983). Assessment and enhancement of functional vocational capabilities: A five-year research strategy. *Vocational Evaluation and Work Adjustment Bulletin* (Monograph No. 1).

Roessler, R., & Bolton, B. (1984). *Vocational rehabilitation of individuals with employability skill deficits: Problems and recommendations*. Fayetteville: Arkansas Research and Training Center in Vocational Rehabilitation.

Scott, T. B., Dawis, R. V., England, G. W., & Lofquist, L. H. (1960). *A definition of work adjustment*. (Minnesota Studies in Vocational Rehabilitation: 10). Minneapolis: Vocational Psychology Research, University of Minnesota.

Tinsley, H. E. A., Warnken, R. G., Weiss, D. J., Dawis, R. V., & Lofquist, L. H. (1969). *A follow-up survey of former clients of the Minnesota Division of Vocational Rehabilitation* (Minnesota Studies in Vocational Rehabilitation: 26). Minneapolis: Vocational Psychology Research, University of Minnesota.

Tseng, M. S. (1975). Job performance and satisfaction of successfully rehabilitated vocational rehabilitation clients. *Rehabilitation Literature, 36*, 66–72.

Walls, R. T., & Tseng, M. S. (1986). Measurement of client outcomes in rehabilitation. In B. Bolton (Ed.), *Handbook of measurement and evaluation in rehabilitation* (2nd ed., pp. 183–201) Baltimore: Paul H. Brookes Publishing Co.

Weiss, D. J., Dawis, R. V., England, G. W., & Lofquist, L. H. (1967). *Manual for the Minnesota Satisfaction Questionnaire*. (Minnesota Studies in Vocational Rehabilitation: 22). Minneapolis: Vocational Psychology Research, University of Minnesota.

Westerheide, W. J., & Lenhart, L. (1973). Development and reliability of a pretest-posttest rehabilitation services outcome measure. *Rehabilitation Research and Practice Review, 4*(3), 15–24.

Westerheide, W. J., Lenhart, L., & Miller, M. C. (1974). *Field test of a Service Outcome Measurement Form: Case difficulty* (Monograph No. 2). Oklahoma City, OK: Department of Institutions, Social and Rehabilitation Services.

Westerheide, W. J., Lenhart, L., & Miller, M. C. (1975). *Field test of a Services Outcome Measurement Form: Client change* (Monograph No. 3). Oklahoma City, OK: Department of Institutions, Social and Rehabilitation Services.

Chapter 6

Outcome Analysis in Independent Living

Margaret A. Nosek

Independent living (IL) has emerged as one of the most promising new developments in the discipline and service system of rehabilitation, yet it has been received more as a maverick and awkward stepchild than as a legitimate component. It had a curious dual genesis in the 1960s and 1970s, with roots in both the social reform/self-help movement and the rehabilitation establishment. While rehabilitationists have tended to fit IL into a scheme of services with discrete outcomes, the equally strong and more holistic influence of the grassroots movement has prevented convenient categorization and blocked attempts at outcome assessment. This chapter traces the interplay of these at times conflicting, at times complementary trends as it presents the state of the art in outcome analysis in IL and a discussion of issues that surround it.

Since the late 1950s, there have been attempts, largely by the National Rehabilitation Association, to incorporate into federal vocational rehabilitation legislation provision for persons who are judged not to have vocational potential (Urban Institute, 1975). "Independent living rehabilitation," as distinct from "vocational rehabilitation," was conceived as those medical and social services that enable persons with disabilities without an immediate vocational goal to live in the community short of being gainfully employed (Humphreys, 1978). Throughout the legislative debate on this issue, a fear has been expressed that IL would dilute the specificity of the vocational outcome. Some professionals feared

that IL services would result in the same charge of nonaccountability often levied against more ill-defined social services, such as those administered under Title XX of the Social Security Act.

Simultaneously and quite separately from these efforts, a movement began among university students with severe disabilities to expand their life options beyond the confines of health care facilities or their parents' homes. Several such students at the University of California at Berkeley successfully moved out of the university health center into an apartment in the community. In 1972 they formed a community-based self-help group called the Berkeley Center for Independent Living. Their purpose was to broaden the approaches and services available to persons with disabilities so that they might acquire the necessary knowledge, skills, confidence, and assistance to participate more fully in society (Brown, 1978; Pflueger, 1977; Zukas, 1975). This program has served as a prototype, seeding similar programs across the country. It also established a philosophical foundation for the movement, based on the principles of self-determination, integration, civil rights, self-advocacy, barrier removal, and quality of life (Nosek, Narita, Dart, & Dart, 1982).

Success along both paths was achieved in 1978 with the passage of the amendments to the Rehabilitation Act of 1973. One of these new provisions, Title VII, allocated funds for the establishment of community-based, consumer-controlled

Preparation of this chapter was supported partially by the ILRU Research and Training Center on Independent Living at The Institute for Rehabilitation and Research (Grant No. G00853C505).

programs based on the model of the Berkeley Center for Independent Living. Eight years later, these funds have been used to establish over 150 such programs. Another section of Title VII, only recently funded, allows for the purchase of independent living support services by vocational rehabilitation agencies. With the expansion of federal funding for independent living services and the increasing demand for accountability for these funds, Congress mandated the development of standards for IL centers and a comprehensive evaluation of the IL center model. Activities in response to this mandate have led to significant advances in outcome analysis for this service delivery area.

According to the *International Classification of Impairments, Disabilities, and Handicaps* (World Health Organization [WHO], 1980; see also Wood & Badley, 1980), traditional physical and mental health care systems can be said to deal largely with impairments and disabilities. Both traditional social service systems and IL programs focus mainly on handicaps in the sense that they attempt to minimize problems with orientation, physical independence, mobility, occupation, social integration, and economic self-sufficiency. Independent living programs are distinguished from traditional social service providers, however, by their 1) emphasis on substantial consumer involvement in the direction and delivery of services; 2) consumer determination of goals; 3) concern with eliminating environmental barriers that produce handicaps; and 4) a comprehensive array of populations and services, including at a minimum peer counseling, information and referral, IL skills training, and advocacy. Further, IL programs place a much stronger emphasis on cognitive and emotional aspects of independence.

Unfortunately, IL services have been viewed primarily as gap-fillers; rehabilitationists have paid very little attention to refining independence as a construct or intervention strategy. In fact, it is a concept that has been discussed and operationalized in several different disciplines, including sociology, education, and psychology, since the early 1950s. The bringing together of these various contributions from a research perspective has occurred only recently (Nosek, 1984).

This chapter first describes the range of IL services available and current service delivery practices. The focus then shifts to outcome analysis methods developed to evaluate programs that deliver these services. The constructs of independence and independent living are then discussed, and methods are reviewed for measuring individual differences. The chapter concludes with a discussion of problems and issues dealing with IL outcomes.

INTERVENTIONS

Services that assist people with disabilities to increase their independence have been offered within traditional health care and social service systems for several decades. Clinical interventions have involved physical and occupational therapists focusing on increasing self-care and mobility skills. Social work techniques are used to help individuals adapt to the realities of living in a basically inaccessible and often economically depressed environment. Vocational rehabilitationists assist in increasing the productivity of persons with a disability by enabling them to acquire the necessary education and adaptive devices for competing in the job market.

However, it was the ineffectiveness of these traditional approaches in addressing the psychological and environmental issues surrounding IL that gave rise to IL programs. These programs draw heavily on the peer role model—the visible example of a person with a severe disability living independently—and the value of peer counseling as an effective technique in motivating persons with disabilities and providing them with information directly relevant to the realities of living with a disability. Services of these programs are directed not only at helping the individual to grow, but also at changing the environment by removing barriers and remediating discrimination, all of which inhibit the individual's ability to realize his or her goals. Differences between the approach taken by IL programs as opposed to traditional programs is clearly presented by DeJong (1979a, 1979b) in his discussion of the locus of the problem and the solution in the medical model/ rehabilitation paradigm versus the IL paradigm.

The centers for IL in Berkeley and Boston established the model upon which a national network of IL programs has been developed and IL funding legislation has been enacted. This model has been defined by Frieden, Richards, Cole, and Bailey (1979) as a community-based, nonprofit, nonresidential program controlled by the consumers with disabilities it serves, which provides directly, or coordinates indirectly through referral, those services that assist individuals with severe disabilities to increase personal self-determination and to minimize unnecessary dependence upon others. The minimum set of services that are provided by an IL center includes housing assistance; attendant care, readers, and/or interpreters; peer counseling; financial and legal advocacy; and community awareness and barrier removal programs. Other services that are either provided or coordinated by IL centers include transportation or registry, peer counseling, advocacy or political action, IL skills training, equipment maintenance and repair, and social/recreational services.

Conceptually, *independent living program* is generic—the most broadly defined term relating to organizations working with disabled individuals who wish to live independently. Several different kinds of IL programs exist in the field in addition to IL centers. They differ from one another in at least six primary areas: the service setting may range from residential to nonresidential; the service delivery method may range from direct to indirect, or a combination of both; the service delivery style may range from professional to consumer; the vocational emphasis may range from primary to incidental; the goal orientation may range from transitional to ongoing; and the disability type served may range from single to multiple. The features of the IL program are determined by the needs of the consumers served, the availability of existing community resources, the physical and social makeup of the community, and the goals of the program itself. Custodial care facilities and primary medical care facilities are specifically excluded from the definition of an IL program.

The typology of IL support services provided, in addition to community-based programs, includes generic IL service providers, transitional programs, and residential programs. Generic IL service providers are organizations that provide several discrete services that can increase an individual's ability or opportunities to live independently. For example, a medical rehabilitation facility may provide outpatient services designed to maintain the physical health of a person who lives independently in the community. However, if the center does not provide or coordinate a full set of services, including transportation, attendant care, and so forth, it is an IL service provider rather than an IL program. Although an IL service provider does not meet the criteria necessary to be classified as an IL program, the services it provides may be used or coordinated by an IL program.

Independent living transitional programs facilitate the movement of people with severe disabilities from comparatively dependent living situations to comparatively independent living situations. The primary service provided by these programs is skill training in such areas as attendant management, financial management, consumer affairs, mobility, educational-vocational opportunities, medical needs, living arrangements, social skills, time management, functional skills, sexuality, and so forth. Additional services may be provided. Transitional programs are usually goal oriented and/or time linked.

Independent living residential programs are live-in programs that provide directly, or coordinate through referral, shared attendant services and transportation. Related services may be provided that increase personal self-determination and minimize unnecessary dependence on others (Frieden et al., 1979).

The diversity of services and service delivery styles that target increasing levels of independence in persons with disabilities makes the task of outcome analysis unwieldy. The following sections illustrate how the constructs of independence and independent living have been operationalized to analyze outcomes for individuals and to determine how individual outcomes reflect the impact of services received.

ANALYZING INDIVIDUAL OUTCOMES IN PROGRAM EVALUATION

Since the beginning of federal funding to IL programs, there have been attempts to develop methods to assess effectiveness through program evaluation (Clowers, Haley, Unti, & Feiss, 1979; DeJong & Hughes, 1982; Muzzio, 1980; Muzzio et al., 1979; Schmidt, Collignon, Stoddard, & Barrett, 1978). Frieden and Nosek (1985) have compiled and analyzed efforts to test the efficacy of the IL program model. Writings on this topic focus primarily on evaluation of context, input, and process, with analysis of consumer outcomes reaching little beyond obvious changes in such areas as living arrangement, mobility, and income.

The California Department of Rehabilitation conducted research in 1980 to develop a measure of client gain to use in assessing the effectiveness of the state's IL programs (Hiehle & Robins, 1982). This very thorough survey compared IL philosophy to measures of client gain in the rehabilitation literature; no instrument was found that adequately covered the goals and needs expressed by the IL movement. To fill this gap, they developed the California Client Gains Scale, a self-reported, multiple-choice questionnaire with items covering financial skills, use of productive and leisure time, activities of daily living, dependence versus independence on a range of health areas, and social and psychological functioning (well-being). Responses to questions include choices reflecting independence by means of assistive devices or personal care assistants. Item analysis and tests of reliability and validity were conducted. Used in a study to determine the effectiveness of IL program services, the scale was found to be sensitive to client change.

The Arkansas Rehabilitation Research and Training Center at the University of Arkansas has made many significant contributions to refining the evaluation process for IL. They list person change—along with environment change, client satisfaction, and project operation—as critical areas for evaluating the effectiveness of IL programs. Roessler and Rubin (1980) stated that program services should contribute to client gains in terms of physical functioning, vocational potential, educational skills, avocational interests, psychosocial functioning, and economic independence. Clark and Rice (1980) listed many assessment instruments that could be used individually in each of these areas. Rice, another

member of the Arkansas team (Rice et al., 1983), drew on Stoddard, Katsuranis, Toms, and Finnegan (1980) and Sigelman, Vengroff, and Spanhel (1979) to develop a list of areas of IL service needs for person change (see Appendix to this chapter). For each of these areas, an analysis of pertinent assessment instruments is given. Similar treatment is given to environmental change, particularly concerning IL services to effect change in the physical, social, economic, and human service environment.

The Research and Training Center on Independent Living at the University of Kansas is developing an IL program evaluation manual (Budde, Petty, & Nelson, 1983). A client-centered evaluation technique is used in which clients list their major goals according to their own definition of independence. Demographic and environmental indicators, like those comprising other evaluation models, are then assigned to the appropriate goal. This instrument is currently being tested and validated.

The University of Washington conducted an evaluation of that state's IL programs in 1982. An IL program evaluation data package was developed that lists the following outcomes categories of services: living arrangement, transportation, attendant care, financial resources, contact with primary medical/health care systems, vocational and educational activities, contact with the vocational rehabilitation system, and satisfaction with the level of independence. Progress toward goals was assessed using a status indicator tool developed by the Rehabilitation Indicators Project (Brown, Diller, Fordyce, Jacobs, & Gordon, 1980).

Wilkerson (1982), a member of the Washington evaluation team, commented on the assessment of consumer outcomes in IL program evaluation, stating that, although many instruments exist for measuring psychosocial characteristics, there is neither the time nor the research orientation to administer them in the IL program environment. Behaviors are easier to assess, but the length of time required for change to occur may be considerable. Behaviors do, however, automatically reflect limitations placed on the individual's IL status by the environment even though these limitations may not be obvious.

"The absence of an independent behavior does not incriminate the environment as the deterrent to independence. On the other hand, while psychosocial or internal orientation to independent living may have been achieved, environmental constraints can still squelch independent living" (Wilkerson, 1982, p. 31). The greatest disadvantage of traditional assessments of skill acquisition is that the possession of a skill does not necessarily mean it will be used.

The most widely used evaluation system for IL programs was developed by the Center for Resource Management (Lachat & Williams, 1984). In close cooperation with the New England Coalition of Independent Living Programs, they identified consumer needs, services generally offered by IL programs to meet those needs based on IL philosophy, and individual outcomes in the areas of knowledge; aids, benefits, and services; daily living skills and procedures; situational or status indicators; and personal/social skills and behaviors. In each outcome category, they list goals commonly identified by consumers in each service content area. Record keeping formats allow responses that indicate whether or not a goal has been targeted and whether or not it has been accomplished. Completion of these forms is done by program staff based on the consumer's report. This system is currently in use by 27 programs and has required little modification in the past 2 years.

The 1984 amendments to the Rehabilitation Act required a comprehensive evaluation of the Title VII, Part B Centers for Independent Living Program. This was conducted by Berkeley Planning Associates (1986) in collaboration with the Center for Resource Management and the Research and Training Center on Independent Living at the University of Kansas. After developing standards for program operation and having them approved by the National Council on the Handicapped, they conducted a comprehensive mail survey of all 156 Part B–funded centers, interviews with staff, consumers, and community agency representatives at 40 programs, and a mail survey of 2,700 consumers from 36 sample centers.

Data on consumers were gathered both directly and indirectly. Because records are not generally kept on severity of disability, this information was determined by proxy, that is, receipt of Social Security Disability Insurance or Supplemental Security Income, reported blindness, use of a Seeing Eye dog or white cane, use of a wheelchair, or use of an attendant. Survey and interview questions presented to program staff and consumers covered achievement of IL goals in 20 different areas listed in the National Council on the Handicapped Standards. Consumers were asked whether they improved or maintained their situation in five key areas (housing, education, employment, income, and transportation) since first contact with the center, and the extent to which the center helped to bring about any improvements. Data were analyzed according to the five outcome areas identified in the Center for Resource Management evaluation system mentioned above. Multivariate analysis was used to determine the effect on outcomes of services received and service characteristics.

THE CONSTRUCTS OF INDEPENDENCE AND INDEPENDENT LIVING

Program evaluation efforts have been hampered by not having an adequately defined construct of independence. Very little empirical research has been conducted to determine a comprehensive definition of independence or independent living. Whereas locus of control, attribution, motivation, perseverence, achievement style, autonomy, learned helplessness, and dependency are well represented in the literature, the affirmative, composite construct of independence has not been the subject of extensive analysis. Independence can be discussed and assessed as a psychological trait, a social state, a set of behaviors, and a level of functional ability. It is also a developmental process; however, this aspect has received very little attention in the literature.

Independence as a Psychological Construct

In the psychology literature, independence is discussed in well-known works by Cattell (1965; Cattell & Schuerger, 1978). He identified independence as the most substantially inherited of source traits; a temperament factor favoring vigor, initiative, and self-sufficiency. He described the independent person as unconventional, assertive, active, alert, and cheerful (Cattell, 1965). Stendler (1954) discussed the learning of both independence and dependence in childhood as basic to the American socialization process. She claimed that successful socialization involves the acquisition of a culturally approved balance between the two. Underlying her theories is the assumption that independence is a learned drive. Beller (1955) viewed the components of independence as taking initiative, overcoming obstacles, persistence, wanting to do something or getting satisfaction from work, and wanting to do things by oneself. Weiss (1981) observed a close connection between independent behavior and moral autonomy.

Nichols and Fine (1980) studied self-concept, expressed value systems, and fantasy production to determine independence, self-support, and responsibility. Kofta (1980) postulated that, by making a choice, individuals shift to an autonomous mode of behavior regulation that produces changes in psychological functioning that include personal control over behavior, increase in perceived responsibility for the outcome of one's actions, greater consistency between internal standards and behaviors, growth in resistance to social pressure, and reorientation of internal criteria for self-evaluation. A very succinct and practical definition of independence is offered by Troutt (1980) in her study of minority adolescent college students' usage of special services. She defined independence as behaviors that reflect the adolescent's ability to make separate and responsible decisions and to assume responsibility for these without immediate parental supervision. This includes the ability to manage life in the areas of one's competence and the capacity to seek help when the realization of one's goals requires assistance.

Independence as a Social and Behavioral Concept

Independent living literature has primarily defined this construct in terms of social status and behaviors, using indices of the individual's level of participation in society and fulfillment of so-

cial roles. Rice and Roessler (1980, p. 2) synthesized several definitions:

> The ability of the severely disabled person to participate actively in society: to work; to own a home; to raise a family; to participate to the fullest extent possible in normal activities; and to exercise freedom of choice and personal control over one's life (Cole, Sperry, Board & Frieden, 1979; Fifth IRI, 1978; Roberts, 1977).

Rice, Roessler, Greenwood, and Frieden (1983) further condensed this definition as: "freedom of choice, personal control of one's life, and participation in significant roles of worker, homemaker, and provider" (pp. 3–4).

The definition created by Independent Living Research Utilization (Frieden et al., 1979), to date the most quoted in the literature, was expanded in the National Council on the Handicapped's National Policy for Persons with Disabilities (NCH, 1983):

> Independent living is control over one's life based on the choice of acceptable options that minimize reliance on others in making decisions and in performing everyday activities. This includes managing one's day-to-day affairs, participating fully in community life, fulfilling a range of social roles, and making decisions that lead to self-determination and the minimization of non-productive physical and psychological dependence upon others. Independence implies an optimally responsible and productive exercise of the power of choice. It further implies that each disabled person, regardless of his or her mental or physical ability, should be encouraged and assisted, with due respect for cultural or subcultural affiliation, to achieve a high quality of life, and to achieve independence and productivity in the least restrictive environment. Independent living is intended to apply to persons with all types of disabilities.

Independence as Functional Autonomy

From the perspective of rehabilitation professionals, IL is judged in terms of the individual's ability to perform activities of daily living autonomously. There have been numerous efforts to develop standardized lists of these activities and to define the line between autonomy and dependence with reference to assistive devices and performance time and quality.

Wilkerson, of the University of Washington, took issue with this in an unpublished manuscript

(1982, p. 27), stating: "Living independently for a severely disabled person, as for anyone, entails much more than an approximation of 'normal' physical functioning. Indeed, physical functioning may play little or no role in the definition of independence for a person who has other priorities." She cited Clowers et al. (1979), DeJong (1979a), DeJong and Wenker (1979), Frieden (1978), Heumann (1977), Muzzio et al. (1979), Pflueger, (1977), and Roberts (1977) as observing that the independent living movement does not suggest the absence of assistance, even in the necessities of day-to-day living. Independence is defined by control or self-direction, not by style or content, and must be determined by each individual in terms that are meaningful to him or her. In describing the components of independence, Wilkerson mentioned two lines of change in one's life: psychosocial characteristics, such as self-esteem, self-direction, and locus of control; and behavior, such as living arrangement, daily activities, participation in family, and community life.

ASSESSING INDIVIDUAL DIFFERENCES

Researchers have used a wide variety of techniques for measuring an individual's level of independence. In the psychology literature, standardized psychometric instruments purport to examine independence along with a list of other personal characteristics. The number of surveys and checklists for functional abilities is large, but evidence regarding reliability and validity is deficient. In IL research, the newness of the field is reflected in the small body of literature and the small number of instruments that have been developed.

Psychological Measures

Among psychometric instruments, the following (as listed in Mitchell, 1983) measure independence along with other characteristics:

California Psychological Inventory (Gough)
Group Environment Scale (Rudolf)
Humor Test of Personality (IPAT)
Jesness Behavior Checklist (Jesness)

Objective Analytic Batteries (Cattell & Schwiger)
Sixteen Personality Factor Questionnaire (Cattell, Eber, & Tatsuoka)
Survey of Interpersonal Values (Gordon)
Triadal Equated Personality Inventory (United Consultants Research Staff)

The California Psychological Inventory and the 16 Personality Factors Questionnaire (16 PF) have been used by Ross (1980) and Nosek (1984), respectively, in studies of independence. The 16 PF Questionnaire has "subduedness versus independence" as a second-order factor determined by a formula using 10 scores on selected primary factors (a different set is used for men and women). The authors describe the independent person as aggressive, daring, and incisive; someone who seeks those situations where such behavior is at least tolerated and possibly rewarded, and is likely to exhibit considerable initiative.

Derdiarian and Clough (1976) studied levels of dependence and independence for patients undergoing total hip or knee replacement. Using Likert-type responses, the authors created two assessment instruments based on Beller's (1955) list of independent behaviors. They addressed questions of whether dependence and independence exist in adults in forms similar to those of children, whether dependence and independence levels change during hospitalization, and whether dependence and independence are separate entities or opposite ends of a bipolar continuum.

Functional Measures

In education and medical literature on functional abilities, there exists a plethora of checklists, inventories, and questionnaires, most of which were either designed for assessing the cognitive and functional abilities of persons with mental retardation, or meeting the intake and closure requirements of programs offering specific services. Most are far too complex and detailed for the purpose of assessing overall independence. Keith (1984) cited poorly conceptualized outcome criteria, lack of standardization, disagreement about methods, multidimensional scales for abilities that are not discrete, and the influence of setting on performance as barriers to effective measurement of functional abilities. Keith called for rehabilitation professionals to "devote thought and resources to the development of useful criteria rather than simply assuming that everyone understands what they are" (p. 75).

The Barthel Index has proven its usefulness in two IL studies (DeJong, Branch, & Corcoran, 1984; Nosek, 1984). It has the virtue of being brief, allowing credit for performing tasks with assistance, and being generally accepted by rehabilitation professionals. The areas of functioning covered include:

1. Feeding
2. Moving from wheelchair to bed and return
3. Personal toilet
4. Getting on and off toilet
5. Bathing self
6. Walking on level surface (or if unable to walk, propelling wheelchair)
7. Ascending and descending stairs
8. Dressing
9. Controlling bowels
10. Controlling bladder

Granger, Albrecht, and Hamilton (1979) published a version of the Barthel Index in which they modified certain items and altered several weightings. Weights were assigned in three categories of responses: "Can do by myself," "Can do with help of someone else," and "Cannot do at all." A person scoring 100 points is continent, feeds him/herself, dresses him/herself, gets up out of bed and chairs, bathes him/herself, walks at least a block, and can ascend and descend stairs. There is no claim that this means the person is able to live alone: He or she may not be able to cook, keep house, and interact with the public, but probably is able to get along without an attendant. A score of 40–60 classified the person as severely disabled, and a score less than 40 as very severely disabled.

Salkind, Beckwith, Nelson, and McGregor (1982) indexed over 130 instruments that are used to assess independence, most of which examine little more than activities of daily living. The diversity in content and level of detail is notable. The majority were geared toward a mentally retarded population. Only seven instruments had been tested for reliability and validity. Thirteen instruments contained some type of measure of control or decision making.

Crewe and Athelstan (1980) developed the Functional Assessment Inventory, a 39-item, normed and validated questionnaire. This instrument is distinguished by the broad range of areas covered, including many that relate to independence, such as learning ability, sensory functioning, physical functioning, health status, economic situation, judgment, problem solving, initiative, and personality characteristics.

Social and Behavioral Measures

Independence as a social status indicator has been operationally defined by the IL movement (Frieden et al., 1979; Muzzio, 1980; Rice et al., 1983; Wilkerson, Weinhouse, & Jamero, 1982). It includes such variables as:

1. Mobility, at home and within the community, including use of public transportation
2. Activities of daily living
3. Use of personal care assistants (attendants)
4. Use of assistive equipment
5. Communication abilities
6. Source and amount of income
7. Living arrangement, including housing and housemates
8. Employment status
9. Education level
10. Use of leisure time
11. Health status, including fulfilling health maintenance requirements
12. Marital status
13. Social life
14. Self-concept

Many of these variables have functional and cognitive components and are broken down into discrete abilities or levels by various assessment instruments used for determining IL outcomes in rehabilitation and IL program settings. Some programs chose four or five as key indicators, usually mobility, employment/income, activities of daily living, and living arrangement. It is noteworthy that these components are among the most functionally oriented on the list. This approach tends to focus on observable behaviors and environmental circumstances with virtually no examination of the personality characteristics underlying such behaviors or of which factors may have led to the existence of such circumstances.

A curious anomaly exists in that, although most IL programs in the country assess independence primarily in terms of functional capacities or environmental circumstances, almost all subscribe to the definition of independence described earlier that focuses on psychological and social factors, developed by Frieden et al. (1979). Undoubtedly, this discrepancy exists because there is currently no practical technique for assessing control in a service provision setting. Rather, it is dealt with somewhat unsystematically under the label of "peer counseling." Nevertheless, this conflict between ideology and practice points out the need for a comprehensive operational definition of the construct.

DeJong et al. (1984) interviewed 111 spinal cord–injured persons from 10 comprehensive rehabilitation centers across the United States 2 years after their discharge in order to determine their IL outcomes. The outcomes were hypothesized to be a function of four sets of variables: sociodemographic characteristics, disability-related variables, environmental barriers, and an interface variable related to the use of assistive devices. The dependent variables were a set of measures reflecting the restrictiveness of the living arrangement (a ranked order of seven outcomes, from living alone or with spouse or friends to living in an institution); the level of productivity (a ranked order of 12 outcomes, including gainful employment, contributions to community organizations, homemaking, participation in school or educational programs, and leisure time activities); and the weighted average of these two. The 42 members of the Massachusetts Interagency Council on Independent Living ranked and weighted the outcomes, assigning a weight of 43% to living arrangement and 57% to productivity (DeJong & Hughes, 1982). The independent variables were sociodemographic and disability related. The main predictors of living arrangement were found to be marital status, transportation barriers, and need for medical supervision. Predictors for productivity were transportation barriers, economic disincentives, and education.

In conducting a needs assessment survey of IL program clients, Jones and Summerville (1983) identified a group they labeled *do-it-yourself independent* persons, those who achieved IL status without the benefit of an IL program. On four out of five indicators of independence (having modified one's home, preferring self-management of finances, using more independent transportation, and ability to perform activities of daily living), this group showed a greater degree of independence than those who achieved independence through an IL program. The authors recommend that IL programs focus as much on the removal of barriers along the avenues to social independence as on the steps toward physical rehabilitation so that more persons with disabilities might pursue independence on their own.

The Use of Multiple Measures

A study by Nosek (1984) examined the relative roles of personality, social status, and functional abilities in assessing independent living status. She asked a sample of 67 persons with severe orthopedic impairments referred by colleges and independent living programs to complete the 16 PF questionnaire by Cattell, Eber, and Tatsuoka (1970), the Barthel Index of Functional Abilities as modified by Granger et al. (1979), and a demographic questionnaire. Using the Independence Scale of the 16 PF as a measure of psychological independence and the Independent Living Scale by DeJong and Hughes (1982) as a measure of social independence, subjects were grouped according to high and low levels of independence, and the common characteristics of each were identified. Nosek's findings showed that certain personality factors and life status indicators distinguished the groups more than functional abilities.

PROBLEMS AND ISSUES

A comparison of definitions of IL and instruments to assess IL outcomes reveals some significant incongruities. The lack of a comprehensive, operational definition incorporating psychological, social, behavioral, and functional elements is reflected in the existence of separate instruments for each of these, but none that validly and adequately combine all four elements. Particularly glaring omissions include psychological traits and stability of personal support systems.

Although research shows that personality characteristics have a significant relationship to successful outcomes in independent living, there is debate about whether or not this factor can be changed through intervention. On one hand, the assertiveness, initiative, and perseverance reflecting an individual's inborn character may be what carries him or her beyond the limitations imposed by disability and society's reaction to it. On the other hand, these same traits may have been irreversibly suppressed by overprotection and learned helplessness from negative environmental influences since an early age. As Jones and Summerville (1983) have stated, it may be more appropriate for IL programs to focus on creating a more accessible and less discriminatory society so that people who have independent personality traits will be freer to realize their potential.

There is general agreement, however, that the use of complex psychometric instruments or detailed, behaviorally oriented assessment instruments for activities of daily living is inappropriate in an IL service setting. As Wilkerson (1982) stated, IL program personnel have neither the time for nor the interest in digging so deeply into an individual's psyche or behaviors when their problems in daily living are so obvious and relatively straightforward to solve. Nevertheless, personality and personal behaviors have a strong influence on levels of independence, and workers in the field must find a valid, convenient method for gathering this type of information for use in providing IL interventions.

Instruments that measure skills gained and changes in social situations rarely allow anything but a dichotomous response. In reality, skill acquisition is a process and stability of social status is a continuum. Although it is expeditious to claim that certain consumers have learned to cook, it is more meaningful to determine whether or not they have reached a level of skill that is useful and satisfactory for them, and whether or not other circumstances in their lives allow them to exercise this skill. Although it is

accurate to claim that an individual acquired an accessible apartment and an attendant, the stability of the situation can be highly variable. If loss of income, injury, or disagreements easily and frequently endanger the viability of this arrangement, then its achievement is hardly a credit. A truer measure of goal achievement is an assessment of the personal support systems that back up individuals and ensure that they will be able to function in their social roles despite changes in circumstances.

Means of outcome analysis used by the rehabilitation establishment and the IL movement differ substantially in two major areas: goal setting and reporting technique. Goal setting is a very sensitive issue for the movement. There is a strong objection to the medical model, in which goals were set without ever consulting the individual. Although IL programs encourage consumers to set their own goals, this is often not as simple as it seems. According to Berkeley planning Associates (1986), "Consumers of independent living services were less likely to have a clear idea of their goals than VR [vocational rehabilitation] consumers, and many found the concept of goalsetting to be unfamiliar if decisions had previously been made on their behalf by someone else. Often goal planning was an evolutionary process rather than a first step. Sometimes the establishment of goals was an outcome in and of itself" (p. 56). Another confounding influence is that, through peer role modeling, programs may present certain life situations as ideal goals, that is, living in an apartment with an attendant and working in an office 9 to 5. Although this may be an attractive and normal-appearing life-style, it may not be attainable or even desirable for some consumers, and it may overshadow more creative and unorthodox options. Again, stability of personal support systems and quality of life should be considered in choosing such goals.

There is also a distinction in the concept of closure. In vocational rehabilitation, for example, the prevailing focus is toward the "26 closure," the point at which the consumer has reached the employment goal and is no longer in need of services. In medical rehabilitation, it is when the individual is medically stable and able to function and need no longer receive out- or inpatient services. Reactivating either of these service relationships is usually based on the occurrence of a major life- or career-threatening change. In independent living, many service needs are lifelong and goals often change with new physical, environmental, or economic circumstances. The approach to goal achievement is ongoing and much more flexible. The implication for both systems is that they should pursue long-term follow-up assessments.

In clinical settings, information is usually gathered by observation. In IL service settings, there is usually total reliance on consumer self-report. Although each is appropriate for its setting, a comprehensive IL assessment instrument should judiciously balance the two. It is important to develop a service plan based on self-reported needs; however, in order to design an appropriate intervention, it may be helpful to observe circumstances and behaviors. Major outcomes, especially those that are situational, can be accurately judged by the consumer. In some areas, particularly those requiring behavioral change, the consumer may not be the most objective judge of his or her progress.

Individual outcome analysis in IL has to date taken a back seat to other aspects of program evaluation. A stronger focus on individual outcomes has the potential to significantly influence directions in the refinement of service delivery content areas and techniques. More discrete and revealing methods for determining needs and gains in psychological aspects of IL and in daily living skills (based on IL philosophy) will lead to a more unified and effective approach to peer counseling and IL skills training, two service areas the national evaluation study (Berkeley Planning Associates, 1986) found to lack consistency.

The impact on public policy is potentially profound. In times of cutbacks in social service spending, the question foremost in the minds of decision makers is the relationship of service cost to consumer benefit. The National Council on the Handicapped has advised Congress that the primary criterion for determining benefit should be the degree to which a service increases an individual's independence (National Council on the Handicapped, 1986). Because of the lack of consensus regarding appropriate and practical assessment instruments, there is currently no means for making this determination.

There have been many pioneering efforts in IL outcome analysis, but, indeed, we are still barely beyond these first steps. A foundation is in place and the field is ready for advancement in the development of both a comprehensive, operational definition of IL and a valid and practical tool for assessing progress and outcomes. Once these advancements have taken place, the mechanism will be available to determine to what degree all disability-related services in fact assist people with disabilities to move toward independence.

APPENDIX: INDEPENDENT LIVING SERVICE NEEDS FOR PERSON CHANGE
(from Rice et al., 1983, pp. 45–46)

1. **Health functions**
   a. Increase the overall physical health of the individual;
   b. Decrease impairments in bodily systems;
   c. Decrease the amount of pain experienced;
   d. Increase the individual's participation in life activities.
2. **Social-attitudinal functions**
   a. Improve the level of acceptance of self and abilities;
   b. Improve the individual's social skills;
   c. Increase the individual's motivation to improve self.
3. **Mobility functions**
   a. Increase the individual's manual skills for manipulating objects and devices;
   b. Increase the individual's capability to move at home, work place, and from place to place in the community;
   c. Decrease the individual's difficulty in participating in other physical activities.
4. **Cognitive-intellectual functioning**
   a. Increase the individual's intellectual ca-

pacity to manipulate symbols and objects;

b. Increase the individual's capability to acquire or store in memory new cognitions and behavior patterns and/or to transfer learning to new situations.

5. **Communication functioning**

a. Decrease the individual's difficulties in sending and receiving messages;

b. Decrease the individual's difficulty in exchanging information and ideas with other persons.

REFERENCES

Beller, E. K. (1955). Dependence and independence in young children. *Journal of Genetic Psychology, 87*, 25–35.

Berkeley Planning Associates. (1986). *Comprehensive evaluation of the Title VII, Part B Centers for Independent Living Program*. Berkeley, CA: Author.

Brown, B. M. (1978). Second generation: West coast. *American Rehabilitation, 3*(6), 23–30.

Brown, M., Diller, L., Fordyce, W., Jacobs, D., & Gordon, W. (1980). Rehabilitation indicators: Their nature and uses for assessment. In B. Bolton & D. W. Cook (Eds.), *Rehabilitation client assessment* (pp. 102–117). Baltimore: University Park Press.

Budde, J. F., Petty, C. R., & Nelson, C. F. (1983). *Independent living center program evaluation (draft)*. Lawrence: University of Kansas, Research and Training Center on Independent Living.

Cattell, R. B. (1965). *The scientific analysis of personality*. Chicago: Aldine Publishing Co.

Cattell, R. B., Eber, H. W., & Tatsuoka, M. M. (1970). *Handbook for the sixteen personality factor questionnaire (16 PF)*. Champaign: Institute for Personality and Ability Testing.

Cattell, R. B., & Schuerger, J. M. (1978). *Personality theory in action: Handbook for the objective-analytic (O-A) test kit*. Champaign, IL: Institute for Personality and Ability Testing.

Clark, W., & Rice, D. (1980). *Implementation of independent living programs in rehabilitation*. Fayetteville: Arkansas Rehabilitation Research and Training Center, University of Arkansas.

Clowers, M., Haley, D., Unti, W., & Feiss, C. (1979). *Independent living project: Final report*. Seattle: Division of Vocational Rehabilitation and University of Washington.

Cole, J., Sperry, J., Board, M., & Frieden, L. (1979). *New options training manual*. Houston: The Institute for Rehabilitation and Research.

Crewe, N., & Athelstan, G. (1980). *Functional assessment inventory*. Minneapolis: Univeristy of Minnesota.

DeJong, G. (1979a). Independent living: From social movement to analytic paradigm. *Archives of Physical Medicine and Rehabilitation, 60*, 435–446.

DeJong, G. (1979b). *The movement for independent living: Origins, ideology, and implications for disability research*. Occasional Paper No. 2. East Lansing: Michigan State University, University Center for International Rehabilitation.

DeJong, G., Branch, L. G., & Corcoran, P. J. (1984). Independent living outcomes in spinal cord injury: Multi-variate analyses. *Archives of Physical Medicine and Rehabilitation, 65*, 66–73.

DeJong, G., & Hughes, J. (1982). Independent living: Methodology for measuring long-term outcomes. *Archives of Physical Medicine and Rehabilitation, 63*, 68–73.

DeJong, G., & Wenker, T. (1979). Attendant care as a prototype independent living service. *Archives of Physical Medicine and Rehabilitation, 60*, 477–482.

Derdiarian, S., & Clough, D. (1976). Patients' dependence and independence levels on the prehospitalization-postdischarge continuum. *Nursing Research, 25*(1), 27–33.

Fifth Institute on Rehabilitation Issues. (1978). *The role of vocational rehabilitation in independent living*. Fayetteville: Arkansas Rehabilitation Research and Training Center, University of Arkansas.

Frieden, L. (1978). IL: Movement and programs. *American Rehabilitation, 3*(6), 6–9.

Frieden, L., & Nosek, M. (1985). *The efficacy of the independent living program model based on descriptive and evaluative studies*. Washington, DC: National Rehabilitation Information Center.

Frieden, L., Richards, L., Cole, J., & Bailey, D. (1979). *ILRU source-book: A technical assistance manual on independent living*. Houston: The Institute for Rehabilitation and Research.

Granger, C. V., Albrecht, G. L., & Hamilton, B. B. (1979). Outcome of comprehensive medical rehabilitation measurement by PULSES profile and Barthel index. *Archives of Physical Medicine and Rehabilitation, 60*, 145–154.

Heumann, J. (1977). Independent living programs. In S. Stoddard Pflueger (Ed.), *Independent living: Emerging issues in rehabilitation* (pp. 60–62). Washington, DC: Institute for Research Utilization.

Hiehle, G., & Robins, B. (1982). *Programs for People: the California independent living centers*. Sacramento: California Department of Rehabilitation.

Humphreys, R. (1978). Putting it all together. *American Rehabilitation, 3*(6), Commissioner's comments.

Jones, B., & Summerville, J. (1983). Avenues and steps to do-it-yourself independence for the physically disabled. *Journal of Rehabilitation, 49*(4), 30–35.

Keith, R. A. (1984). Functional assessments measures in medical rehabilitation: Current status. *Archives of Physical Medicine and Rehabilitation, 65*, 74–78.

Kofta, L. (1980). Freedom of choice and automous regulation: Outline of a theory. *Polish Psychological Bulletin, 11*(1), 13–21.

Lachat, M. A., & Williams, M. (1984). *The evaluation system for independent living*. East Kingston, NH: Center for Resource Management.

Mitchell, J., Jr. (Ed.). (1983). *Tests in Print 3*. Lincoln: Buros Institute of Mental Measurement, University of Nebraska.

Muzzio, T. C. (1980). Independent living programs and evaluation, basic principles for developing a useful system. *Issues in Independent Living*. Houston: Independent Living Research Utilization.

Muzzio, T., LaRocca, J., Koshel, J., Durman, E., Chapman, B., & Gutowski, M. (1979). *Final report: Planning for independent living rehabilitation: Lessons from the*

Section 130 demonstrations. Washington, DC: The Urban Institute.

National Council on the Handicapped. (1983). *National Policy for Persons with Disabilities*. Washington, DC: Author.

National Council on the Handicapped. (1986). *Toward independence: An assessment of Federal laws and programs affecting persons with disabilities—with legislative recommendations; Appendix*. Washington, DC: U.S. Government Printing Office.

Nichols, R., & Fine, H. (1980). Gestalt therapy: Some aspects of self support, independence and responsibility. *Psychotherapy: Theory, Research and Practice, 17*, 124–135.

Nosek, M. A. (1984). *Relationships among measures of social independence, psychological independence, and functional abilities in adults with severe orthopedic impairments*. Doctoral dissertation, University of Texas.

Nosek, M. A., Narita, Y., Dart, Y., & Dart, J. (1982). *A philosophical foundation for the independent living and disability rights movements*. Occasional Paper No. 1. Houston: The Institute for Rehabilitation and Research.

Pflueger, S. S. (1977). *Independent living: Emerging issues in rehabilitation*. Washington, DC: Institute for Research Utilization.

Rice, B. D., & Roessler, R. T. (1980). *Introduction to independent living rehabilitation services*. Fayetteville: Arkansas Rehabilitation Research and Training Center, University of Arkansas, Arkansas Rehabilitation Services.

Rice, B. D., Roessler, R. T., Greenwood, R., & Friedan, L. (1983). *Independent living rehabilitation program development, management and evaluation*. Fayetteville: Arkansas Rehabilitation Research and Training Center, University of Arkansas, Arkansas Rehabilitation Services, The Institute for Rehabilitation and Research.

Roberts, E. V. (1977). Foreword. In S. Stoddard Pflueger (Ed.), *Independent living. Emerging issues in rehabilitation* (pp. ii–iv). Washington, DC: Institute for Research Utilization.

Roessler, R. T., & Rubin, S. (1980). *Goal setting: Guidelines for diagnosis and rehabilitation program development*. Fayetteville: Arkansas Rehabilitation Research and Training Center, University of Arkansas.

Ross, H. (1980). The relationship between level and object relations and degree of autonomy in mothers and their adult daughters. *Dissertation Abstracts International, 41*(5), 1894A–1895A.

Salkind, N. J., Beckwith, R. M., Nelson, C. F., &

McGregor, P. A. (1982). *A summary of instruments that assess independence*. Report No. 1. Lawrence: Research and Training Center on Independent Living, University of Kansas.

Schmidt, B., Collignon, F., Stoddard, S., & Barrett, L. (1978). *In search of standards for independent living*. Berkeley, CA: Berkeley Planning Associates.

Sigelman, C., Vengroff, L., & Spanhel, C. (1979). Disabilities and the concept of life function. *Rehabilitation Counseling Bulletin, 23*(2), 103–113.

Stendler, C. B. (1954). Possible causes of overdependency in young children. *Child Development, 25*, 125–146.

Stoddard, S., Katsuranis, F., Toms, L., & Finnegan, D. (1980). *Evaluation report on the state's independent living centers funded by AB 204: Final report*. Berkeley, CA: Berkeley Planning Associates.

Troutt, B. (1980). Independence and ego identity reflected in minority students' utilization of the support services in an academic special program. *Dissertation Abstracts International, 41*(5), 2029A.

Urban Institute. (1975). *Report of the comprehensive needs study*. Washington, DC: U.S. Department of Health, Education, and Welfare, Rehabilitation Services Administration.

Weiss, W. W. (1981). Independent behavior and moral judgment in primary school pupils. *Psychologic in Erziehung und Unterricht, 28*(6), 334–343.

Wilkerson, D. (1982). *A measure of independence: Perspectives on evaluation on independent living*. Unpublished paper, Seattle: University of Washington.

Wilkerson, D. L., Weinhouse, S., & Jamero, P. M. (1982). *Independent living center evaluation: Washington state data system and data from the first year of Title VII*. Seattle: Independent Living Evaluation Project, University of Washington.

Wood, P. H. N., & Badley, B. M. (1980). *People with disabilities: Toward acquiring information which reflects more sensitively their problems and needs*. New York: World Rehabilitation Fund.

World Health Organization. (1980). *International classification of impairments, disabilities, and handicaps: A manual of classification relating to the consequences of diseases*. Geneva: Author.

Zukas, H. (1975). CIL history. *Report of the State of the Art Conference, Center for Independent Living* (RSA Grant 45-P-45484/9-01). Berkeley, CA: Center for Independent Living.

SECTION II
Methodology in Outcome Analysis

Chapter 7

Design and Statistical Considerations in Rehabilitation Outcomes Analysis

Diana H. Rintala

The goal of this chapter is to acquaint or reacquaint the reader with some of the issues that must be considered in the design and statistical analysis of rehabilitation outcomes studies. It is not intended to replace the many excellent books that cover program evaluation, research design, and statistics. On the contrary, the reader is directed to several of these sources as various issues are discussed. Some books that cover many aspects of outcome analysis include Franklin and Thrasher (1976), Posavac and Carey (1980), Riecken and Boruch (1974), and Struening and Guttentag (1975).

The approach and goals of outcome analysis will be somewhat different, depending on which stage the program is in when assessment begins. Ideally, planning for the measurement of outcomes should start when a program is beginning to be developed and continue into maturity. In this way, outcome analysis can play a role in each developmental stage by encouraging developers to specify the goals of the program in measurable terms and by providing more or less continuous feedback to the program developers as measurement of outcomes proceeds. However, formal outcome analysis does not begin until after a program has been in operation for quite some time. It is much harder to effect changes in a fully established program because those involved in its implementation may resent or resist change. Sometimes goals may not be clearly specified or stated in terms that allow for direct measurement. The goal of "better adjustment" is one example.

It is the job of the person directing the outcome analysis to help program implementors see the value of the feedback to be provided and to engage them in planning the analysis by specifying measurable goals.

Analyzing outcomes of a major program usually should involve a series of studies, each with its own specific goals. If the person responsible for the analysis has not been an integral part of the program's development or implementation, his or her first step, of course, is to become as familiar as possible with each program component. The next task is to specify the questions to be answered by the research. Investigatable issues may emerge not only through questions from program staff, but also through conducting a series of studies that build upon each other to facilitate selection of a final set of outcome variables and a feasible design. This series may include descriptive studies, correlational analyses, and finally, hypothesis testing.

Descriptive studies can be useful to characterize the clients involved (e.g., provide demographic data), the services delivered, and the status of the clients on a wide range of outcome variables using frequency distributions, means, standard deviations, and the like. By formalizing and quantifying various aspects of the program, one can begin to generate or refine the specific questions to be answered by later phases of the assessment.

Exploratory correlational studies are often a good next step. They can help explicate relationships between various aspects of the program while further refining and focusing questions yet to be answered. For example, correlations between services delivered and outcomes can begin to suggest causal hypotheses to be tested. Techniques such as factor analysis can help to group outcome variables to aid in selecting a few representative key variables for further examination.

Finally, formal hypothesis testing of the effects of the program on the desired outcomes can be undertaken. This type of study is best undertaken when the program is in a fairly mature stage of development. It is inefficient to formally test the effects of a program that is changing rapidly. By the time the results are reported, the program, as it was at the time of evaluation, will no longer exist.

The analytical strategy described is elucidated in the remainder of this chapter. Among the topics discussed are: 1) description of the program and the outcomes, 2) the functions of correlational analyses, 3) assessment of whether the desired outcomes have been achieved, 4) selection of the sample, and 5) selection of the measures. An attempt has been made to keep jargon to a minimum to increase readability for people from a variety of backgrounds. However, where appropriate, reference is made to the widely used terminology of Campbell and Stanley (1966), Cook and Campbell (1979), and others regarding threats to internal validity—bases for attributing results to causes other than those being studied—and external validity—constraints on the generalizability of the results to other times, places, or clients.

BEGIN WITH DESCRIPTION

To evaluate outcomes of a program, one must first obtain a thorough knowledge of both the process by which the program is conducted and the expected and actual outcomes. To do this, one must gather many kinds of data from multiple sources in a systematic fashion. Discussions with project administrators and staff and with the clients receiving the services are essential to begin to sort out what is happening and what are the important outcome variables. In the first of a series of studies, it is important to gather both quantitative and qualitative data on a wide array

of different aspects of the program and its outcomes to eventually select an efficient set of key outcome variables (Cronbach et al., 1980). For information that is quantifiable, descriptive statistics can be used to help make sense of the data. These include frequency distributions, percentages, cross-tabulations, mean, median, mode, and standard deviation.

Each service variable (e.g., type and amount of service) and outcome measure (e.g., functional status, vocational status, health status) can be described across all clients or by subgroups based on variables such as age, race, sex, diagnostic category, and severity of disability. Case studies and anecdotal incidents can aid in fleshing out the information gained from the quantitative data. By describing many different aspects of the clients, services, and outcomes, individual bits of information can be understood in the context of the whole program. An initial broad approach is more likely to promote insightful thinking about the program than would a premature narrower focus only on selected quantitative outcome measures.

EXAMINE CORRELATIONAL RELATIONSHIPS

Two major functions of exploratory correlational analyses are relevant to outcome evaluation: data reduction and accounting for the variance in certain variables. This type of analysis can be performed on the same data set used in the descriptive analysis and usually should be undertaken as an exploratory step in evaluating the outcomes of a program prior to formal hypothesis testing. Data reduction techniques such as factor analysis (Rummel, 1970), multidimensional scaling (Shepard, Romney, & Nerlove, 1972), and cluster analysis (Everitt, 1977) all "explore associations among variables in an effort to detect groups of variables sharing common sources of variance" (Cleary, 1983, p. 771). Factor analysis is appropriate for use with interval and ratio data but not for dichotomous or ordinal data. Multidimensional scaling and cluster analysis can be used when factor analysis is inappropriate. Based on these analyses, weights can be assigned to the variables so that a composite score represents each group of variables for each individual measured. For example, suppose that 50 variables were analyzed using one of these techniques and five groups of related variables were formed. Each subject then would have a single score for each group, a total of five scores rather than 50. This makes interpretation more manageable.

Correlational analyses can also illuminate relationships between variables that help to account for variance in some outcome measures. For example, a variety of demographic (e.g., age, sex) and service (e.g., amount of therapy, time in hospital) variables may be used to account for the variance in functional status. Multiple regression is appropriate if a single outcome measure is to be accounted for by several demographic and process variables or if a group of outcome measures are each to be accounted for separately (Cohen & Cohen, 1975). Multivariate analyses account for variance in a group of several outcome measures simultaneously (Tatsuoka, 1971). These relationships can be used to generate hypotheses about causal relationships that can be tested in later research.

DECIDE IF THE DESIRED OUTCOMES OCCURRED

Once a clearly delimited program has been identified or developed, more than simple description may be desired. There are a variety of methods for determining whether the outcomes of interest have occurred. Some require only minimal resources to conduct. Others are more elaborate and require a relatively large commitment of resources.

Single System Designs

Research designs that are relatively easy for rehabilitation professionals to implement in conjunction with full-time clinical practice are known as single system designs. The essential distinguishing characteristic of these designs is that no control or comparison group is required. Practitioners can evaluate each client independently as they provide services, and they can aggregate findings across many clients. Two helpful books devoted to single system designs are those

by Bloom and Fischer (1982) and Kazdin and Tuma (1982).

Goal attainment, single time series, and time series with repeated introduction of the treatment are examples of single system approaches to outcome research.

Goal Attainment Design One straightforward approach to program evaluation is assessment of whether preset goals have been attained. Cook and Campbell (1979) referred to this as a preexperimental, one-group, posttest-only design. A number of recording and scoring schemes have been devised to facilitate use of this approach. These include Concrete Goal Setting, Goal Attainment Scaling, Goal-oriented Automated Progress Note, and the Patient Progress Record (Davis, 1973; Franklin & Thrasher, 1976). The goal attainment approach involves, as a regular part of the program, setting and recording goals for each client, and later, after services have been provided, assessing the extent to which each goal has been met. Some schemes include identifying the relative importance of each goal for the particular client in question. The goals either can be negotiated between the program staff and the client or may be set by the staff alone. The methods to be used to attain each goal sometimes are recorded as a routine part of the assessment process. Aggregating the results for many clients helps to evaluate the success of the services offered by the program.

The major advantages of the goal attainment approach are its simplicity and the provision of constant feedback to the service providers, which in turn allows continuous adjustments in the services offered. When the methods used are recorded, comparisons of the outcomes attained when using various methods can be made. A typical use of this approach would be a vocational rehabilitation program that set paid employment as a goal for its clients. The percentage of clients who attained this goal would be a measure of the program's success.

The major drawback of this approach is that it does not establish a cause-and-effect relationship between the services given and the goals attained. The clients possibly would have done as well, nearly as well, or even better in meeting the goals without receiving the services. The lack of a comparison group who did not receive the services makes it impossible to determine the actual impact of the services on client outcomes. Ironically, the results of this approach are of greater value if they are negative rather than positive. If goals are not being met, service providers are informed of this fact in a systematic and continuous manner. They can try to modify the services until the rate of goal attainment reaches acceptable levels.

Single Time Series Design   Another design that does not require a comparison group but that does allow some determination of program outcomes (i.e., is quasi-experimental) is the single time series. The variables to be affected by the program are measured at several points in time both before and after the program is implemented. In essence, preprogram baseline measures serve as comparison data for postprogram outcome measures. Evaluating the trend over time of the preprogram measures makes it possible to estimate the changes that would have occurred without the program. Such changes are referred to as maturation by Cook and Campbell (1979). For example, one would expect some improvement in functional status over time in persons recovering from recent serious physical injuries (e.g., spinal cord injury) even without a comprehensive rehabilitation program. Healing would occur in any case, assuming basic medical and nursing care were provided. Any additional improvement beyond that normally expected after implementation of the program can then be attributed to the effects of the program if there is no other plausible reason for the abrupt change, such as some simultaneous event. Potential threats to internal validity include the main effect of history (i.e., some external event), a change in instrumentation (i.e., way of measuring or recording data), and a change in the composition of the sample (i.e., selection bias due to dropouts).

This design can be used in evaluating change over time in a single client. For example, a client's level of activity could be measured for 2 weeks before, and 2 weeks after, instituting a treatment for pain. It can also be used to measure change in the outcomes of consecutive groups of clients receiving the services of an organization. An example of the latter would be measuring each year the proportion of clients institutionalized for several years before and after the implementation of a new service program aimed at reducing the need for institutional care. In this case, outcomes for different groups of clients are measured each year.

To allow evaluation of a program's effect, a time series on a single individual or sequential groups served by a single organization should include measurements at a minimum of 20 to 30 points. However, if the changes are assessed by using a time series design for each of many individuals and then aggregating the results, far fewer measurement points will suffice; as few as two before and two after implementation of the program may be needed. Computerized statistical packages are available to aid in analyzing the data. Cook and Campbell (1979) recommend using the autoregressive integrated moving average (ARIMA) models developed by Box and Jenkins (1976). Special adaptations must be made in analyses of aggregated time series data to account for the dependence between the repeated measures of each individual. Bloom and Fischer (1982) described several analytical techniques for single system designs.

Time Series Design with Repeated Introduction of the Treatment   Time series designs can be modified to improve the interpretability of results and to answer more complex questions. In some cases, it may be possible to introduce a treatment, stop it for a time, and then reintroduce it. This pattern of treatment–no treatment–treatment can be extended indefinitely. Measurement of outcome variables is done before and after each switch. This design is best used when a treatment is expected to have an immediate effect in one direction and removal of the treatment is expected to have an immediate effect in the opposite direction. To prevent resentment over discontinuing the treatment, the subject should be convinced of a logical reason for its removal. For example, this design might be used when too many clients in a rehabilitation program want to try the few available assistive devices undergoing assessment. Each person might be allowed to try the equipment for one day until all have had the opportunity, then everyone has a second chance, and so on. If an individual's functional status improves greatly only on days when the equipment is in use but decreases each time the equipment is removed, it is possible to attribute the improvement in function to the use of the equipment. Care must be taken in scheduling to avoid linking the timing of the interventions to some preexisting cyclical pattern such as treatment in the morning, no treatment in the afternoon. Results can be aggregated across a number of clients. A variation on this design involves comparing two different treatments; the second treatment is introduced and stopped between repetitions of the first treatment. Bloom and Fischer (1982) extensively discussed a number of variations of single system designs.

Multiple Group Designs

Although single system designs are relatively simple and useful, it is often desirable to be able to make comparisons between two or more groups who are treated differently. Before discussing some designs for multiple groups, a discussion of the way individuals are assigned to the various groups is necessary.

Randomized Groups If observation of more than one group is desirable and feasible, it must be determined whether individuals will be assigned to the various groups on a random basis. Random assignment can be accomplished by using a table of random numbers or a computerized random number generator. Relevant subgroups (e.g., male, female) can be identified and random assignment can be made from within each subgroup.

There are both advantages and disadvantages to random assignment. The major advantage is that, when comparing a group who received the services being evaluated and a group who did not, the groups are initially more likely to be similar in all respects if group membership is assigned randomly. Using a stratifying procedure for subgroups prior to random assignment further increases the comparability of the groups. Because the groups are comparable except for receiving the services being evaluated, it is possible to be highly confident in the conclusions drawn regarding the effect of treatment. For this reason, randomization is considered to be the most scientifically acceptable method of group

assignment in research and is the only true experimental approach.

There are, however, drawbacks to random assignment. For example, a long-existing program may be so revered by the clients, staff, or community at large that any attempt to deny an otherwise eligible group access to the program may cause strong negative reactions to the research and researchers by one or more of these groups. This in turn could have an effect on the implementation of the program itself and on the evaluation of the impact of the program. Initially comparable groups could become dissimilar because of resentment about group assignment and consequent withdrawal from the study by many of the control group members. The political and ethical implications of denying treatment to some people may be far too severe for random assignment to be part of the evaluation design.

Under some circumstances, there are ways to overcome the problems associated with random assignment. For example, if the intervention permits only a limited number of people to be accommodated at one time, assignments can be made randomly to groups that will receive the services in question at various points in time. The groups not yet served function as control groups until their turns begin. Another solution is possible if whole groups of people can be used as the unit of analysis, such as consecutive groups enrolled in a month-long educational program designed to facilitate reentry into the community after rehabilitation. Random assignment of a whole class to one of two or more program types can be made. The sample size in this case is the number of classes receiving each type of program, not the number of people. If program participants are unaware of the differences between the two programs or have no prior preference, resentment over group assignment should not occur.

Nonrandomized Groups When use of a randomly assigned control group is impossible, other types of comparison groups can be used. Often these are naturally occurring groups who for one reason or another did not receive the services being evaluated or received a different type of service. Sometimes group membership is based on the preference of the individuals involved. Other times, the comparison groups are composed of persons who were not eligible for the services; for example, they were in the wrong geographic area, income bracket, diagnostic category, or age group. Sometimes the reasons for inclusion in the unserved groups vary from individual to individual, some based on voluntary considerations, others based on eligibility considerations.

Difficulties in interpreting results often occur when using comparison groups formed without random assignment. This is because it is not known whether the groups are equivalent on all relevant dimensions prior to the implementation of the program. Without this assurance, it is impossible to unequivocally attribute differences in outcomes to the effect of the program. The known or unknown initial differences between the groups may have caused differences in the outcomes even without the program. Simply matching the groups on pretest measures of interest does not counteract this problem. This is because the groups may differ in an unknown manner on other variables that are related to the outcomes.

Three types of difficulties that arise when matching is used warrant discussion. First, suppose there is a program designed to improve the functional independence of persons with disabilities. Persons self-select themselves into the group who receive the service. Those who did not choose to participate in the program are recruited as the comparison group. A pretest of independence is performed on both groups. Each member of the treatment group is then matched with a person in the nontreatment group based on the similarity of their pretest scores. Tests of independence are then administered to the matched groups following completion of the program. Because of their act of electing to be in the treatment group, it is reasonable to wonder whether the treatment group was representative of a more highly motivated or better informed population than was the nontreatment group. If there were initial differences of this type, any posttest differences in independence between the two groups could be attributed to initial differeences on these other relevant variables even though they were matched on initial level of independence. In other words, the group with higher initial motivation would have become more independent even

without the program than would the less motivated comparison group. Matching on more than one pretest measure still does not assure that some other relevant initial difference in the group does not exist. This is often labeled a selection–maturation interaction.

Second, suppose persons are selected for the program based on severity of disability as measured by a functional assessment scale. The most disabled persons are selected for the program. Those in the treatment group just below the cutoff score and those in the nontreatment group just above the cutoff score are compared on postprogram outcomes. This is done so that the groups being compared are as similar as possible before the treatment. Because the high scorers in the treatment group are members of the whole treatment group and the low scorers in the nontreatment group are members of the whole nontreatment group, a statistical phenomenon called regression toward the mean occurs. The pretest high scorers in the treatment group will be likely to have posttest scores closer to the whole treatment group's average posttest score. In other words, they are not likely to be the highest scorers of their group on the posttest. Conversely, the low scorers in the nontreatment group will be likely to have posttest scores closer to the average for the whole nontreatment group. These occurrences can make the program appear detrimental regardless of its actual impact.

Third, other problems that accompany nonequivalent comparison groups include floor and ceiling effects where one group has very little room for improvement. If this happens to be the treatment group, it can make the program appear to have a negative impact since the nontreatment group may improve more than the treatment group. Similarly, if the nontreatment group has less room for improvement than the treatment group, the apparent impact of the program, if any, could be exaggerated. These problems are caused by flaws in the instruments used to measure the variables of interest. The intervals at the ends of a scale may be wider or narrower than in the middle.

To help overcome these difficulties in finding a satisfactory comparison group, one must have an in-depth knowledge of how the groups were formed and use only those groups for which the method of determining group membership was likely to result in equivalent or nearly equivalent groups. In addition, use of a combination of research designs (e.g., time series and comparison group) or a program of studies can help sort out the impact of initial differences from the impact of the program.

Pretest–Posttest Design Whether assignment to groups is done on a random basis or not, one basic multiple group approach that can be used is the pretest–posttest design. With random assignment, this is the classical control group design. Each group is measured on the relevant variables once before and once after the program; however, one or more groups either do not receive the program or get a different kind of program. The pretest assesses the initial comparability of the groups on the measures in question. If they are initially comparable, the posttest comparison provides the desired information on the impact of receiving the services or the relative impact of two or more types of services. Many variations of this basic design can be devised to answer research questions and to improve the interpretability of the results.

If the groups, in fact, are comparable initially, because of either randomization or other selection criteria, and no resentment toward group assignment exists, there are few problems with interpretation. However, when initial group differences exist, as noted above, there can be a number of explanations for the findings other than the effect of the program. Cook and Campbell (1979, pp. 103–112) provided a detailed discussion of interpretations of various patterns of outcomes using this design. The statistical analysis of the results using a pretest–posttest design is not an easy task when randomized groups are not used. Each of the techniques available has its own source of bias. Even with extensive knowledge of any selection differences, absolute confidence cannot be placed in the conclusions drawn.

Analysis of variance (ANOVA) is appropriate for analyzing results of randomized group designs. For nonrandomized groups, ANOVA does not adjust for any known initial differences between the groups. Analysis of covariance (ANCOVA), with one or more variables used as covariates, can compensate for some known initial differences between the groups. However, not all differences are known, and those that are known are probably not measured without some error. Both of these factors bias the results of ANCOVA. Any influence besides the treatment capable of producing the difference between groups can also bias analysis of variance using gain scores (i.e., change scores, improvement measures) as outcomes. Such influences may include ability or motivation differences (i.e., selection–maturation interaction), floor and ceiling effects (instrumentation), and statistical regression to the mean. To minimize bias as much as possible, the researcher must carefully evaluate the situation in question and choose among the available analytic techniques. Even then, caution is advised with regard to the confidence placed in the results.

Multiple Time Series Design The multiple time series approach combines the strengths of both the single time series and the pretest–posttest designs. This design can be used whether group assignment is random or not. Each group is measured on relevant variables at several points in time both before and after the program is implemented. Each group's preprogram measures serve as its own comparison data on the postprogram measures. As with the single time series, this provides a forecast of each group's future performance without the program. Comparing two or more time series can supplement this forecast by showing the actual outcomes for the two groups. If the trends for the two or more groups are very similar before the program but abruptly become different after implementation of the program, the difference in outcome usually can be attributed to the program. One must verify, however, that some other event that could have caused the change did not occur to only one group at the time of the treatment (i.e., history–selection interaction). As with the single time series, the time series for each group can be analyzed using the ARIMA model.

Recurrent Institutional Cycle Design A useful approach when randomization is impossible is a design that measures the outcomes of interest before and after each of several consecutive groups receives the services in question. This situation arises when new groups of people periodically begin a program offered by a rehabilitation facility. The ending scores of one group are compared with both their own beginning scores and the beginning scores of the next group who enter the program. If the two groups have approximately the same average score before the program and the same improved average score after the program, the improvement can often be attributed to exposure to the program. However, the possibility that the change would have taken place even without the program needs to be considered. If there is no plausible reason to believe that the change would have occurred anyway, then conclusions about the impact of the program are valid. Understanding the method of group assignment is also important. For example, if the more severely disabled were more likely to be in the earlier group (i.e., selection effect), biased results would be obtained.

Regression–Discontinuity Design Another approach that can be used when random assignment is not feasible is the regression–discontinuity design. This design should be used when a definite cutoff score on some pretest is used to determine who receives the treatment. For example, a program for persons with mental retardation uses a score of 70 as a cutoff point on an intelligence test. Only those with a score of 70 or below are admitted into the program. Pretest and posttest measures are obtained on both those qualified and those not qualified. Imagine plotting on a graph the pretest score against the posttest score for each individual. A line is drawn through the center of the range of points below the cutoff on the pretest and another line is drawn through the range of points above the cutoff. The position of each line within its range of points is mathematically calculated to minimize the sum of the squares of the distances from the line to each point. This is called a regression line. If the two regression lines do not meet at the cutoff point, the discontinuity can be attributed to an impact of the program, since one continuous line would be expected if no program was implemented. The major threat to internal validity is that one or both of the regression lines may actually be curvilinear rather than straight. The ap-

propriate statistical technique for testing group differences with this design is analysis of covariance with the pretest score as a single covariate. Cook and Campbell (1979) provided an excellent discussion of this design and its analysis.

SELECTING THE SAMPLE

Sample Composition

The first step in sample selection is to set up criteria for including potential subjects in the study. Examples of such criteria include minimum and/or maximum age, sex, ethnicity, diagnostic category, and severity of disability. These criteria should be the same as those expected to be used to select persons for the new treatment or program, if adopted in the future. In other words, the sample must represent the population of interest.

The second step is to decide on the desired proportion of various subgroups to be selected. Each eligible category may be represented in proportion to its actual size in the eligible population. In some cases, however, it may be desirable to include some types of people in the sample in a disproportionate manner. For example, only a relatively small proportion of persons with spinal cord injury are female (20%). However, the impact of a program on females may be of special interest. To acquire a sufficiently large sample for inferring treatment impacts on women, one may choose a higher proportion of women than found in the spinal cord injured population. When statements are meant to generalize to the entire eligible population, weights can be assigned to the findings for each subgroup to reflect the true proportions in the population.

The third step is to randomly select participants from the population, thereby increasing the external validity of results. This should not be confused with the random assignment to treatment groups that is done subsequently. Suppose it was decided the sample size should be 100, and 40% of the participants should be female. If the population of interest includes 300 female potential candidates, then 40 of them should be randomly chosen from among the 300. If there are

1200 male potential candidates in the population, then 60 of them should be randomly selected.

Random selection is essential to enable generalizing the results from the sample to the population (i.e., to attain external validity). Often investigators do not have the luxury of a large pool of individuals from which to sample. In that case, every eligible person is recruited until the desired sample size has been obtained or until some time limit has been reached. It is then necessary to estimate the extent to which the obtained sample is representative of the population of interest. One way to circumvent this problem is to arrange interinstitutional studies that provide a larger and more representative sample.

Sample Size

The sample size needed is in part determined by the research design selected. The larger the sample size, the more statistical power is available to detect relationships between variables, such as group differences on outcome measures. Also, assuming unbiased sampling techniques, the larger the sample, the more accurate the estimate of the mean of the population will be. This is because the standard error of the mean decreases as the sample size increases. These benefits of large samples have to be weighed against the resources available to carry out the study. Having a larger sample may mean a reduction in the richness of the data collected about each individual. This could result in the loss of some important information.

From a statistical point of view, there are some rules of thumb about sample size to use for various types of analyses (Cleary, 1983). For multiple regression, at least 100 subjects are suggested, and at least 25 subjects for each independent variable. In factor analysis, at least four or five subjects per variable are required. Tables of power analysis aid in calculating the sample size necessary for testing differences between groups (Cohen, 1969; Myers, 1972). To use them, one must decide how large a difference in outcomes will make a meaningful difference in program planning. For example, suppose that the score on a functional assessment scale is the outcome variable of interest, and a new treatment aimed at

improving function is tested against the usual treatment. One needs to decide by how many points the average score of the group receiving the new treatment must exceed the average score of the group receiving the usual treatment before a decision will be made to replace the old treatment with the new treatment.

Three other factors are involved in using the tables. First is the acceptable probability of incorrectly identifying an effect of treatment when none exists. This is known as alpha, Type I error rate, or *specificity*. Most studies use .05 or .01. If many tests are done, as is common in exploratory studies, the more stringent .01 should be used to reduce the possibility of chance findings. Second, the probability of detecting an effect of the chosen size, if there is one, must be selected. This is known as power or *sensitivity*. The conventional probability used is .80. Third, an estimate of the standard deviation of the outcome variable can be obtained from previous research using the same or a very similar variable. When the required magnitude of the effect is large relative to the standard deviation, a smaller sample size is required than when the situation is reversed. Similar calculations of required sample size can be made when proportion of variance or magnitude of a correlation coefficient are of interest rather than differences between means.

Samples of the size recommended by statistical theory may not be available in many applied situations within the time limitations of a study. In that case, recognize that using a small sample increases the probability of coming to the incorrect conclusion that there was no effect.

SELECTING THE MEASURES

Number of Outcome Measures

The number of outcome measures to choose depends on several issues. First, what variables are hypothesized to be affected by the program being evaluated? If the program is broad in scope, many aspects of the participants' lives may be affected and each needs to be measured. Second, whenever possible, more than one method of collecting data on a given aspect should be included. This is particularly true if the concept of interest is not directly measurable but must be inferred from one or more indices. For example, the number of trips to friends' houses per week is one index of social participation, but it does not represent every aspect of social participation. Other indices might include phone calls to and from friends and family, attendance at club meetings, or visits by family and friends. By getting several measures, a more complete picture of social participation can be obtained in order to increase construct validity. Third, the arguments for many measures must be weighed against the cost of collecting and handling large amounts of data. Fourth, as mentioned in the section on sample size, greater numbers of participants are needed as the number of measures increases if various statistical analyses are to yield acceptable estimates of relationships between variables. Thus, although gathering a great many variables is tempting in order to more fully understand the effects of a program, certain resource and statistical constraints need to be considered.

Sensitivity, Reliability, and Validity of Measures

The measures selected must be sensitive to differences among subjects at a point in time and within subjects over time. They should be equally sensitive across all points along the continuum of scores. For example, the measuring instrument should be capable of detecting small differences in independence between persons with quadriplegia as well as it detects differences between those with paraplegia if the instrument is intended for use with both groups. The measures chosen should also be reliable in that, given the same actual or true situation (i.e., participant status) and the same measurement instrument and methods, the same scores would be obtained on the measures at a different time or when rated by a different investigator. Even if one is using standardized measuring instruments with published reliability figures, it is frequently desirable to reestablish their reliability in one's own study. To do this, a clear and unambiguous set of procedures must be developed for collecting and coding the data to ensure sufficient consistency across participants and across data collectors and coders.

The measures must also be valid in that they must be good representatives of the concepts in question. As noted above, several independent measures may be needed to obtain a valid representation of some concepts. Validity depends, in part, on choosing the appropriate type or types of measures. Outcome measures should be closely linked to the goals of the program, and good rehabilitation program goals should generally be stated in terms of specific measurable behaviors. Thus, behavioral outcomes are generally the best type of measures to answer the questions of interest (Brown, Gordon, & Diller, 1984; Rintala et al., 1984). Less often, attitudinal and physiological measures may be appropriate.

Method of Obtaining Measures

There are six major methods of obtaining the necessary data: 1) interviews (structured, free form, or a combination); 2) questionnaires; 3) direct observation of behavior (e.g., watching performance by the client of some learned task) or appearance (e.g., physical exam); 4) physiological samples (e.g., blood, urine); 5) mechanized measures (e.g., heart rate monitor, activity monitor); and 6) existing records kept for some other purpose (e.g., medical records, attendance records, school records). The choice of methods depends on which will give the most reliable and valid answers to the questions of interest and which are feasible in view of monetary and other resource limitations.

Interviews and questionnaires elicit only verbal responses to questions. These answers can sometimes be misleading for a variety of reasons, including desire to give socially acceptable responses, poor recall of past events, inaccurate or incomplete perceptions, and lack of knowledge. The amount of distortion also depends on the relative subjectivity versus objectivity of the required information. Questions about specific current behaviors are more likely to elicit reliable and valid responses than requests for global ratings. The major benefit of interviews and questionnaires is that they are relatively cost-effective methods of gathering large amounts of data.

Direct observation by trained independent observers, physiological tests, and mechanized measures are all excellent methods of obtaining reliable and valid information. The major drawback of these types of measures is their cost for personnel and/or equipment.

A warning regarding use of data from existing records is in order. The records must contain the desired data, and this information must be in a form applicable to the evaluation. The reliability of such data is often questionable, since the recording of data may be inconsistent from time to time or recorder to recorder. The evaluator usually has little control over the quality of these data. The benefits of using existing records include relatively low cost of data collection and no reactivity to the study.

CONCLUSION

Outcome assessment can provide insights into not only how a program seems to work, but also how it can be improved. Results can be obtained by means of a series of studies ranging from simple description to elaborate hypothesis testing. In any case, investigations should be as methodologically rigorous as possible.

No matter how statistically valid, the information supplied is only one of many considerations in deciding what program changes should be made. Franklin and Thrasher (1976) observed that the findings of outcome studies often have no influence on ultimate decisions. They point out that decision makers such as program managers or policymakers may have a very different orientation from that of the evaluator. Decision makers must deal with bureaucratic concerns that include funding cycles, deadlines, and politics, whereas assessors often are concerned primarily with methodological issues such as reliability, causal inference, and generalizability. The only solution to these differences in perspective is for managers and evaluators to work closely together to educate each other regarding their respective values and constraints and to arrive at a negotiated agreement. In this way, pragmatism and scientific rigor can be reconciled.

REFERENCES

Bloom, M., & Fischer, J. (1982). *Evaluating practice: Guidelines for the accountable professional.* Englewood Cliffs, NJ: Prentice-Hall.

Box, G. E. P., & Jenkins, G. M. (1976). *Time-series analysis: Forecasting and control.* San Francisco: Holden-Day.

Brown, M., Gordon, W. A., & Diller, L. (1984). Rehabilitation indicators. In A. S. Halpern & M. J. Fuhrer (Eds.), *Functional assessment in rehabilitation* (pp. 187–203). Baltimore: Paul H. Brookes Publishing Co.

Campbell, D. T., & Stanley, J. C. (1966). *Experimental and quasi-experimental designs for research.* Chicago: Rand McNally.

Cleary, P. D. (1983). Multivariate analysis: Basic approaches to health data. In D. Mechanic (Ed.), *Handbook of health, health care, and the health professions* (pp. 766–790). New York: Free Press.

Cohen, J. (1969). *Statistical power analysis for the behavioral sciences.* New York: Academic Press.

Cohen, J., & Cohen P. (1975). *Applied multiple regression/correlation analysis for the behavioral sciences.* New York: John Wiley & Sons.

Cook, T. D., & Campbell, D. T. (1979). *Quasi-experimentation: Design and analysis issues for field settings.* Chicago: Rand McNally.

Cronbach, L. J., Ambron, S. R., Dornbusch, S. M., Hess, R. D., Hornik, R. C., Phillips, D. C., Walker, D. F., and Weiner, S. S. (1980). *Toward reform of program evaluation.* San Francisco: Jossey-Bass.

Davis, H. R. (1973). Four ways to goal attainment: An overview. *Evaluation, 1*(2), 43–48, 95.

Everitt, B. S. (1977). Cluster analysis. In C. R. O'Muir-cheartaign & C. Payne (Eds.), *The analysis of survey data* (pp. 63–68). New York: John Wiley & Sons.

Franklin, J. L., & Thrasher, J. H. (1976). *An introduction to program evaluation.* New York: John Wiley & Sons.

Kazdin, A. E., & Tuma, A. H. (Eds.). (1982). *Single case research designs.* San Francisco: Jossey-Bass.

Myers, J. L. (1972). *Fundamentals of experimental design* (2nd ed.). Boston: Allyn & Bacon.

Posavac, E. J., & Carey, R. G. (1980). *Program evaluation: Methods and case studies.* Englewood Cliffs, NJ: Prentice-Hall.

Riecken, H. W., & Boruch, R. F. (Eds.). (1974). *Social experimentation: A method for planning and evaluating social intervention.* New York: Academic Press.

Rintala, D. H., Uttermohlen, D. M., Buck, E. L., Hanover, D., Alexander, J. L., Norris-Baker, C., Stephens, M. A. P., Willems, E. P., & Halstead, L. S. (1984). Self-observation and report technique (SORT): Description and clinical applications. In A. S. Halpern & M. J. Fuhrer (Eds.), *Functional assessment in rehabilitation* (pp. 205–221). Baltimore: Paul H. Brookes Publishing Co.

Rummel, R. J. (1970). *Applied factor analysis.* Evanston, IL: Northwestern University Press.

Shepard, R. N., Romney, A. K., & Nerlove, S. B. (Eds.). (1972). *Multidimensional scaling: Vol. 1.* New York: Seminar Press.

Struening, E. L., & Guttentag, M. (Eds.). (1975). *Handbook of evaluation research: Vol. 1.* Beverly Hills: Sage.

Tatsuoka, M. M. (1971). *Multivariate analysis: Techniques for educational and psychological research.* New York: John Wiley & Sons.

Chapter 8

Cost–Benefit Methodologies in Rehabilitation

Mark V. Johnston

Rehabilitationists have long spoken of the cost–benefits and cost-effectiveness of rehabilitation. To judge from historical records, vocational rehabilitation (VR) was explicitly begun as an economic proposition. In the last 15 years, benefit–cost analyses attempting to show that vocational rehabilitation is justified on purely economic grounds have become "virtually a cottage industry" (Bureau of Economic Research, 1985b). In medical rehabilitation too, interest in benefit–cost analysis (BCA) and cost-effectiveness analysis (CEA) has risen as pressures for fiscal accountability have risen, and a few BCAs and CEAs have been attempted (M. V. Johnston & Keith, 1983).

In the last decade or so, hundreds of works on BCA and CEA have been published in the literature of health care, education, and social program evaluation (e.g., Office of Technology Assessment, 1980; Thompson, 1980; Warner & Luce, 1982). Methodological works have been common. Some problems seem to remain intractable, although slow progress has been made with others. Substantial advances have been made in statistical methods and research designs applicable to field studies (Cook & Campbell, 1979). This entire book is testament to the progress that has been made in outcome measurement. A large number of highly informative BCAs and CEAs can now be found in fields related to rehabilitation.

So many BCAs and CEAs have been attempted in rehabilitation and closely related fields that we should be able to learn more from them than from the study of theory alone. This chapter presents lessons drawn from the experience of these studies. These lessons will be presented in the form of 10 *sutras*—points that need to be understood to facilitate appropriate applications of BCA/CEA in rehabilitation. The Sanskrit word "sutra" is used because of its precision: A sutra is a point or lesson that is explicitly not meant to stand by itself. Rather, a sutra (root meaning—stitch or suture) covers a gap and binds together parts of a wider whole. Similarly, the 10 sutras to follow are not meant to be a systematic or complete introduction to BCA or CEA. Rather, they are intended to orient rehabilitation professionals to BCA or CEA and to help analysts adapt benefit–cost and cost-effectiveness methodologies to the particular requirements of medical and vocational rehabilitation. And just as a stitch carries tension but does not relax it, the sutras to follow are not without controversy and even contradiction. The aim is to present promising approaches, not theoretical nicety.

DEFINITIONS

A few basic terms and concepts need to be explained to give readers the conceptual tools they need to begin to understand BCA/CEA. For a more thorough understanding, readers are referred to books on cost–benefits analysis in health care (Office of Technology Assessment, 1980; Warner & Luce, 1982), program evaluation (Thompson, 1980), business (Henry & Haynes, 1978), and vocational rehabilitation (Bureau of Economic Research, 1985b), and to reviews by

Nobel (1977) and M. V. Johnston and Keith (1983).

Monetary Analyses

Cost in economics is the difference in monetary return between the use of a scarce resource in one way and its use in a promising alternative. For example, an economist might estimate the value of donated resources in computing the cost of a program to society. Such *opportunity costs,* however, rarely need to be computed for all monetary items in a real BCA or CEA. In practice, ordinary accounting costs and monetary gains are quite serviceable. Biases in accounting practices have been less problematic in the literature of rehabilitation than the absence of any empirical cost data.

Costs are not the same as charges. The most common procedure is to apply a ratio (e.g., costs = .75 times charges for Medicare patients). In some circumstances, however, charges can actually yield a better estimate of social costs and resource consumption than accounted costs. For example, cost allocation schemes in hospitals have been manipulated for over 15 years to maximize reimbursement, while charge rates may have been set to cover what hospital management believes services cost across payment classes.

Direct costs are typically the costs of operation for personnel, facilities, and so on. *Indirect costs* are those due to mixed causes or related to more than one cost objective (Anthony & Reece, 1979; Henry & Haynes, 1978). Lost earnings are an indirect cost of many educational programs and illness, but they are not an indirect cost of inpatient medical rehabilitation programs, since patients in such programs are too ill for return to work to be an option.

Economists calculate *social costs and benefits.* These are monetary costs and benefits accruing to clients, taxpayers, program personnel—that is, to everyone. The analytic techniques of BCA, however, are equally applicable to subsets of society. For instance, benefit–cost techniques may be used to estimate the relative attractiveness of management options in an individual firm (Henry & Haynes, 1978).

Incremental costs and benefits are typically crucial for both BCA and CEA. Incremental costs are the difference in cost between the program in question and a viable or promising alternative. Costs that do not vary across alternatives, called *invariant costs,* should be excluded from the computation of net costs and benefits. *Fixed costs,* those that cannot be changed over the short run or over the temporal horizon of the analysis, also may be excluded.

Techniques have been developed to estimate the *cost of illness.* For instance, Berkowitz's group (Bureau of Economic Research, 1985a) estimated that "medical care and other direct costs of spinal cord injury amounted to more than one-half billion dollars in 1977." Indirect costs of lost earnings were much greater—approximately $2.4 billion. These figures imply that substantial savings to society are possible by saving the lives of spinal cord–injured patients and returning them to work. In contrast, the National Survey of Stroke (Weinfeld, 1981) found that the direct costs of stroke—primarily hospitalization—were about $3.26 billion in 1976. Indirect costs were $2.9 to $4.8 billion. M. V. Johnston (1983a) found that nonrehabilitation medical costs comprised the majority (55.8%) of illness-related costs after discharge for stroke rehabilitation patients. Rehospitalization costs were a large percentage (45.5%) of these postdischarge medical expenses. Including the costs of rehabilitation, hospitalization costs were 74.3% of illness-related costs. These studies imply that, aside from prevention, the greatest potential savings to society in caring for stroke patients may be decreasing utilization of hospital care. Cost-of-illness studies are useful for prioritizing research expenditures toward areas of greater potential social benefit. However, because cost-of-illness studies do not specify whether there is any current or future technology for altering the course of illness, they are of little practical value for improving current efforts to deal with disability.

Benefit–Cost and Cost-Effectiveness Analysis

Benefit–cost analysis (called cost–benefits analysis by some authors) provides a method by which all monetary factors relevant to a decision can be synthesized into a single number. An economic BCA balances short-run costs of an investment against long-run gains. The results of a BCA are summarized in terms of net benefits (benefits minus costs) or a benefit–cost ratio. In BCA, an attempt is made to analyze an investment in rehabilitation just as if it were an investment in anything else. This method is important because the direct costs of rehabilitation are misleading in that they are, wholly or in part, recouped by subsequently increased earnings (vocational rehabilitation) or decreased institutionalization (medical rehabilitation).

Since a dollar in the future is not worth as much as a dollar now, the value of future monetary flows must be reduced by a certain percentage for each year in the future. The percentage is called the *discount rate* and the procedure is called *discounting to present value*. Figures such as 10%, 12%, or the expected inflation rate plus 3% are used for the discount rate. Uncertainty about what discount rate to use subjects benefit–cost analysis to uncertainty.

Cost-effectiveness analysis is distinguished from BCA in that costs and effectiveness are not expressed in the same metric. Monetary factors are expressed in monetary terms whereas improvements in health status, functional independence, and so on are measured and presented in their own terms. Studies of cost-effectiveness generally compare two or more programs that have similar objectives. For instance, a CEA in rehabilitation might compare two programs or treatments that have equal funding to see which has the greater impact on patient or client outcomes. Or it might determine which of two treatments could bring randomly assigned patients up to the same level of functional independence at discharge. Since rehabilitation programs have outstanding non-monetary goals and outcomes, CEA is essential to their analysis.

Although BCA and CEA have a different focus, they are not mutually exclusive. These two methods can be combined into a more embracing analysis aggregating all items that have a clear monetary value using BCA while presenting prominent non-monetary outcomes in terms of accepted disability-related measures. This chapter refers to such a broad analysis as BCA/CEA.

Rigorous study of therapeutic or program effectiveness is fundamental to both BCA and CEA. If a program is not effective, it cannot be cost-effective or cost-beneficial. Since the efficacy of most programs and treatments in rehabilitation has not been proven by rigorous experimental designs, great savings should be possible by weeding out ineffective approaches and fostering the adoption of more effective treatments.

Now that key terms have been explained, the 10 sutras will be examined.

FORMULATION OF THE STUDY: SUTRA 1. MAKE IT A COMPETITION

The purpose of BCA and CEA is to provide information to aid choice between alternatives. Meaningful BCAs and CEAs compare the costs and outcomes of one program or treatment with a viable alternative. Most frequently, a new program is compared with an established practice, but unproven treatments also deserve rigorous evaluation. Examples of meaningful comparative studies include those of Cummings, Kerner, Arones, and Steinbock (1985); Garraway, Walton, and Akhtar (1981); Hendricksen, Lund, and Stromgard (1984); Rubenstein et al. (1984); Smith, Garraway, Smith and Akhtar (1981); and Weissert, Wan, and Livieratos (1979).

Studies that purport to demonstrate the cost–benefits or cost-effectiveness of a program may not in fact measure or even discuss an alternative program. Such claims are logically unjustified, because without an alternative opportunity costs or incremental costs do not exist. Close study of such writings may reveal that they use a judgmental alternative (i.e., invent numbers) or attribute the entire pre–post difference in outcomes (e.g., earnings) to the rehabilitation program. This has been a frequent problem in BCAs of vocational rehabilitation (Bureau of Economic Research, 1985b; M. V. Johnston & Keith, 1983).

Control Group Methods

Identifying the faster runner in a race requires that all runners start the same distance from the finish line. Similarly, comparing the costs and outcomes to reveal cost-effectiveness requires that the alternative programs begin with comparable populations. Control group methods are required to disentangle the effects of rehabilitation from those of natural healing or from the help clients receive in the community without formal rehabilitation. Control group methods include randomized experiments, quasi-experimental designs (Cook & Campbell, 1979), and statistical controls. These methods are reviewed in Chapter 7. The problems of valid inference in BCA/CEA are the same as in other areas of biomedical and social science research.

Choice of Alternatives

The program or treatment chosen as the comparison is crucial. To maximize the chance of obtaining statistically significant results, the alternatives chosen should be as different as possible in cost and treatment strategy but as similar as possible in client types and goals. Economists write that the alternative should be the "next best" use for the resource in question (e.g., Henry & Haynes, 1978, p. 23) but, in practice, the alternative needs to be socially and technically viable. Political and practical considerations severely limit the choice of alternatives. It is not possible to deny rehabilitation to a client for mere research purposes even if the effectiveness of that rehabilitative treatment has never been demonstrated. Imagination is needed even to begin the search for an alternative.

FORMULATION OF ALTERNATIVES: SUTRA 2. GO HUNTING

Opportunities for BCA/CEA—even control groups—can be found, but it is necessary to hunt for them. Rehabilitation in our society is not homogeneous. Admission practices, treatment approaches, and available funding differ substantially across states and types of impairments. The geographic distribution of rehabilitation facilities is highly uneven. Some insurance policies exclude inpatient rehabilitation. Clearly, persons who are very similar in disability to clients in conventional rehabilitation programs may receive very different kinds or amounts of services. The most salient barrier to identifying such

groups is the tendency of researchers to stay in their offices rather than to network and establish contacts in different settings.

Data Systems

Hunting involves preparation and lying in wait. Similarly, BCA/CEA in rehabilitation frequently requires the establishment of long-term program evaluation monitoring systems.

Almost any professional familiar with rehabilitation programs can think of a large number of factors relevant to assessing their cost-effectiveness and cost–benefits. An attempt to define the absolute minimum set of such factors is displayed in Table 1. The list overlaps 90% with the proposed Uniform National Data System presented in Chapter 10 and variables contained in the R-300, used in vocational rehabilitation. The primary changes recommended are addition of a measure of vocational skills to the R-300, improved measures of cost, and compensation for missing data (Bureau of Economic Research, 1985b). Desirable but less essential measures are in parentheses.

Although simplified, the list in Table 1 is presented to emphasize that measuring a small number of variables reliably is much better than measuring a large number haphazardly. Continuity in gathering data over time is necessary to detect the effect of new policies. The variables chosen need to be those with the highest correlations with cost and outcome variables. Given the limited budgets of program monitoring systems, leaving room in the budget for special studies and links with other data bases is better than attempting to measure all factors of likely importance.

Statistical methods allow a limited amount of information on cost–benefits or cost-effectiveness to be extracted from typical data-monitoring systems. In medical rehabilitation, improvement–cost ratios provide a handy tool to identify areas of probable higher versus lower efficiency. For instance, Harasymiw and Albrecht (1979) and Hamilton and Granger (1985) found that improvement per dollar was greatest for stroke patients of intermediate severity on the Barthel index. Pitfalls in the analysis of such ratios are discussed under the sixth sutra on process measurement.

Table 1. Basic measures for BCA/CEA in rehabilitation

Medical rehabilitation	Vocational rehabilitation
Input measures	
Functional status at admission	Functional skills levels
Self-care and mobility ADL[a]	Earnings at acceptance
Communication	Earnings at history
Vocational status	Education
Impairment class	Disabling condition
Primary diagnosis	Demographics, e.g., age, sex
Demographics, e.g., age, sex	
(Family help available)[b]	
Cost measures	
Length of stay	Service units and type
Charges	Estimated costs
Outcome measures	
Functional status at discharge	Earnings at closure
Discharge destination: home vs. board & care vs.	Vocational status
nursing home vs. hospital vs. death	(Long-term follow-up of earnings)
Vocational status	
(Follow-up measures)	
(Functional status)	
(Rehospitalization days)	
(Vocational status)	

[a]ADLs, activities of daily living.
[b]Measures in parentheses are desirable but less essential.

Data-monitoring systems only do half the job. Such systems usually need to be augmented by special in-depth studies to yield information on cost–benefits or cost-effectiveness. The most serious limitation on many data-monitoring systems is that they are established only in programs that are very similar. Indeed, their function is often to ensure that participating programs are as similar as possible. This can make it impossible to detect definite differences in client outcomes or costs. A data system will reveal clear information on cost–benefits or cost-effectiveness only if the *same* measures are taken across *different* programs.

INPUT MEASUREMENT: SUTRA 3. ALL OUTPUT DEPENDS ON INPUT

Outcomes attained by rehabilitation clients depend as much on client potential or case severity as on the treatment program. An outcome that is easy for one client to obtain may be difficult or impossible for another. Cost–benefits and cost-effectiveness vary as a function of initial severity (e.g., Bureau of Economic Research, 1985b; Ha-

rasymiw & Albrecht, 1979; M. V. Johnston, 1983a). Without measures of the severity of disability, it is impossible to adjust statistically for variation in client potential at admission, to reduce error variance by stratification techniques, or even to assess the success of randomization. Measurement of outcome alone is then useless. We must also measure input.

The need for input measurement is implicit in much current rehabilitation research that measures improvement in patient function, but improvement scores are insufficient. First, there are technical problems with the use of change scores. Residual change scores—the scores that result when input measures are regressed on the outcome measure—are better (Cohen & Cohen, 1975). More importantly, the initial potential of clients depends on more than initial functional level or initial earnings. With stroke rehabilitation, for instance, functional outcomes in self-care and mobility are predicted by preadmission improvement, patient age, and hemorrhagic etiology as well as functional severity (M. V. Johnston, 1983a). In vocational rehabilitation, earnings at closure are predicted by (in descending order) sex, Minnesota Functional Assessment Inventory (FAI), "vocational qualification" score, FAI physical condition score, FAI cognition, FAI motor, intermediate age (a curvilinear function), earnings at acceptance, FAI judgment, FAI vision, race, and education (Dean & Milberg, 1985).

Measuring Client Potential

A five-step strategy is recommended to develop an index of client potential or severity:

1. Think! What client characteristics, program descriptors, or ecological variables should logically have the greatest impact on cost-related variables or patient outcomes?
2. Search the research literature. In virtually all fields of rehabilitation there are studies that identify predictors of patient/client outcomes.
3. On the basis of logic, judgment, and prior research, it is then possible to discriminate between well-established predictors of outcomes, promising or controversial predictors, and long shots. This threefold classification forms the basis for a hierarchical hypothesis and analysis, which may be essential to conserve degrees of freedom in a study with a large number of variables and a small number of subjects (e.g., less than 10–15 subjects per variable.
4. The likely predictors can then be correlated with key cost and outcome variables using hierarchical multiple regression/correlation analysis (Cohen & Cohen, 1975), log-linear analysis, or other techniques. These analyses will reveal which variables are the strongest predictors of outcomes. These strong predictors are the key input variables for which one must control.
5. By weighting these input variables, indices of case severity or difficulty can be developed (e.g., M. V. Johnston, 1983a).

Better measures of potential for rehabilitation will aid in developing admission criteria, help practitioners plan their therapeutic strategies, and provide invaluable assistance in calculating BCA/CEA. A great deal of work needs to be done to develop better objective measures of job potential. Even more work needs to be done to

develop ecological measures (see seventh sutra on experimental design).

Targeting Services

Rehabilitative programs are unlikely to achieve cost-effectiveness or net cost savings unless they target their services to those likely to benefit most from them.

Over the last decade, seven dozen demonstration programs have been launched to lessen reliance on nursing homes for geriatrics and other disabled persons by providing augmented home care, rehabilitation, and day care. In many of these demonstration programs, total costs increased. For instance, Weissert et al. (1979) studied the effects of randomly expanding Medicare coverage to include day care and homemaker chore services. Costs increased dramatically because program benefits were offered as an entitlement rather than strictly targeted to persons most at risk of institutionalization.

In contrast, more targeted geriatric evaluation and case management programs have been found to be cost-effective. For instance, a special hospital assessment, treatment, and rehabilitation program not only reduced 1-year mortality from 48% to 24%, but also saved money by reducing rehospitalization (Rubenstein et al., 1984). This program strictly screened out patients who were not at risk for reinstitutionalization or who had progressive fatal diseases.

Measurement of client input characteristics will enable us to increase the cost-effectiveness of our programs by improving admission policies. This same information will tell us how to improve net benefits to society by reaching out to clients who respond most to our treatments.

ECONOMIC UTILITY VERSUS HUMAN GOOD: SUTRA 4. MONEY IS A LOT, BUT IT ISN'T EVERYTHING

Monetary saving has never been the primary motive of rehabilitationists. The endeavor to improve the quality of life of disabled persons has always been preeminent. Underlying the measured abstractions of BCA/CEA is the crying of human needs. The increasing frequency with which disabled persons are dumped into under-staffed nursing homes or found disoriented, even dying, in the back alleys of our society testifies to what is at stake. Taking care of severely disabled persons costs money. I have heard it said that "The cheapest thing to do with any of these people is to shoot them"; monetary savings through increased suffering and shortened life are entirely possible. Compassion and ethics are at issue in BCA and CEA.

At the same time, rehabilitation clients are not the only persons with needs. Could more human good be done by giving food and shelter to several homeless persons than by spending tens of thousands of dollars on one rehabilitation client, with unsure results? Furthermore, the needs of different rehabilitation clients must be balanced against each other. We cannot avoid the necessity for economic choice, and so we need to balance benefits against costs.

Conditions of scarcity force choice and thereby reveal relative human values. Monetary transactions give a number to this value. Money is a human good, too.

Methodological Implications

The need to balance monetary and non-monetary utility has concrete methodological implications.

Non-monetary Outcomes

Non-monetary outcomes are prominent in medical rehabilitation (Table 1). Even in vocational rehabilitation, outcomes such as improved function, improved homemaking skills, and psychological benefits may be substantial (Cardus, Fuhrer, & Thrall, 1980). Non-monetary outcomes need to be measured and reported in BCA/CEA in rehabilitation.

Shadow Pricing This method of pricing is used to input a monetary value to goods and services that are not actually transacted on a monetary basis. Shadow pricing is useful when a nearly equivalent good or service is transacted in a market. For instance, the value of a home-maker's productivity can be estimated as at least equal to the value of housekeeping and child care. However, economists' attempts to assign a monetary value to goods that are not actually transacted on a market (e.g., suffering, severe

disability, or human life itself) are on shaky grounds. In actual policy forums, any exact monetary value for human life is likely to be attacked on ethical and technical grounds and thus discredited. Clearly, non-market outcomes are best measured in their own terms.

The ethical BCA/CEA analyst needs to attempt to distinguish monetary savings due to increased suffering and early death from gains due to greater efficiency. Some analysts have even recommended that monetary gains due to increasing numbers of deaths be excluded from the analysis. Although this strategy demonstrates compassion, it risks violation of analysts' professional responsibility to present the facts accurately.

The ideal of rehabilitation is not charity. Its ideal is to enable the disabled to do for themselves. From this ideal stems its cost-effectiveness: If disabled persons can do for themselves, they are less of a burden on society. The aim of rehabilitation can be seen as achieving the best balance between the needs of the disabled and the needs of society. BCA/CEA helps to define this optimum.

OUTCOME MEASUREMENT: SUTRA 5. A STEW, NOT A PUREE

A stew is eclectic enough to provide a complex taste. A puree is composed of so many tiny pieces that it becomes an indiscriminate, uniform mass. This sutra argues for an optimal level of complexity; ordinarily, we need to use a modest number of non-monetary outcome measures (e.g., three to seven) and avoid temptations to use hundreds of outcome measures or reduce everything to a single number.

Simplification

The very term *effectiveness* in "cost-effectiveness analysis" implies that there exists some entity or non-monetary outcome that one needs to measure. The idea of effectiveness implies clarity, even simplification of purpose. Data reduction and simplification are essential to reduce the complexity of measurement in BCA/CEA. The greatest barrier to cost-effectiveness research in rehabilitation is probably the difficulty of simplifying complex human outcomes.

The author knows of a number of well-funded data systems that failed to live up to their promise because they attempted to measure hundreds of inputs and outcomes. Data involving dozens of outcome measures, and hence thousands of relations with input measures, could not be analyzed. The number of statistical tests performed exceeded limits imposed by the sample size. The usual technique for reducing hundreds of items to a single score—the creation of additive indices (e.g., average of functional independence in self-care items)—failed. The large number of items increased the chance of missing data. Because deletion of cases with missing data was the only defensible statistical procedure, the majority of the sample had to be thrown out.

Even if the data could have been fully analyzed, who would have time to read the thousand-page report that would result, or to discern an overall pattern or conclusion from the hundreds of statistical tests? In sum, it is essential to limit the number of variables in a study.

Data Reduction Techniques

A number of techniques are available to reduce the number of variables one needs to measure in a study.

1. Measure at the level of disability or major events (e.g., return to work, reinstitutionalization) rather than at the level of specific impairments. Activities of daily living measures, for instance, reflect the involvement of a variety of impairments—cognitive, physical, psychological, and metabolic.

2. Use factor analysis to group many separate measures (e.g., functional items) into a smaller number of scales. With stroke patients, for instance, factor analysis showed the presence of a general factor, labeled "physical disability," which was distinct from continence and communication abilities (J. E. Johnston, 1975; M. V. Johnston, 1983a).

3. Use cluster analysis to group many categorical items (e.g., diagnoses) into a small number of groups according to an index of similarity (e.g., similarity in cost).

4. Convert items with market prices to dollar values rather than leaving them in terms such as number of treatments. Adding together costs with similar generic purposes—defining a "cost objective"—is basic to accounting (e.g., Anthony & Reece, 1979) and needs to be done when aggregating and presenting monetary data. Such BCA techniques as discounting to present value should be used to balance current costs against long-term future monetary gains.

5. Reduce several non-monetary outcome measures into a single composite index of effectiveness using judgmental techniques. DeJong and Hughes (1982) found that a panel of judges of consumers and professionals agreed well on the relative importance of different measures as indices of independence of living arrangements and productivity outcomes, including non-monetary outcomes. Important implications for disability policy can be drawn even from such global indices (DeJong, Branch, & Corcoran, 1984). In the hands of less skilled researchers, however, such procedures could easily obscure important relationships. Outcomes that are factorially and conceptually distinct need to be analyzed separately.

To See the Forest, Look Down from Afar

To identify the most outstanding outcome measures, one needs to start from above or outside the specifics of the program. Generally, this means starting with the outcomes expected by clients and families and funding sources rather than with the treatment objectives of professionals. Clients and funding sources typically have much simpler, grosser expectations than do professionals. For instance, funding sources may evaluate a rehabilitation program entirely on financial grounds. Patients may expect general functional improvement and return home. Successful BCA/CEA involves educating professionals to distinguish between the short-term goals of their treatments and the overall, longer term goals of the entire program, which includes the efforts of many professions. Before meeting the needs of professionals to understand and justify their work, BCA/CEA meets the needs of society to make programs more accountable.

Optimal Complexity Oversimplification, too, needs to be avoided. Any BCA/CEA that treats cost–benefits or cost-effectiveness in rehabilitation as a single number obscures as much as it reveals. Oversimplification may be seen in studies that consider the outcomes of medical rehabilitation only in terms of physical restoration while ignoring communication, psychosocial functioning, and reduced occurrence of institutionalization. Similarly, reduction of the outcomes of vocational rehabilitation to monetary earnings is questionable. The inputs and outcomes of rehabilitation are multivariate.

Ratio Analysis Perhaps the most common method of analyzing and presenting data on cost-effectiveness involves the use of ratios (e.g., dollars per closure, cost per patient day). Such ratio indices are extremely useful for identifying areas of probable cost-effectiveness versus inefficiency. However, by themselves they do not provide sufficient information to allow definitive conclusions about cost-effectiveness or waste. More information is needed.

M. V. Johnston (1983a, 1983b) found that improvement–cost ratios are useful. Correlating a variety of factors with improvement–cost ratios facilitated identification of disequilibrium in program functioning. For instance, improvement–cost rates were lower for left hemiplegic stroke patients, probably because of deficiencies in screening for constructional apraxia and spatial problems. However, improvement–cost ratios can have three meanings. One group can have a higher improvement–cost ratio than another because 1) cost is lower, 2) improvement is greater, or 3) the improvement scale is noninterval (e.g., ceiling and floor effects exists in the scale of functional performance). Improvement–cost ratios must be used heuristically; they identify areas of concern, but further investigation is required to determine which of their three meanings is most likely. Arraying major elements of costs and effectiveness is recommended over attempts to reduce all to a single number (Doherty & Hicks, 1977; Office of Technology Assessment, 1980; Warner & Luce, 1982).

PROCESS MEASUREMENT: SUTRA 6. OPEN THE BLACK BOX

A black box model is often used to perform BCA and even CEA: inputs and outputs are measured, but what goes on in between is not. Although a black box approach is sometimes necessary, the approach has limited utility. An approach that

ties outcomes to processes is more likely not only to advance the science of rehabilitation but also to gain political acceptance.

Rehabilitation has grown more out of the needs of disabled persons and those who must deal with them than out of any technological discovery. Rehabilitation is eclectic. It draws from physical, occupational, and speech therapy; prosthetics and orthotics; bioengineering; internal medicine; nursing; psychology; and education—any techonology that will help restore function to the disabled individual. Cost–benefits and cost-effectiveness are likely to vary substantially across such different technologies since some are of proven effectiveness and others are not. Process measures are necessary to distinguish cost-effective client treatment combinations from ineffective ones.

Even within a specific program, lack of cost-effectiveness or monetary losses can be due to many possible causes. Such a result might be due to the ineffectiveness of a particular treatment strategy, specific problems with admission screening procedures, or high staffing and wages. Unless a reason is identified, program personnel cannot respond constructively to results of a BCA/CEA.

Moreover, people do not believe statistics alone—and with good reason. Any single empirical study is subject to numerous threats to validity (e.g., Cook & Campbell, 1979). Everyone has heard of studies with contradictory and questionable results. Furthermore, people reason from ideas and images more than from numbers and facts. An unexplained result is likely to be perceived as an anomaly and forgotten. Process management makes explanation possible and persuasion more likely.

TECHNIQUES OF EXPERIMENTAL DESIGN: SUTRA 7. IN THIS FLUX, CHAOS, DISCERN THIS PATTERN, ORDER

BCA/CEA shares with all science the difficulty of finding order in a complex, changing world. Research in rehabilitation is particularly challenging because the interventions do not aim at cures, which are easy to substantiate. Instead, the objective is the achievement of limited yet very real improvements in functioning. Powerful research techniques are commonly required to quantify the effects of rehabilitation.

Techniques to increase the power and precision of research include control group methods, measurement of input, measurement of processes, and search for treatment–client interactions, as discussed above. Other proven techniques are outlined below.

Using More Reliable Measures

Reliability of a rating scale can be increased both by clarifying what is measured and by increasing the number of intercorrelated items used in a scale (Cook & Campbell, 1979; Nunnally, 1967).

Increasing Sample Size

The importance of a large sample is frequently overrated by professionals who have never studied research design. Representativeness and randomness of sampling and care in measurement are far more important than a large sample per se. Nonetheless, a moderate-to-large sample size is probably necessary to detect the effects of typical rehabilitation programs. For instance, it takes a sample of 1308 to have a 95% chance of detecting a small effect (one with a population $r = .10$) using a t-test at alpha $= .05$ (Cohen & Cohen, 1975, p. 480). A moderate-sized effect (population $r = .30$) takes a sample of 139.

Looking for an Effect
Where One is Likely to be Found

One example of this concept is that many rehabilitative treatments involve learning, and learned behaviors are known to extinguish over time if they are not practiced. Clients are exposed over time to more and more causal factors, making rehabilitation an increasingly small part of the totality that influences them. The effects of rehabilitation will probably be strongest near termination of service and weaker after discharge or in long-term follow-up. Conversely, if no effect of rehabilitation is found in the short run, it is unlikely that one will be found in the long run.

Another example is provided by studies that have tried and failed to find effects of administrative or organizational changes (e.g., establish-

ment of a stroke unit in a hospital) on client outcomes. The negative result is not surprising, since these studies have failed to demonstrate that clients or patients received different treatments after the reorganization. Administrative changes should have administrative effects (e.g., better communication, education, less wasted time, cost savings). Changes in client outcomes are most likely to occur as a response to changes to client treatments.

Ecological Measures

The outcomes of rehabilitation depend upon social-environmental and ecological factors as much as on the treatment program itself. For instance, nursing home institutionalization following stroke rehabilitation is correlated as highly with family help available as with the functional status of the patient (M. V. Johnston, 1983a, 1983c). The chance of finding a job following vocational rehabilitation depends on the general unemployment rate, financial disincentives, and employer and union willingness to modify jobs. Considerable increase in experimental power and predictability can be expected if these factors are measured. Furthermore, the analyst will be less likely to blame the disabled person for outcomes that are really under the control of the larger society.

Weighting Outcome Indices

Current models for CEA involve creation of an additive index of client outcomes. For instance, several related items are added together to create an index of independence in activities of daily living (e.g., in the Katz or Barthel scales), or functional improvement might be weighted along with other goals to create an index of overall program effectiveness. Although such procedures are valid and useful, they suffer from imprecision. Therapists may, for instance, be working actively only on those one or two functional activities that are the most important to that client. An outcome that is crucial to one client may be trivial to another. Rapid progress may occur on these key items, but global progress may result more from general physiological recovery than from specific rehabilitation treatments. An effectiveness index that weights specific outcomes equally across patients measures more questionable factors than a more targeted index, and thus increases error variance.

Experimental power and relevance to clinical goals can in principle be improved by weighting outcome measures by their importance. Mathematically, effectiveness E could be defined as the sum of the product of a vector of outcomes O times a vector of individual goal weights G, $E = \Sigma(O \times G)$, where G values ranged between 0 and 1 and sum to 1. Full use of this model would entail creation of standards for the goal weights. Although difficult, objective research on the goal definition process for clients is needed anyway. The proposed model would allow one to distinguish between waste resulting from ineffective technology and waste resulting from poor prioritization of goals.

Follow-Up Methodology

A neglected problem is the technical difficulty of distinguishing relevant costs and benefits in a follow-up questionnaire from thousands of other economic transactions occurring with the patient and family. This is most crucial for measuring relevant monetary expenditures to the patient and family after discharge; patients and family will not reveal their total family budget. Procedures are available to ameliorate such problems. For instance, asking only about disability-related costs, medical costs, or increased support costs after medical rehabilitation programs is quite feasible (M. V. Johnston, 1983a).

THE BOUNDARIES OF EMPIRICAL ANALYSIS: SUTRA 8. LOOK IN THE SHADOWS, SEE IN THE LIGHT

Using BCA/CEA is like hiking in the hills at night with a dim flashlight: You can see clearly only with the aid of empirical analysis—the flashlight—but to perceive the larger picture—the great slopes and cliffs—you must use broader, less precise methods.

The success of any empirical study depends on astute marshalling of limited research resources, but the problem is more acute in BCA/CEA because the analysis is exceptionally ambitious for problems in rehabilitation. Strictly speaking, one needs to measure all program outputs, both monetary and non-monetary, for years, even decades. Not only will client earnings and physical dependence be affected by rehabilitation, but there are also likely to be changes in specific impairments, self-esteem, psychological function, and in the lives of family members. As discussed above, input measures are essential, and process measures are desirable. Sophisticated control methods are needed to disentangle the effect of rehabilitation from other processes affecting clients. No study in the literature does all of these things. In reality, it is impossible to measure *all* of the factors relevant to BCA/CEA in rehabilitation.

Successful BCAs and CEAs have used a variety of methods to circumvent these limitations.

Judgment

The bounds of knowledge are greater than the bounds of data. Rehabilitation, like so many other fields of human endeavor, is based on accumulation of experience, which is more qualitative than quantitative. Tapping into this accumulated store of qualitative knowledge is a key to successful, practical BCA/CEA.

In fact, elaborate quantitative BCA/CEA is only justifiable under certain circumstances, for instance, when the "folk wisdom" in rehabilitation is ambiguous or contradicts findings from other fields and when those who pay for rehabilitation begin to question its value.

Panel Designs One method used to tap into the qualitative knowledge of experienced practitioners is the panel study, which includes the "Delphi" method. In this design, the query of experts is used instead of direct empirical measurement. Although panel studies give much less reliable information than direct empirical measurement, they are less expensive, more timely, and often quite informative. Results are most questionable when panel members are asked about matters in which they have no experience (e.g., asking hospital physicians about family costs after discharge), or for which they have a clear bias (e.g., asking rehabilitation personnel to estimate the value of rehabilitation). The best uses of panel studies in cost–benefit research are probably in defining what factors most need to be measured, defining outcome goals, estimating small factors that are not worth the expense of exact empirical measurement, and defining issues most worthy of study.

Methods of Simplification

Successful studies use a variety of methods to bound and simplify their empirical analysis, as outlined below.

Limiting the Scope of Analysis   Even the best studies answer only one or two questions. In vocational rehabilitation, the scope of study might be limited to assessing only monetary costs and benefits. Although the exclusion of non-monetary benefits can be questioned, policymakers may attend only to monetary factors anyway. In medical rehabilitation, a CEA might focus on improved functional outcomes and direct costs (Hamilton and Granger, 1985; Harasymiw and Albrecht, 1979; M. V. Johnston, 1983a, 1983b). A greater understanding of how to increase improvement per dollar would be valuable, even if it raised as many questions as it answered.

Using Data from Other Sources   Many BCAs do not collect their own data but only synthesize data from other studies (e.g., Bureau of Economic Research, 1985b; Eazell & Johnston, 1981). Using data from a variety of sources is essential to estimate long-term effects such as survival rates and long-term employment rates, to extrapolate cost savings over the whole country, and to estimate the price of some items.

Sensitivity Analysis   Sensitivity analysis is used to test the effects of crucial uncertain parameters on conclusions. It involves replacing the uncertain parameter with highest likely and lowest likely values and calculating the effect on costs and benefit estimates. Sensitivity analysis is most frequently used in BCA to estimate the effect of different time discount rates on estimates of long-term benefits, but the approach is equally applicable to any uncertain but highly important element of BCA or CEA. For instance, M. V. Johnston (1983a) found that conclusions were the same regardless of whether very high or very low estimates of rehospitalization were used. On the other hand, estimates of long-run

benefits are frequently highly sensitive to the discount rate employed (e.g., Bureau of Economic Research, 1985b; Office of Technology Assessment, 1980; Warner & Luce, 1982).

Limiting Follow-Up

All ongoing data collection effects must strictly limit the number or period of follow-up measurements. Studies are always limited but not invalidated by these limits.

In choosing a follow-up period, one should wait long enough after the program (e.g., more than a month) to avoid the greatest instability of outcomes. However, long-run follow-up (e.g., 1 year) is expensive, increases missing data because of the difficulty of tracking clients over long periods, and delays reporting the results. Sample size must also be increased with long-term follow-up since effects of educational programs have usually been found to decrease over time, as ensuing experiences diminish the effects of the past. For instance, Garraway and colleagues (1981) found that the favorable effects of a stroke rehabilitation unit on patient independence, which were quite significant at discharge, had declined to nonsignificant by 1 year post-stroke.

One should adhere to conventions for follow-up so that the results of one program can be compared to the results of another. The 60-day follow-up period for earnings in the R-300 data set is useful because it permits comparison of one program with another. Medical rehabilitation would benefit from establishing similar conventions, such as a 3-month follow-up period for program evaluation.

Long-term follow-up studies are still needed on samples of rehabilitation clients. Extrapolation would be subject to far fewer dangers if we had better survival curves, curves showing typical decay of functional skills over time, and data on long-term unemployment of rehabilitation closures.

Proxy Variables

Although direct measurement of costs is preferable to use of proxies, even rigorous studies use proxy variables to some degree. For instance, M. V. Johnston (1983a) found that even cooperative families using diaries usually could not report all disability-related expenses in exact dollar terms. Typical prices were used to convert item descriptions into dollar values. That study also showed that hospital length of stay (LOS) can be an excellent proxy for resource consumption costs: LOS and charges correlated at $r = .98$.

In medical rehabilitation, the most frequent problem is that cost data are unreported or unavailable (M. V. Johnston & Keith, 1983). Subtle biases in cost estimation pall by comparison.

Looking for Major Effects

Most methodological problems in BCA/CEA are avoidable by studying effects that are more likely to be sizeable than subtle. Experienced practitioners can often make informed guesses about whether treatment strategies and policies are likely to be wasteful. Such assertions are almost invariably controversial and worth resolution by empirical study. One might, for instance, compare outcomes of two rehabilitation programs known to differ markedly in price but claiming to offer comparable services (e.g., nursing home versus hospital-based rehabilitation).

UTILIZATION OF BCA/CEA: SUTRA 9: YOU CAN LEAD A HORSE TO WATER, BUT YOU CAN'T MAKE HIM DRINK

Reviews have concluded that the main role of BCA/CEAs in health care has been educational (Office of Technology Assessment, 1980; Warner & Luce, 1982). Specific policy decisions have not been affected appreciably. One reason for this was a lack of technically solid and clear findings, but even definite findings have not affected decisions. However, in the author's opinion, this conclusion is limited to academic, published BCAs and CEAs.

The literature on BCA and CEA in business management (e.g., Henry & Haynes, 1978) leaves little doubt that management decisions are affected by the results of sound investment analyses. This conclusion generalizes to rehabilitation. The author has observed that managers listen eagerly to even the most informal BCA/CEA—

provided that the benefits and costs are those to the organization, that is, provided the study relates to profitability. In contrast, findings that rehabilitation appears to be ineffective for a class of clients are greeted with indifference or hostility, because Medicare will pay anyway and beds must be filled.

Under cost-based reimbursement, hospitals did little to cut costs, but diagnostic related groups have had a dramatic effect. Lengths of stay have been slashed, personnel cut, and the rate of growth of hospital expenditures finally controlled. Cost-cutting now saves hospitals money.

People need a concrete monetary motive, not a theoretical one, to act on results of a study. Academic BCAs and CEAs most frequently deal with costs and benefits to society and disabled persons, rather than with any specific organization's pocketbook. Such studies inform the community, but one can no more expect them to determine policy changes than one can expect a horse to drink at a certain place after having let him drink elsewhere at will. The way to make a horse drink is to limit his water intake—that is, establish a water budget. Similarly, managers are likely to respond directly to a BCA or CEA if it tells them how to do more with their budget. The horse drinks when it's thirsty.

CONCLUSIONS: SUTRA 10. SEEK AND YE SHALL FIND

Past BCA/CEA in rehabilitation has had such blatant holes (Bureau of Economic Research, 1985b; M. V. Johnston & Keith, 1983; Nobel, 1977) that one cannot help but wonder whether the aim was to find out if rehabilitation is cost-effective or to prove that it is. Although rhetoric has its place, the need for scientific information on the cost–benefits and cost-effectiveness of rehabilitation remains. Without information on cost-effectiveness, there is no good way of deciding which rehabilitative programs are worth expanding and which are lower priorities. Without information on cost–benefits to society, there is no alternative but to throw money at programs, or brusquely cut them, depending on the winds of politics rather than contributions to society.

Our government is devoting increasing efforts to devising payment systems that will give managers strong incentives to cut costs (e.g., development of prospective payment systems). Information on cost–benefits and cost-effectiveness is needed *now* so that such systems can be designed in such a way as to increase cost-effectiveness and cost–benefits to society, rather than to simply cut costs regardless of other considerations. Information on cost–benefits and cost-effectiveness will be needed even more to enable rehabilitation managers to respond intelligently when new reimbursement systems are implemented.

Although there are many pitfalls in the conduct of BCA/CEA, there are also many paths toward progress. Substantial progress is being made in measurement of outcomes and in research designs suitable for BCA/CEA. Multivariate techniques are now highly developed and well tested, but even simple designs can contrib-

ute. Effectiveness studies alone have potent implications for BCA/CEA. Greater public availability to cost data would be very useful. Almost any honest study presenting empirical data connecting costs and patient or client outcomes is a contribution today.

Confronted by the pressing needs of their clients, professionals have developed methods that appear to help. However, in the absence of rigorous study, we cannot know which of these methods are effective—and which are no more effective than the loving care of families or unskilled helpers. In all probability, the technology of rehabilitation today is both ridden with waste and graced by treatments worthwhile not only to the client but also to society. The chief problem with benefit–cost and cost-effectiveness analysis in rehabilitation today is that serious studies are rarely attempted. The chief remedy is greater effort.

REFERENCES

Anthony, R. N., & Reece, J. S. (1979). *Accounting* (6th ed.). Homewood, IL: Irwin.

Bureau of Economic Research, Rutgers University (M. Berkowitz, Ed). (February, 1985a). *Economic consequences of spinal cord injury.* New Brunswick, NJ: Rutgers University.

Bureau of Economic Research, Rutgers University (M. Berkowitz, Ed.). (December, 1985b). *Analysis of costs and benefits in rehabilitation.* Final report (Department of Education Contract No. 300-84-0259). New Brunswick, NJ: Rutgers University.

Cardus, D., Fuhrer, M. J., & Thrall, R. M. (September, 1980). *A benefit-cost approach to the prioritization of rehabilitation research* (Report grant HEW 12-P-59036/6-03). Houston, TX: Baylor College of Medicine, The Institute for Rehabilitation and Research. (NARIC call no. 495)

Cohen, J., & Cohen, P. (1975). *Applied multiple regression/correlation analysis for the behavioral sciences.* Hillsdale, NJ: John Wiley & Sons.

Cook, T. D., & Campbell, D. T. (1979). *Quasi-experimentation.* Chicago: Rand McNally.

Cummings, V., Kerner, J. F., Arones, S., & Steinbock, C. (1985). Day hospital service in rehabilitation medicine: An evaluation. *Archives of Physical Medicine and Rehabilitation, 66,* 86–91.

Dean, D., & Milberg, W. (December, 1985). Using better measures of disability status. In M. Berkowitz (Ed.), *Analysis of costs and benefits in rehabilitation* (pp. 353–434). New Brunswick, NJ: Rutgers University, Bureau of Economic Research.

DeJong, G., Branch, L. G., & Corcoran, P. J. (1984). Independent living outcomes in spinal cord injury: Multivariate analyses. *Archives of Physical Medicine and Rehabilitation, 65,* 66–73.

DeJong, G., & Hughes, J. (1982). Independent living: Meth-

odology for measuring long-term outcomes. *Archives of Physical Medicine and Rehabilitation, 63,* 68–73.

Doherty, N., & Hicks, B. (1977). Cost-effectiveness analysis and alternative health care programs for the elderly. *Health Services Research, 12,* 190–203.

Eazell, D. E., & Johnston, M. V. (1981). *Cost-benefits of stroke rehabilitation* (Monograph Series 4). Washington, DC: National Association of Rehabilitation Facilities.

Garraway, W. M., Walton, M. S., & Akhtar, A. J. (1981). Use of health and social services in management of stroke in community: Results from a controlled trial. *Age and Aging, 10,* 95–104.

Hamilton, B. B., & Granger, C. V. (1985). Multicenter prospective estimate of stroke rehabilitation efficiency (Abstract). *Archives of Physical Medicine and Rehabilitation, 66,* 541.

Harasymiw, S. J., & Albrecht, G. L. (1979) Admission and discharge indicators as aids in optimizing comprehensive rehabilitation services. *Scandanavian Journal of Rehabilitation Medicine, 11,* 123–138.

Hendriksen, C., Lund, E., & Stromgard, E. (1984). Consequences of assessment and intervention among elderly people. *British Medical Journal, 289,* 1522–1524.

Henry, W. R., & Haynes, W. M. (1978). *Managerial Economics* (4th ed.). Dallas, TX: Business Publications.

Johnston, J. E. (1975). *A short-term follow-up of stroke patients using factored measures of functioning.* Master's thesis, Claremont Graduate School, Claremont, CA.

Johnston, M. V. (1983a). *The costs and effectiveness of stroke rehabilitation: Measurement and prediction.* Doctoral dissertation, Claremont Graduate School, Claremont, CA.

Johnston, M. V. (1983b). Improvement/cost indices as indicators of cost-effectiveness (Abstract). *Archives of Physical Medicine and Rehabilitation, 64,* 501.

Johnston, M. V. (1983c). Family help available: Development

of a measurement scale (Abstract). *Archives of Physical Medicine and Rehabilitation, 64,* 498.

Johnston, M. V., & Keith, R. A. (1983). Cost-benefits of medical rehabilitation. *Archives of Physical Medicine and Rehabilitation, 64,* 147–154.

Nobel, J. H., Jr. (1977). Limits of cost-benefit analysis as a guide to priority-setting in rehabilitation. *Evaluation Quarterly, 1,* 347–380.

Nowak, L. (Spring, 1983). A cost-effectiveness evaluation of the Federal-State vocational rehabilitation program using a comparison group. *American Economist, 27,* 23–29.

Nunnally, J. C. (1967). *Psychometric theory.* New York: McGraw-Hill.

Office of Technology Assessment, U. S. Congress. (1980). *Implications of cost-effectiveness analysis of medical technology.* Washington, DC: U. S. Government Printing Office.

Rubenstein, L. Z., Josephson, K. R., Wieland, G. D., English, P. A., Sayre, J. A., & Kane, R. L. (1984). Effective-ness of a geriatric evaluation unit: A randomized clinical trial. *New England Journal of Medicine, 311,* 1664–1670.

Smith, M. E., Garraab02way, W. M., Smith, D. L., & Akhtar, A. J. (1982). Therapy impact on functional outcome in a controlled trial of stroke rehabilitation. *Archives of Physical Medicine and Rehabilitation, 63,* 21–24.

Thompson, M. S. (1980). *Benefit-cost analysis for program evaluation.* Beverly Hills, CA: Sage Publications.

Warner, K. E., & Luce, B. R. (1982). *Cost-benefit and cost-effectiveness analysis in health care: Principles, practice, and potential.* Ann Arbor, MI: Health Administration Press.

Weinfeld, F. D. (Ed.). (1981). *National survey of stroke. Stroke, 12*(Suppl. 1), 11–191.

Weissert, W. G., Wan, T. T. H., & Livieratos, B. B. (1979). *Effects and costs of day care and homemaker services for chronically ill: randomized experiment.* Hyattsville, MD: National Center for Health Services Research.

Chapter 9

Outcome Analysis
for Program Service Management

Stephen Forer

The integration of outcome analysis with other management information systems provides an effective management tool. This chapter discusses how research and gathering of such outcome information can be influenced by internal and external pressures such as changes in program emphasis or reimbursement. The first section addresses some of the more pragmatic considerations such as political, funding, organizational, and administrative factors that influence both the development and use of outcome analysis. The primary focus of this chapter is on management and clinical applications of evaluation research in a medical rehabilitation setting. However, many of the principles discussed may also be relevant to other settings, such as sheltered workshops, drug and alcohol abuse programs, transitional living centers, and long-term care facilities, as well as to psychiatric and vocational rehabilitation.

Outcome analysis concentrates on the results of services, programs, and treatment or intervention strategies generally following termination of services or during a predetermined follow-up period. Outcome analysis allows an evaluator, administrator, or program manager to systematically evaluate the outcome of rehabilitation efforts in terms of the operation, provision of services, appropriateness and effectiveness of services, efficiency of the system, and adequacy of serving the needs of the clients. Some of the benefits a facility may gain through outcome assessment are: 1) better community acceptance, 2) informed decision making for future planning,

3) persuasive data for marketing purposes, 4) cost-effectiveness information (the costs of a program are compared with the benefits or outcomes achieved by clients), 5) identification of problem areas requiring more detailed investigation, and 6) better alignment of internal program goals and objectives with client needs. Despite these inherent benefits, the majority of rehabilitation facilities resist doing outcome analysis. A purpose of this chapter is to shed light on why this resistance exists and how it can be overcome.

USES OF OUTCOME EVALUATION

Outcome information can be encouraging to the treatment staff. Most professionals dislike working in an ambiguous environment where standards used to evaluate their performance are unclear. Outcome analysis can alleviate some of this ambiguity by specifying the desired client outcomes. Through the use of outcome analysis, management can provide staff with the resources needed to achieve desired results. Inpatient staff often lose touch with clients after their discharge from inpatient care. Feedback of outcome results can provide staff with an opportunity to evaluate the success of their treatment and to use this information to modify treatment strategies or develop new programs better suited to meet clients' needs. This follow-up can identify clients who are having substantial adjustment problems at home or in the community and communicate such postdischarge problems to rehabilitation staff.

Quality Assessment
and Program Modification

Feedback reports indicate when the outcome of treatment has not met previously established criteria and expectancies. The reports may prompt individual chart audits and special studies to assist further in problem resolution. By identifying problem areas that need further investigation, outcome evaluation can provide a more specific direction for quality assurance committees. The intention of outcome evaluation is to provide an overall picture of performance and outcome. In its most simplistic form, however, it does not provide specific answers to problem areas, but merely identifies that the problem exists. Typical problems that have been identified through various outcome studies include lack of anticipated improvement, deterioration in functional abilities of clients, preventable secondary medical complications, excessive program costs or length of stay, insufficient treatment, substantial adjustment problems encountered at home or in the community, unexpected mortality, rehospitalization, poor motivation, psychosocial maladjustment, self-imposed social isolation, issues regarding discharge placements, movement into more restrictive environments during follow-up, regression to maladaptive behaviors, and inadequate use of community and outpatient services.

As outcome information is processed and analyzed, suggestions are frequently made for the revision of existing programs, treatment techniques, or intervention strategies. One of the important benefits of outcome evaluation is that it allows a facility to monitor the impact of revised programs and techniques. It provides a baseline to which results can be compared before and after change is implemented. Through this process of testing various approaches, the most effective techniques can be selected. As both problems and predictors of outcomes are identified, the treatment team can modify a program to better meet the needs of clients.

When recommendations are made from outcome studies, they should be followed up by an activity report. The nature of the recommendation, date for implementation, and person responsible for implementing the recommendation should be specified. Actions to improve program performance or resolve an identified problem should be documented. Follow-up monitoring is then necessary to determine whether the actions taken have successfully improved performance or ameliorated the problem.

Results from outcome studies, both positive and negative, should be fed back to the entire staff. A feedback of outcome evaluation results can be encouraging to staff because it supplies information on client outcomes that can be attributed directly to treatment rendered. Studies have shown that patients continue to improve after discharge from a comprehensive medical rehabilitation unit and that their functional level is typically higher than at discharge (Anderson et al., 1978; Feigenson, Githlow, & Greenberg, 1979; Feldman et al., 1962; Forer & Miller, 1980a; Granger, Albrecht, & Hamilton, 1979; Lehmann et al., 1977; Mor, Granger, & Sherwood, 1983; Scranton, Fogel, & Edman, 1975; Susset, Vobecky, & Balck, 1979; Weddell, Oddy, & Jenkins, 1980). Similar postdischarge results have been obtained in skilled nursing facilities (Gabow et al., 1985; Hemenway, 1983; Linn, Gurel, & Linn, 1977; Weissert & Scanlon, 1985), alcohol and drug abuse halfway houses (Booth, 1981; Van Ryswyk, Churchill, Velasquez, & McGuire, 1981–1982), psychiatric day treatment programs (Reihman, Wolford, Knapp, MacCallum, & Murray, 1983), and state psychiatric hospitals (Byers & Cohen, 1979; King, Houghland, Shepard, & Gallagher, 1980; Mattes, Klein, Millan, & Rosen, 1979).

When clients are released from these various rehabilitation settings, staff members may lose contact with them and never know whether their efforts were successful. This lack of feedback or follow-up results can discourage staff into feeling that their work was futile (Carey & Posavac, 1978). Staff are concerned about what happens to their clients after discharge. Although some clients may return for outpatient treatments, day care treatment, or follow-up evaluations at some facilities, the return rate is less than 40% of the inpatient caseload (Forer & Miller, 1980b). In addition to feedback on functional outcomes, staff are often interested in feedback on client satisfaction.

Individual Care Modification

When outcome data indicate a specific client is in need of professional intervention, prompt action may reduce the severity of the problem and resulting complications. To achieve this goal, criteria should be established for screening both inpatient and outpatient outcome data to trigger immediate review of the potential problem by the appropriate person.

Outcome Data for Research Studies

Functional outcome information can be useful for research and comparative studies. Special studies are often needed to further refine outcome information for management purposes. Outcome data can be regrouped and compared according to various factors. Some of the more common types of comparative analyses of functional outcomes are: 1) clients staying for different lengths of rehabilitation, 2) different treatment techniques or different rehabilitation settings, 3) clients discharged home versus to long-term care facilities, 4) different quarters of the year (3-month intervals), and 5) those clients treated in a comprehensive rehabilitation center and those treated in facilities with less extensive programs.

Some investigators have used functional outcome data in attempts to identify the best predictors of successful outcome for disabled persons following medical rehabilitation. Several studies have shown that the age at onset and duration of initial hospitalization tend to be the best predictors (Carey & Posavac, 1978; Johnston & Keister, 1984; Miller & Miyamato, 1979; Susset et al., 1979). Another study (Forer & Miller, 1980a) suggested that bladder management and cognition are the best predictors of successful home placement. Several studies (Cope & Hall, 1982; Gilchrist & Wilkinson, 1979; Jennette & Bond, 1975; Rappaport, Hall, Hopkins, Teodoro, & Cope, 1982; Teasdale & Jennette, 1975) have shown that duration of coma is the best predictor of functional recovery and outcome for traumatic brain-injured individuals. Others (Feinberg, Mackey, Steer, Unger, & Fierstein, 1979; Hertran, Dernopoulos, Yang, Calhoun, & Feningstein, 1984; Hertran & Yang, 1980; Miller &

Miyamoto, 1979; Rao, Jellinek, Harvey, & Flynn, 1984; Rappaport, Hall, Hopkins, & Belleza, 1981; Timming, Orrison, & Mikula, 1982) have related the findings of computerized axial tomography (CT scans) to the prediction of functional recovery following a stroke or head injury. Another study (Miller, Miyamoto, & Forer, 1980) related carotid artery occlusion to stroke outcomes. Still other studies (Jellinek, Torkelson, & Harvey 1982; Rao, Jellinek, & Woolston, 1985; Reyes & Heller 1981) have related levels of distress, agitation, and restlessness to head injury outcomes. All of the aforementioned are examples of how outcome data can be used for research and comparative studies in medical rehabilitation facilities.

Similar attempts have been made to identify the best predictors of functional recovery and outcome in other rehabilitation settings. In one study, the one factor consistently related to patient outcomes in nursing homes was RN hours (Linn et al., 1977). Another study (Gabow et al., 1985) examined predictors of mortality in nursing home versus community residents. Another study (Wachtel, Derby, & Fulton, 1984) found the most important predictors of successful home placements for nursing home residents to be presence of spouse at home, number of previous admissions, mental disorder, and musculoskeletal disorder. A similar study (Weissert & Scanlon, 1985) found that younger, married, less dependent, non-Medicaid patients are considerably more likely to go home.

In drug and alcohol treatment programs, studies (Vaillant, 1966; Zahn & Ball, 1972) have found that social class, age, education, employment history, and marital status are related to treatment outcomes. Another study of psychiatric hospital patients (Watson, Daly, & Zimmerman, 1980) found that high scores on the Protective Benevolence Scale were associated with improvement. Others (Byers & Cohen, 1979; King et al., 1980) have found that institutional or organizational variables such as status at admission, type of separation, size of staff, structure, and characteristics tend to be the best predictors of psychiatric rehospitalizations. These are also examples of how outcome data can be used for research or comparison purposes.

Planning for Future
Program Development

Outcome data can be used for planning future program development as well as projecting various growth rates or changes in client programs. Outcome evaluation provides a basis for monitoring changes in: client characteristics or needs, diagnostic composition of caseload, number of clients treated, number of treatments rendered per patient, average length of stay, average cost per case, program interruptions, age of clientele, sex and race distribution, referral patterns, time from onset to rehabilitation admission, utilization of outpatient or other community services, and many other variables. When these types of outcome and descriptive data are effectively integrated with various management information systems such as productivity statistics, revenue statistics, staffing, census, and daily treatment records, projecting a growth rate based on retrospective and concurrent data is possible. Facility, staffing, equipment, and treatment techniques can be modified to serve the current and anticipated needs of patients. Innovative programs such as community outreach and follow-up programs, case management, and patient recovery and retrieval mechanisms can be implemented. One facility (Forer & Miller, 1980a) has developed a case management program to assess the client's social support system (family, friends, neighbors, etc.) with the goal of identifying and removing obstacles to successful home placement.

Marketing

Outcome data can also be used in marketing the rehabilitation programs and services to current and potential referral sources and clientele, as well as in promoting better community awareness and acceptance. One of the major purposes of outcome evaluation is to justify, maintain, or expand funding and general community support. The Commission on Accreditation of Rehabilitation Facilities (CARF) strongly advocates reporting of outcome data in marketing and public relations (CARF, 1981).

There is a definite need for elaborate and appropriate comparative data, from which sound marketing decisions can be made. Comparative data from other similar rehabilitation facilities will be covered in more detail later in this chapter. To market a rehabilitation program effectively and to enhance the image of the program in the community, it is helpful to know the costs, length of stay, and functional outcome of various conditions treated in the program and how these figures compare to similar programs or to different types of rehabilitation settings that may also treat the same type of clientele. However, there are often differences in the type and intensity of services provided, philosophy and goals of the program, staffing patterns, and acuity or severity of disabilities and conditions treated that can affect both costs and outcome (Forer & Miller, 1983). Having an overall sense of the characteristic differences between programs and care settings is essential. Several studies have attempted to identify the characteristic differences among programs and different care settings (Granger, Hamilton, & Forer, 1985; Keith & Breckenridge, 1985; King et al., 1980; Linn et al., 1977; Mullner, Nuzum, & Matthews, 1983; Udin & May, 1982; Weissert & Scanlon, 1985).

Knowing the costs of rehabilitating various types of disabilities or conditions in a particular facility is also crucial. Since costs fluctuate greatly according to the severity of the condition, age, time from onset, services rendered, program interruptions, length of stay, and many other factors, it is often more feasible to estimate the average total charge and daily charge for each disability or condition. For facilities that do not have a set daily rate that includes all services, one useful method is to audit a representative sample of bills for clients with a specific disability or condition and then determine the breakdown of charges by service and the typical utilization pattern. For example, in a medical rehabilitation facility, a sample of 10 acute stroke cases could be selected that approximate the average age, time from onset, severity, length of rehabilitation hospitalization, functional outcome, and discharge disposition for strokes treated in that facility. By auditing the hospital bills of these 10 cases and isolating rehabilitation charges from acute medical/surgical charges, one can determine the average total charge and daily charge for stroke rehabilitation. Then the breakdown of charges in terms of the room rate, physical therapy, occupational therapy, speech pathology, psychology, recreation therapy, and other ancillaries (laboratory, X-ray, CT scans, medications, hospital supplies consumed, etc.) can be determined. Based on the typical unit charge (e.g., for 30-minute treatment sessions) it is possible to estimate how much therapy patients received. Finally, since use of ancillaries varies considerably from case to case, expressing them as a percentage of the total bill is perhaps simpler.

After estimating the costs (average daily charge) of rehabilitating a stroke patient in one facility, the same percentage and utilization statistics can be used to determine the daily charge estimates at other rehabilitation facilities using their rate structure. This method allows for differences in the characteristics, level of severity, and degree of impairment of rehabilitation patients treated in other care settings. Results of this analysis will indicate the relationship of one facility's charges to those of other competing facilities. This type of information can be used not only for marketing, but also for adjusting one's own rates to remain competitive.

Outcome information should be presented in a simple format that is easily understood. The use of graphs and tables can be helpful to display functional improvement, average length of stay, and costs of rehabilitation by disability, as well as percentages of different discharge dispositions. Often a narrative summary is also beneficial. Facilities may wish to publish quarterly or annual outcome information for marketing purposes.

DESIGNING AN OUTCOME ANALYSIS SYSTEM

A number of administrative considerations in developing an outcome analysis system are discussed in this section.

Inside versus Outside Evaluation

One of the first administrative issues to be considered in designing an outcome analysis system is whether the evaluation should be done by trained research or management staff within the facility (i.e., inside evaluation) or by an outside firm or consultant (i.e., outside evaluation). The development of an evaluation system often requires skilled and expensive staff. A specialized agency or outside consultant have the resources readily available, staff are usually on salary, and the facility only pays for the effort needed. Conversely, staff hired by the facility remain on the payroll beyond the time their evaluation skills are needed. An outside group has broader expertise and provides continual updating of the evaluation procedures at a minimal cost. The availability of expert staff on call provides capability for problem solving and special studies. In addition, having contact with a wide variety of programs enables sharing of experiences, which assists in program improvement and grant preparation. Quality control and integrity of results are assured by unbiased staff. Since outside consultants are often considered more objective, they have more credibility with third-party reviewers and licensing, accreditation, and funding agencies.

On the other hand, inside evaluators offer the following advantages:

1. They are familiar with the organization and are usually able to delineate program objectives and plausible outcome measures in a timely fashion.
2. They are familiar with information currently available in various records of the institution.
3. They are readily available to meet with management and staff during both the development and implementation of the outcome evaluation system to gain input and make adjustments accordingly.
4. They are available to do continuing research and program development.

According to Franklin and Thrasher (1976), the major argument in favor of internal evaluation and against external evaluation is the external evaluator's relatively incomplete knowledge of the program's history and circumstances. A reasonable compromise is to have an evaluator who is inside the system but outside the program, thereby reaping some of the benefits from both approaches.

Role of the Evaluator

To accomplish these goals, the evaluator must establish sufficient credibility to influence the chief administrators' decisions about programming and overcome expected staff resistance while limited to an advisory role. According to Caro (1972), "the evaluator's prestige and power are considered to be positively related to the likelihood that his findings will be implemented" (p. 21). Therefore, the inside evaluator should have a prestigious position within the organization, whereas the outside evaluator should have strong professional and organizational credentials.

The role of the evaluator in developing, implementing, and interpreting outcome evaluation should be clearly defined before an institution attempts to design a system. The reporting relationship and accountability of the evaluator should be well established. Outcome evaluation should create an image of "potential" and focus on improving program effectiveness. Inevitably, management and staff at all levels will perceive the evaluator as a "policeman." However, as the evaluator develops relationships, gaining the trust of key staff members and administration, the negative stigma of being a policeman will begin to seem less important. The evaluator can gain positive support by emphasizing the potential of the program and improving its effectiveness rather than criticizing its deficiencies. Nevertheless, program management is a high-risk occupation with an average of less than 5 years' tenure in any one institution (Franklin & Thrasher, 1976). This rapid turnover may discourage administrators from incorporating ongoing evaluation. Therefore, neither the administrator nor the evaluator is likely to witness the full evolution of an outcome evaluation system within a given institution.

Funding and Costs

Development and implementation of a comprehensive and workable outcome evaluation system generally takes a minimum of 6–9 months per program. The costs of designing and implementing an evaluation system are directly related to its complexity, design, number of objectives, types of measures, data analyses, methods of collecting follow-up data, use of existing data sources, involvement of staff, and many other factors. In some medical facilities, especially those that have research and training functions, an extensive data base may be needed and justified. However, a facility can also operate and maintain a highly useful outcome evaluation system at very little cost. The costs of using inside evaluators to develop and implement a system depend upon these persons' professional training, expertise, and position in the organization. According to a national study in 1982, most evaluators make between $18,000 and $29,000 annually, although their time may not be entirely dedicated to outcome evaluation. In contrast, consultant costs range from $200 to $500 per day. The cost of a total product contract ranges between $3,000 and $7,000 depending on the complexity and extensiveness of the evaluation system.

The costs of training data gatherers, whether they are volunteers, clerical staff, or evaluation staff, to obtain client information through structured telephone interviews with former rehabilitation clients, family members, significant others, or attending nurses, is approximately $75 to $100 per follow-up worker. This estimate is based on Forer and Miller's (1980b) description of 12 hours in intensive training plus ongoing supervision.

The salaries of the staff physical therapists, occupational therapists, speech pathologists, audiologists, rehabilitation nurses, social workers, and psychologists, including fringe benefits, required to contact and interview 500 former rehabilitation patients by telephone was approximately $28,000 per year in 1980–1981. This estimate is based on an average hourly wage of $12.50 plus benefits.

According to Forer and Miller (1980b), the costs of using trained volunteers to conduct telephone interviews was $33.60 per patient or $1.40 per patient day. All of these estimates reflect only the cost of obtaining follow-up information and do not include the developmental costs or report preparation.

There is, as expected, very little state, federal, or private funding available for outcome evaluation. Some of the demonstration or model project types of grants may partially fund outcome evaluation. For the most part, the costs are assumed by the institutions and passed on to their clients as part of the operating expense.

Potential Impact on the Organization

Before developing an outcome evaluation system, one should carefully assess the potential impact on the organization in terms of costs, additional documentation requirements, staff time and commitment, and receptivity of staff and management to the entire concept of outcome evaluation. Other considerations are how the results will be used and by whom, and the likelihood that outcome data will in fact influence decision making about programs, services, equipment, staff, facilities, and future planning. The institution must be strongly committed to evaluating outcome; satisfying a mandate by a licensing, accreditation, or funding agency should not be the primary motivation. The institution and its staff should remain cognizant of both the benefits and potential impact of such an evaluation system.

Many institutions with a secret desire to maintain the status quo are not ready for outcome evaluation. They merely seek data to prove that their programs are cost-effective. As with any social program, the possibility of change can be extremely threatening. Administrators usually prefer to conceal inefficiency for which they may be held responsible and to resist disruptive change. Not only is knowledge of outcomes in and of itself threatening, but the evaluator who collects, analyzes, and disseminates this information can be perceived as a threat to the institution. Outcome evaluation may be viewed as obstructive by administrators who are more concerned about political constraints, budgetary problems, and limitations of staffing and facilities.

Existing Documentation Requirements

Before proceeding further, an evaluator should identify what information is already available in the institutional or client records. This review should include all management information systems, quality assurance, case records, daily treatment records, billing records, outpatient and follow-up reports, plus reports from other community agencies. Since most outcome evaluation systems assess a client's functional status at admission, discharge, and follow-up, it may be revealing to take a careful look at the evaluation forms and treatment plans used by the clinical services.

Once existing documentation has been identified, additional information can be easily built into routine record keeping and reporting systems. According to Franklin and Thrasher (1976), unless evaluation can be built into a routine documentation, the quality and accuracy of the information are no better than the unaided expert judgment of the program manager. Economy of documentation should be of utmost concern to the evaluator. Every attempt should be made to streamline documentation and integrate it with existing documentation requirements.

Minimizing Disruption to the Organization

Organizational resources must be used efficiently in the development of an outcome evaluation in order to minimize the disruption to the organization. After a program has been selected for evaluation, the evaluator and administrator should carefully select the appropriate committee structure and composition, the disciplines to be involved, and the meeting schedule and target completion dates.

Data should not be cumbersome for staff to collect. Data that are already available in case records can be abstracted without interfering with clinical operations. Needed information such as functional assessments can be obtained by using simple checklists or worksheets initially placed in the charts and removed upon discharge or follow-up. The use of an abstract or coding sheet can greatly simplify data collection.

Involvement of Staff

The single most common reason for failure of evaluation efforts is the lack of staff involvement in the development and implementation of the system (CARF, 1976a, 1976b, 1979, 1980, 1981; Lorber & Lundstrom, 1981; Weiss, 1972). This is not to imply that the treating staff are uninterested in the outcomes of their efforts. Administrators typically find that the development of an outcome evaluation system does not necessarily require extensive staff involvement. However, direct involvement of staff is both prudent and necessary. The first reason is that staff must have a commitment to the evaluation system since they are the ones responsible for providing the services and in part for supplying the data. Second, staff participation can greatly increase the technical quality of the evaluation system. Furthermore, staff can contribute to setting realistic expectations of program outcomes and goals. Results are then much more meaningful to staff, and more apt to enhance morale, initiative, and cooperation.

Staff often fear that an evaluation system will not adequately measure the quality and outcome of services provided. A typical comment about functional assessment is that the instruments are not sensitive to small increments of improvement and do not show patient progress. Therefore, staff should be involved in developing the outcome evaluation system and measures. They need to be reassured that outcome measures will be used to evaluate programs and not their individual performance. Staff participation in evaluation system development may appear time consuming and costly. However, when viewed from the perspective of technical soundness and the need for proper installation and maintenance of the system, staff involvement during system development will likely reduce the long-term cost of the evaluation system. More detailed information on managing staff resistance will be presented later in this chapter.

Design

There are a number of methodological issues to consider in designing an outcome evaluation system. Outcome evaluation should monitor not only progress during in-hospital stay, but also progress after discharge, which is often a much more realistic measure of actual outcomes. Evaluation systems that monitor only inpatient progress from admission to discharge are not sufficient to meet CARF program evaluation standards (CARF, 1979).

A facility may consider two basic evaluation approaches. The first is to view outpatient services as an extension of an inpatient program and

to measure outcome or improvement by combining these two time frames into one. Facilities using this approach may elect to measure outcome at termination of outpatient services or at some prearranged time after discharge from inpatient care (usually 90, 120, or 180 days postdischarge). The disadvantage of combining inpatient and postdischarge progress into one measure is that data analysis is delayed until all follow-up information is obtained. Often this is many months after inpatient services have been provided. In some cases, patients may still be receiving outpatient services, and their gains, therefore, are not yet complete (CARF, 1979). Other patients may not receive any outpatient services at all. Furthermore, during the time interval between discharge and the follow-up contact, patients may suffer from secondary medical complications or other disabilities that will reduce their functional competency at follow-up. Conversely, spontaneous recovery may also occur during this period and confound the results. The influence of these two divergent factors may be minimized by early follow-up so that the results are more attributable to rehabilitation services provided.

The second evaluation approach is to separate inpatient progress (improvement from admission to discharge) from postdischarge progress and provide two separate reports, one for each time frame. The advantages to this approach are:

1. Clear information, more easily traceable to treatment strategies, separating out some of the spontaneous recovery.
2. Immediate and more time-efficient reporting of results. If reports are prepared on a quarterly basis, a report of inpatient progress should be available within 6 weeks from the last patient's discharge, which is consistent with CARF Standards (CARF, 1979).
3. Taking into account mortality of patients, which tends to bias the results, since those patients who are more impaired on admission are usually the ones to expire (Miller & Forer, 1983).

Follow-up contact success is rarely 100%, but tends to average 60%–86%. Evaluators cannot report on patients lost to follow-up, but, with two separate reports, at least inpatient progress for these patients can be reported.

Functional Assessment Instruments

Evaluators in the field of rehabilitation are continually searching for objective, sensitive, and reliable functional assessment instruments for clinical, research, or program evaluation purposes. It is important to describe the functional level of clients upon entry into the program, the amount of functional gains made while in the program as well as after discharge, and the final functional level attained by clients at follow-up. Generally this information is obtained using a functional status rating instrument to assess a client's functional competency and independence in a variety of parameters such as activities of daily living (ADL), mobility, communication, psychosocial adjustment, cognitive abilities, and vocational adjustment.

Rating instruments assessing the degree of independence have ranged from a 3-point scale to a 10-point scale (Forer, 1985). In most cases, assessment of the level of independence takes into account the amount of assistance required to complete the activity. The amount of assistance can be specified, for example, maximum, moderate, minimal, standby assistance, or supervision. The 3-point scales tend to divide performance into: unable to do the activity, can complete the activity with help, or can complete the activity independently. Several rating instruments (Carey & Posavac, 1978; Sarno, Sarno, & Levita, 1973; Susset et al., 1979) also take into consideration whether special equipment or preparation is needed. One rating instrument (Carey & Posavac, 1978) also assesses the speed and overall efficiency with which a client is able to complete the activity. Table 1 lists some of the published functional assessment instruments.

Functional status inventories have ranged from as few as 20 to as many as 200 items. The selection of instruments and appropriate items really depends on the population (diagnostic group) being evaluated. Several rating instruments yield a total or composite score for all of the items in the inventory, whereas others provide subscores in each major category such as self-care or mobility. When selecting a functional assessment inventory, the evaluator should remember that the instrument is intended to be an evaluation tool to assess outcome, not a refined clinical instrument. Oftentimes clinical staff exert great pressure on the developmental process to mold or pattern the instrument after clinical tests and measures. Functional assessment instruments generally provide a global overview of performance and outcome (Granger & Gresham, 1984).

Standardization, Reliability, and Validity of Measures

Many of the outcome measures used in rehabilitation lack rigor in terms of standardization, scaling, discriminative power, methods of weighting, reliability, and validity (Keith, 1984). An often overlooked requirement for standardization is a manual for test administration that contains specific instructions for administering the measures, normative data, precautions and limitations, and guidelines for interpretation. Normative data are often absent. The heterogeneity of a rehabilitation caseload makes comparisons difficult, but not insurmountable. Most functional status scales purport to have the characteristics of an interval scale, that is, equal-appearing intervals between the various levels of functions. The evaluator must be prepared to defend the position, for example, that the difference between maximum assistance and moderate assistance is the same as the difference between minimal assistance and supervision.

Reliability refers to the consistency of scores obtained by the same person when reexamined with the same test on different occasions, with different sets of equivalent items, or under variable examining conditions. Scale developers attempt to minimize error variance due to time sampling, content or item heterogeneity, and interinformant and interrater differences. Despite all efforts to control these conditions, however, *no test is a perfectly reliable instrument*. For this reason, evaluators should continually monitor and report reliability data on instruments used to assess a client's functional abilities and limitations.

One of the most important steps that can be taken to enhance interrater reliability is training.

Table I.　Functional assessment instruments

Instrument	References
Barthel Index	Mahoney & Barthel (1965)
	McGinnis, Seward, DeJong, & Osberg (1986)
Colorado Client Assessment Record	Reihman, Wolford, Knapp, MacCallum, & Murray (1983)
Disability Rating Scale	Rappaport, Hall, Hopkins, Teodoro, & Cope (1982)
ESCROW	Granger, Albrech, & Hamilton (1979)
Fairview Self Help Scale	King, Hougland, Shepard, & Gallagher (1980)
Functional Assessment Inventory	Crewe & Athelston (1981)
Functional Life Scale	Sarno, Sarno, & Levita (1973)
Functional Limitation Scale	Williamson (1971)
Functional Status Index	Jette (1980)
Geriatric Resident Goals Scales	Cornbleth (1978)
Goal Attainment Scale for Psychiatric Inpatients	Guy & Moore (1982)
Hospital Utilization Project	HUP (1974)
Katz Index of Independence	Katz, Ford, Moskowitz, Jackson, & Jaffe (1963)
Kenney Self-Care Evaluation	Iverson, Silberberg, Stever, & Schoening (1973)
Level of Rehabilitation Scale	Carey & Posavac (1978)
One Hundred Point Scale	Miller & Johnston (1985)
Patient Evaluation Conference System	Harvey & Jellinek (1981, 1983)
Psychosocial Functioning Inventory	Feragne, Longabaugh, & Stevenson (1983)
PULSES	Granger, Albrecht, & Hamilton (1979)
Rapid Disability Rating Scale	Linn, Gurel, & Linn (1977)
Rehabilitation Indicators	Brown, Gordon, & Diller, (1984)
REHABIS	Harasymiw & Stahl (1979)
Revised Functional Status Rating Instrument	Forer (1982)
Scaled Outcome Criteria in an Extended Care Facility	Howe, Coulton, Almon, & Sandrick (1980)
Self Assessment of Disability Outcomes	Susset, Vobecky, & Balck (1979)
Social Functioning Examination	Robinson, Bolduc, Kubos, Starr, & Price (1985)
Telephone Structured Interview	Alexander & Halstead (1979)
Uniform National Data System	Granger, Hamilton, & Forer, (1985)

During training of data gatherers, evaluators can monitor interrater reliability. For example, trainees can be given the opportunity to observe interviews with clients conducted by professional staff, and functional assessment scores obtained by trainees and professional staff can be compared and discussed. Differences in ratings can be pointed out and resolved. Often videotapes are helpful in this type of training. Educating staff on functional assessment and goal setting can also enhance interrater reliability. After training, professional staff can audit several interviews done by them to ensure they consistently adhere to the follow-up protocol and probe for information correctly.

Establishing validity involves conceptual as well as methodological issues. The three more commonly used types of validity are criteria-related validity, content validity, and construct validity. Criteria-related validity concerns whether functional assessed scores are related to some external criterion such as successful home placement. Content validity is concerned with how well the measure samples the domains of interest. According to Keith (1984), most functional assessment scales used in rehabilitation are designed to measure a narrow range of self-care, mobility, communication, psychosocial, and cognitive skills pertinent to a disabled population. Construct validity requires relating the measure to a network of similar measures that form a theoretical construct. A sensitive functional assessment measure will discriminate between diagnostic categories, impaired versus normal subjects, institutionalized and noninstitutionalized, socially adjusted and maladjusted, and many other dichotomies. Some researchers (Crewe & Athelston, 1981; Katz, Ford, Moskowitz, Jackson, & Jaffe, 1963; Sarno et al., 1973) have reported correlations between clinical judgments and functional assessment.

Methods of Collecting Follow-Up Data

The three follow-up procedures that have been used most often by rehabilitation facilities are follow-up return visit, mailed follow-up survey, and telephone interview.

Follow-Up Return Visit Some facilities choose to obtain follow-up information during return visits to the facility. These visits are often scheduled at the time of the client's discharge. The reevaluations may be comprehensive and completed by the entire rehabilitation team or by one representative (usually a physician or case worker). The more comprehensive evaluations can take as long as 1½ hours to complete. However, when completed by one or two rehabilitation team members, they can be done in less than 30 minutes.

One of the drawbacks of depending on return visits is that funding is not always available. Additionally, the cancellation rates are high and clients may move out of the area and not be accessible. Consequently, the potential for sampling biases arises.

If return visits are used, some consideration should be given to who conducts the evaluation. Although using previous service providers as evaluators offers the advantage of establishing rapport with former clients, this approach often brings into question the objectivity and credibility of data collected.

Mailed Follow-Up Survey This follow-up procedure requires mailing a questionnaire to clients that is returned to the facility upon completion. This approach provides little control for accuracy of information, and return rates are rather low. One method of enhancing the response rates is to explain to clients upon discharge that they will be contacted for follow-up information. Follow-up letters and phone calls may also be necessary. Despite such efforts, the return rates generally average 60% of questionnaires mailed out. Most experts agree that return rates under 75% can present problems of sam-

pling bias. Evaluators should ask themselves how results would have changed if all clients returned completed questionnaires.

When instructions and questions are clearly written and simple direct answers required, a mailed questionnaire of 30 items can be completed in less than 30 minutes. However, respondents often have questions regarding the interpretation of various items. Combined with occasional language barriers or reluctance to divulge information, response times can be two to three times as long.

Telephone Interview The telephone interview is the most commonly used method for obtaining follow-up data, especially when the majority of clients do not live near a facility. Facilities using the telephone interview find it necessary either to use professional staff (occupational therapists, physical therapists, social workers, psychologists, or nurses) who are experienced in interviewing techniques, or to rely on some type of well-structured interview protocol. However, carefully selected and trained paraprofessional volunteers can also obtain follow-up data through structured telephone interviews (Forer & Miller, 1980b). Experience shows that former clients or their relatives are quite responsive to providing information over the phone.

Some evaluators have chosen to rely on a personal interview/observation, conducted by visiting nurses (Linn et al., 1977; Susset et al., 1979), nurse–social worker teams (Granger et al., 1979), trained interviewers (Feragne, Longabaugh, & Stevenson, 1983; Jette, 1980; Reihman et al., 1983), friendly visitors (Mor et al., 1983), and evaluation staff (Carey & Posavac, 1978). These approaches are generally more expensive than telephone interviews.

As a general rule, telephone or personal interviews should be brief and well structured and require no more than 20–30 minutes to complete. The telephone interview can provide an inexpensive means of collecting accurate information from a large sample of clients in a relatively short period of time. The telephone interview, therefore, appears to be the most efficient method of collecting follow-up information.

Time Delays In past research, the time interval between discharge and the collection of follow-up data has varied greatly. In one report (Anderson et al., 1978), follow-up data were collected as long as 12 or 13 years postdischarge. Others have restricted the time lag to 1–2 years (Byers & Cohen, 1979; Forer & Miller, 1980a; Granger et. al., 1979; Mor et al., 1983; Susset et al., 1979), 6 months (Linn et al., 1977; Robinson, Bolduc, Kubos, Starr, & Price, 1985), 4½ months (Carey & Posavac, 1978), 90 days (Ives, Lounsbury, & Tornatzky, 1976; Reihman et al., 1983), or 2 months (Cummings, Kerner, Arones, & Steinbock, 1985) postdischarge. The decision about when to collect follow-up data should depend on how the information will be used. For research purposes, longer time intervals between discharge and follow-up may be desirable. For evaluation purposes, however, the time interval needs to be shorter, such as 3–6 months.

Development of a Follow-Up Protocol

As mentioned previously, a follow-up protocol is needed to accompany functional status rating instruments when follow-up information is to be obtained through a structured telephone interview. Protocols usually consist of a series of probe questions designed to elicit the information required to make accurate judgments of a client's status. Questions should always be framed in language that is simple and clear. It is also important to ascertain whether the respondent actually has the information sought.

General Probes The follow-up protocol should begin with a few general probe questions that take no longer than 2–5 minutes. After the interviewer has an idea of which activities (items) the client is limited in or requires assistance with, more specific questions can follow. Follow-up interviewers often find that, when they begin with a brief series of general questions, respondents provide more information in a short period of time and the interviewer can probe further for elaboration and clarification.

Branching Questions Some evaluators choose to use a carefully laid out pattern of branching questions, where one response given by a client leads the interviewer to ask more specific questions until an accurate assessment of the client's abilities and limitations can be reached (Kaufert, 1983). In some areas of functional as-

sessment branching questions are quite helpful, whereas in other areas they can be cumbersome and time consuming. Whichever method is used, care should be taken in developing a follow-up protocol so that clients and their significant others can reply easily, the time required to get the information is minimal (less than 30 minutes), and complete and accurate information is obtained.

Advantages of Allowing for Comments The follow-up protocol should allow for comments from respondents. These comments often provide important information for supplementing or clarifying functional status ratings. Clients can be identified who are having substantial adjustment problems at home, secondary medical complications, or maladaptive behavior patterns.

Comparison with Program Data Reliability of functional status ratings also depends in part on the data source (e.g., client, family member, employer, or attending nurse). Some evaluators have studied interinformant reliability (Carey & Posavac, 1978; Mor et al., 1983). Frequent differences occur in reported functional levels of clients, depending upon whom is being interviewed. A client may distort or exaggerate functional abilities or limitations when interviewed at follow-up. Conversely, it is sometimes easier and less frustrating for family members to provide direct assistance to clients rather than watch them struggle. Therefore, when interviewed, family members may indicate that clients require help with a self-care activity when in fact the individuals are capable of doing it themselves. As another example, a visiting nurse does not have the opportunity to observe clients during many of the activities for which functional assessment is desired. In the absence of personal observations, the nurse may underestimate a client's capabilities.

It is recommended that, prior to interviewing a former client, family member, or significant other, follow-up workers should familiarize themselves with background information obtained while the client was in the program. This information may assist in identifying false or exaggerated information about clients' abilities and limitations. Information obtained from several sources (client, family member, and significant others) can also be compared. Occasionally, information obtained during outpatient reevaluation is available at the time of follow-up contact. Information obtained from these multiple sources should be compared whenever possible, especially when the reliability of the information obtained is in question.

IMPLEMENTING AN OUTCOME EVALUATION SYSTEM

Acceptability of Results

Outcome evaluation results must be clear, concise, relevant, meaningful, palatable, and understandable for staff and management. Staff and management need to be able to synthesize the results into meaningful patterns and apply them to clinical practices. Practitioners are always suspicious of evaluation results and rarely find the information to be completely adequate. Particularly in functional assessment, clinicians will criticize that the instruments are not sensitive enough to measure small increments of change or client progress. The results may conflict with staff members' preconceived expectations, notions, or clinical values. When the results turn out to be entirely different from those expected, they question the reliability and validity of the instruments, integrity of the data and data sources, and adequacy of the information. Fears related to technical aspects of the evaluations system are usually expressed in terms of doubts about the validity and reliability of the entire evaluation system (Lorber & Lundstrom, 1981). These fears are expressed in general terms by saying "what we are doing can't easily be measured," or by claiming that the evaluation system is a useless bureaucratic procedure that demands considerable time and effort but ultimately has little value.

A related concern often expressed by program managers is that their program will show poor outcome results because the functional assessment instruments are not sensitive enough to measure small increments of client improvement. Some managers are also fearful that the indices and measures will not conform with the objectives of the program. This is particularly true in programs that focus on maintaining acquired skills and abilities, providing a sheltered work environment, enriching life experiences, or preventing further deficits or deterioration.

An evaluator should be aware of potential resistance to accepting the outcome results and take steps to manage this resistance. The means of accomplishing this goal are discussed in a subsequent section of this chapter.

Integration with Other Management Information Systems

Quality Assurance The essential components of quality assurance are: 1) identification of potential problems, 2) objective assessment of possible causes, 3) implementation of decisions or actions designed to eliminate identified problems, 4) monitoring activities to ensure desired results have been obtained, and 5) documentation to substantiate that quality assurance has led to enhanced patient care. Recent developments in quality assurance indicate a trend or expansion to include some of the issues and methods of outcome evaluation. It appears that the Joint Commission on Accreditation of Hospitals (JCAH) is placing more emphasis on ongoing efforts to monitor appropriateness of treatments and clinical judgments.

Outcome evaluation should be integrated with various management information systems, including quality assurance. Outcome evaluation reports can indicate areas in which performance is substandard and outcomes of treatment have not met previously established criteria or expectancies. Management reports based on the outcome data may prompt individual chart audits and special studies to further assist in problem resolution. The intention of outcome evaluation is to provide an overall picture of performance and outcome. However, in its most simplistic form, outcome evaluation does not provide specific answers to problem areas, but merely identifies that problems exist. Special studies and audits are necessary outgrowths from outcome evaluation. Several researchers (Bartilotta and Rzasa, 1982; Dentino, 1983; Forer, 1981; Wellington, Benditsky, Taintor, & McCleery, 1985) have demonstrated how outcome evaluation can be integrated with various management information systems, including quality assurance, to assure effective application of results.

Other Management Information Systems Outcome evaluation should also be integrated with other management information systems such as productivity studies and revenue statistics, as well as staffing, census, and budget reports. When these types of feedback data are effectively integrated, it is possible to project growth rates for the program. As shown in Figure 1, outcome, billing, cost allocation, medical record, case mix, and census data can be integrated into one information system to produce management reports, planning reports, marketing reports, financial reports, and special studies. Staffing, budgeting, equipment acquisitions, treatment techniques, and operating procedures can be modified to serve current and anticipated needs of clients. The extent to which different reporting systems can be integrated into a single system is a complex issue. The following factors must be considered when developing an integrated system: duplicate information, controlling and integrating data from multiple sources, timing requirements, external approval from funding and regulatory agencies to modify source documents, computer limitations and costs, types of reports that are likely to be useful, and ready availability of data required. Data integration can reduce the overall reporting costs.

Despite the advent and ready availability of computers, published literature is sparse on integrated management information systems in the field of rehabilitation. Wellington et al. (1985) discussed general principles for use of an integrated management information system for a psychiatric population. Administrative decision making regarding staff–patient ratios based on a patient classification system has been introduced by Schroder and Washington (1982). A computerized patient information system has been developed that combines concurrent and retrospective monitoring while providing an interactive system for quality assurance and utilization review (Bartilotta & Rzasa, 1982). For nursing homes, Romaniuk and Blanks (1984) discussed administrative considerations in the development and implementation of an automated management information system. One management information system can assess the input of seasonal changes on case mix and efficiency while providing cost information (Hinnant, 1983). Dentino (1983) contrasted financial information systems with patient medical information systems and described the Rose System of Patient Care Management. A more extensive literature search of computerized hospital information systems was recently conducted by the American Hospital Association (1986). A listing of 30 publications up through 1983 is provided.

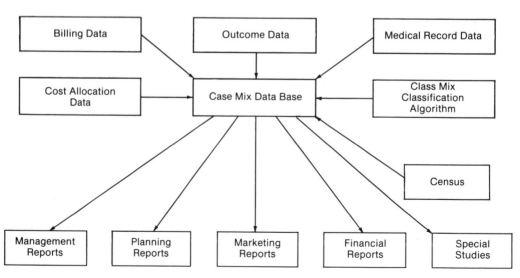

Figure 1. Information systems model.

Data Management Services

There is a definite need for a data bank or common repository to store and consolidate information supplied by individual facilities. A data management service can provide: 1) a collection of primary data for user facilities on standardized formats, 2) verification of accuracy of data and quality control, 3) automated and computerized data analysis, 4) report generation for user facilities, 5) aggregate reporting of results from all user facilities, 6) data storage for future retrieval and analysis, and 7) special studies for research purposes.

There are several companies currently providing various types of data management services to rehabilitation facilities. They include: Hospital Utilization Project (HUP), Monitrend, Commission on Professional and Hospital Activities (CPHA), Level of Rehabilitation Scale (LORS), Patient Evaluation Conference System (PECS), Shared Medical Systems (SMS), and National Easter Seal Society Data Management Service. The majority of these services are designed for medical rehabilitation, but some may also have application to other settings. Traditionally, such services have emphasized financial information. More recently, there has been a growth of data management services providing client demographic and outcome information (Powell & Scott, 1983). Because each system is different, there is presently no way to combine and compare information. Costs of participating in these data management services vary. There is usually an initial and annual fee plus a charge per abstract submitted. Some of the charges are based on client volume or revenue.

ANALYZING AND REPORTING OUTCOME RESULTS

Methods of Presenting Feedback Information

Both positive and negative results from outcome studies should be fed back to the entire staff. Outcome information also should be presented to program managers, administration, governing bodies, third-party payors, referring professionals and agencies, potential consumers, and the community. Those persons and organizations who are in a position to make decisions and facilitate change or improve performance and outcome should have access to outcome information (CARF, 1981). Outcome information should be presented in a manner that is clear, concise, timely, understandable and relevant to those receiving this feedback information. The more commonly used methods of presenting feedback information are statistics, graphs, matrices, narrative descriptions, and client satisfaction comments. Different methods of providing feedback information should be used for different audiences.

Statistics In the feedback reporting of results, there are several methods of summarizing and collecting statistical data. The two more commonly used methods are criteria-oriented measures and improvement measures (Forer & Magnuson, 1984).

The criteria measure identifies in absolute terms the specific outcome (either at discharge or follow-up) desired. Criteria-oriented measures are usually expressed in terms of the percentage of clients who have reached a previously established level of performance by a specific point in time. Some (CARF, 1979; Keith, 1984) claim that the advantage in using a criteria-oriented measure is that the information presented has more meaning and a greater likelihood of impact on changing or modifying client programs and outcomes. Criteria-oriented measures can be easy to interpret.

The improvement measure assesses change in a client's functional abilities or limitations over time. An improvement measure can provide information on the amount of change and can also describe functional outcome of clients. Anderson et al. (1978) compared estimates of outcomes with actual patient records and follow-up interviews. In another study (Lehmann et al., 1977), evidence was found that progress gained through rehabilitation was retained after discharge and that the functional level was typically higher at follow-up.

The use of criteria-oriented measures (percentages) versus improvement measures (amount of gain) is still an area of considerable controversy. The use of improvement measures allows evaluators to describe the functional level of clients upon entry into the program, the amount of functional gains made in the program as well as after discharge, and the final functional level attained by the client at follow-up. However, the evaluator must remember that the rating scale used in the functional assessment instrument may not approximate the characteristics of a true interval scale, making the use of mean and standard deviation statistics inappropriate. Therefore, care and rigor must be taken in the development of the scale and of reliability and validity data. For most evaluators, the advantages of using improvement measures far outweigh those for alternative methods of summarizing data, and the disadvantages are minimal.

Graphs The use of graphics can also be helpful to display functional improvement. The technique may add perceptual clarity to the statistics because reviewers are presented with a visual presentation of the data. Histograms (bar graphs) and polygrams (line graphs) should be used whenever possible to display functional outcome data. Figure 2, based on hypothetical data, provides an example of a histogram used to display means and standard deviation of functional outcome information in a medical rehabilitation setting.

Matrices Another useful technique for displaying functional outcome data is through the use of a matrix. The matrix in Figure 3 displays the admission and discharge scores for 26 patients on the item of dressing. For example, of those patients who had a score of 2 at admission, two had a discharge score of 2, 11 a discharge score of 3, and four a discharge score of 4. The two heavy diagonal lines separate those who improved from those who stayed the same.

Narrative Descriptions Staff and administration are often more interested in a narrative description or summary of results than they are in actual statistics, graphs, or matrices. Quantifiable data or scores are needed for statistical or comparison purposes, whereas a description of abilities is needed for more practical and clinical applications. Narrative descriptions should accompany outcome data whenever possible because they help to interpret data and are more easily understood by staff.

Client Satisfaction Comments The structured interview and functional status rating instrument should encourage comments. Such comments from former clients, family members, or significant others can supplement or clarify functional status ratings. Additionally, it is advisable to query former clients and family members about their satisfaction with the rehabilitation program and services and to solicit any concerns they may have. Since this information is not easily quantified, comments are usually reported separately from outcome data. One technique is to separate positive and negative comments and provide specific departments with feedback pertinent to their areas only. The evaluator consequently avoids creating resentment among staff members for sharing confidential and potentially threatening negative information. Also recommended, however, is a built-in accountability system to respond to comments and accusations from former clients and family members.

Comparison Data

Many management decisions require the availability of comparable data from other facilities. We need to look toward standardization and uniformity of evaluation and management information systems to allow comparisons among facilities and regions.

Several states have organized data-sharing activities. Two basic methods of data sharing are used: annual surveys providing aggregate or summary results and individual client abstracting and data reporting. The California Association of Rehabilitation Facilities (Cal-ARF) conducts an annual survey of member facilities to collect information on staff composition and salaries, therapy charges, caseload composition, average length of stay, outcome and costs of inpatient medical rehabilitation by diagnoses, and other important information. This association also conducts special surveys such as "Impact of Prospective Payment on the Delivery of Rehabilitation Services" as needed. These surveys provide statistical information needed to support or oppose pertinent legislation and regulations and also provide participating facilities with comparative data that can be used for planning and

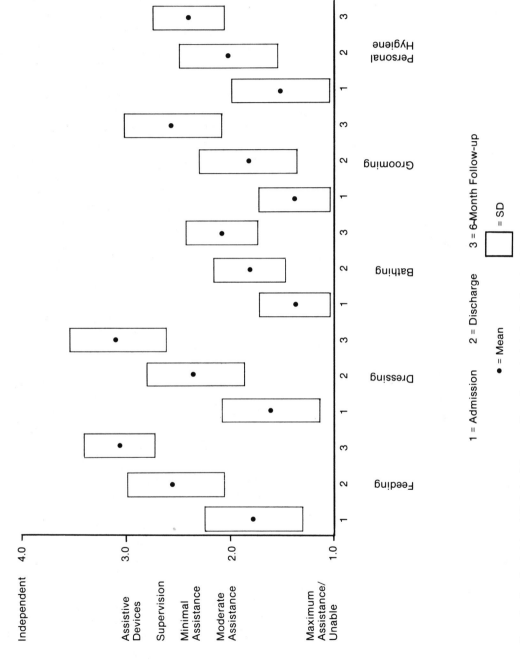

Figure 2. Functional status of 50 stroke victims on self-care items at admission, discharge, and 6-month follow-up.

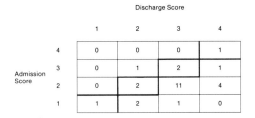

Figure 3.　Functional status in dressing on admission and discharge of 26 patients.

management purposes. Other states, including Illinois and Pennsylvania, are engaged in similar data-sharing activities.

On the national level, collecting comparable data has been attempted but without widespread participation (HUP, 1974; Keith & Breckenridge, 1985; Mullner et al., 1983; NARF, 1985; Udin & May, 1982). More recently, Kane et al., (1986), in a collaborative study involving the Rand Corporation and the Medical College of Wisconsin, attempted to identify the predictors of resource consumption and costs of medical rehabilitation.

The rehabilitation industry, including freestanding rehabilitation hospitals, distinct rehabilitation units, psychiatric hospitals, children's hospitals, and long-term care facilities, has been granted a temporary exemption from the Medicare DRG (diagnostic related group) Prospective Payment System. The challenge to the industry is to be able to justify the cost-effectiveness of rehabilitation and the need for a separate and more appropriate Medicare reimbursement system. Since there is a paucity of data and no common language, perhaps the only way this can be accomplished is through development of a uniform national data system. This monumental task has been attempted several times before. However, never before has there been such a desperate need for such a system. Rehabilitation professionals need to unite in attempting to reach agreement on what type of information (data) is needed and feasible to collect (Forer et al., 1984). (See Chapter 10 for a more detailed discussion of the development of such a system.)

Overcoming Obstacles and Managing Resistance to Evaluation

According to Lorber and Lundstrom (1981), resistance to outcome evaluation can occur on three

different levels: the organizational level, the technical level, and the personal level. At the first level, one of the most influential resistance factors is lack of clarity of the purpose of the organization. Outcome evaluation is predicated on a complete understanding of the organization, purpose, philosophy, goals, and objectives. The relative work of an agency as perceived by society may also influence the level of resistance to evaluation if it is perceived to influence ability to obtain public funding. In addition, the organization's own perceived level of success in accomplishing its purpose will affect the level of resistance to evaluation. A final organization factor is the justification for the cost of outcome evaluation and its potential benefits.

At the technical level, several aspects of an outcome evaluation system can affect resistance. The added burden of another reporting system, the complexity or simplicity of the evaluation system, and inflexibility to changes in program emphasis, as well as fairness, comprehensiveness, and objectivity of the evaluation system, can affect the level of resistance. Fears related to the evaluation system are usually expressed in terms of doubts about its validity and reliability. Outcome evaluation is often criticized for neglecting the issue of quality of care.

On the personal level, two fears seem to be more apparent. Staff members who are threatened by outcome evaluation are fearful that a poor rating for their program will be a reflection on their performance. Another fear is that evaluation is invalid because it cannot adequately measure client progress. Weiss (1972) also wrote about some of the personality factors causing friction and resistance. The evaluator is likely to be a detached individual, more interested in ideas and abstractions, whereas the practitioner is likely to be warm, outgoing, and more concerned about clients, concrete specifics, and the here and now. They may have conflicting goals, values, interests, and frames of reference. The evaluator's lack of clear role definition may be an additional source of resistance.

How does an evaluator overcome these obstacles and manage resistance to outcome evaluation? The first step is to realize that resistance is a normal occurrence. It is likely that every attempt to introduce outcome evaluation into an organization will meet with some form of resistance. With good communication and careful planning, most evaluators can proceed in a calm and cooperative atmosphere. The next step is to educate and train management and staff about outcome evaluation. A more thorough understanding of its purposes and operations can help to reduce resistance. Staff participation in the early development, implementation, and ongoing maintenance of an evaluation system is vital to the success of the evaluation effort. It is equally important to realize the limits of the evaluation staff and consultants and resources available in the facility to produce an evaluation system.

Flexibility in the design and implementation of the evaluation system can help to alleviate resistance by staff. Another area in which flexibility can help is in setting outcome expectations. Providing information that staff view as useful can be effective in circumventing resistance. Once the outcome evaluation system has been designed, staff and management may make numerous requests to modify the format of reports, to change the method of presenting feedback information, or to add or delete data.

Resistance can also be minimized by making sure the evaluation results are attributable to rehabilitation program efforts and not extraneous variables. Constructing or choosing functional measures that are sensitive enough to detect small increments of client progress will help to minimize fears of practitioners. It is important to explain to the program managers that the development of accurate and sensitive functional assessment tools is part of the implementation phase while assuring them that each measure will be continually evaluated. Finally, the evaluator can avoid resistance by identifying and using existing documentation and minimizing disruption to the program and organization. The support of top administration is also crucial to getting and maintaining the cooperation of staff.

REFERENCES

Alexander, J. L., & Halstead, L. S. (1979). Functional outcome assessment: A practical, new approach to follow-up. Official program of the American Congress of Rehabilitation Medicine, 56th Annual Session, p. 73.

American Hospital Association. (1986). Management information systems in acute hospitals. Chicago: Author.

Anderson, T. P., McClure, W. J., Athelstan, G., Anderson, E., Crewe, N., Ardts, L., Ferguson, M. B., Baldrige, M., Gullickson, G., & Kottke, F. J. (1978). Stroke rehabilitation: Evaluation of its quality by assessing patient outcomes. Archives of Physical Medicine and Rehabilitation, 59, 170–175.

Bartilotta, K., & Rzasa, C. B. (1982, March). Quality assurance utilizing a computerized patient information system. Quality Review Bulletin, 17–22.

Booth, R. (1981). Alcohol halfway houses: Treatment length and treatment outcome. The International Journal of Addictions, 16, 927–934.

Brown, M., Gordon, W. A., & Diller, L. (1984). Rehabilitation indicators. In A. S. Halpern & M. J. Fuhrer (Eds.), Functional assessment in rehabilitation (pp. 187–204). Baltimore: Paul H. Brookes Publishing Co.

Byers, E. S., & Cohen, S. H. (1979). Predicting patient outcome: The contribution of prehospital, in-hospital, and post hospital factors. Hospital and Community Psychiatry, 30, 327–331.

Carey, G., & Posavac, E. J. (1978). Program evaluation of a physical medicine and rehabilitation unit: A new approach. Archives of Physical Medicine and Rehabilitation, 59, 330–337.

Caro, F. G. (1972). Readings in evaluation research. New York: Russell Sage Foundation.

Commission on Accreditation of Rehabilitation Facilities. (1976a). Program evaluation in rehabilitation: Hospital based facilities. Chicago: Author.

Commission on Accreditation of Rehabilitation Facilities. (1976b). Program evaluation: A first step. Tucson: Author.

Commission on Accreditation of Rehabilitation Facilities. (1979). Program evaluation in inpatient medical rehabilitation facilities. Tucson: Author.

Commission on Accreditation of Rehabilitation Facilities. (1980). Program evaluation in outpatient medical rehabilitation facilities. Tucson: Author.

Commission on Accreditation of Rehabilitation Facilities. (1981). Program evaluation: Utilization and assessment principles. Tucson: Author.

Cope, N., & Hall, K. (1982). Head injury rehabilitation: Benefits of early intervention. Archives of Physical Medicine and Rehabilitation, 63, 433–437.

Cornbleth, T. (1978). Evaluation of goal attainment in geriatric settings. Journal of the American Geriatrics Society, 26, 404–407.

Crewe, N. M., & Athelston, G. T. (1981). Functional assessment in vocational rehabilitation: A systematic approach to diagnosis and goal setting. Archives of Physical Medicine and Rehabilitation, 62, 299–305.

Cummings, V., Kerner, J. F., Arones, S., & Steinbock, C. (1985). Day hospital service in rehabilitation medicine: An evaluation. Archives of Physical Medicine and Rehabilitation, 66, 86–91.

Dentino, J. (1983). The role of computers in managing patient care: The Rose system of patient care. Journal of American Health Care Association, 9, 10–13.

Feigenson, J. S., Githlow, H. S., & Greenberg, S. D. (1979).

The disability oriented rehabilitation unit: A major factor influencing stroke outcome. *Stroke, 10*, 5–7.

Feinberg, S., Mackey, F., Steer, H., Unger, P., & Fierstein, S. (1979). Stroke outcome prediction by computer tomography. Official Program of the American Academy of Physical Medicine and Rehabilitation, 41st Annual Assembly, p. 77.

Feldman, D., Lee, P., Unterecker, J., Lloyd, K., Rusk, H., & Toole, A. (1962). Comparison of functionally oriented medical care and formal rehabilitation in management of patients with hemiplegia due to cerebrovascular disease. *Journal of Chronic Disease, 15*, 297–319.

Feragne, M. A., Longabaugh, R., & Stevenson, J. F. (1983). The psychosocial functioning inventory. *Evaluation and the Health Professions, 6*, 25–48.

Forer, S. K. (1981) Integrating program evaluation and quality assurance. *Journal of the Organization of Rehabilitation Evaluators, 2*, 15–21.

Forer, S. K. (1982). Functional assessment instruments in medical rehabilitation. *Journal of the Organization of Rehabilitation Evaluators, 2*, 29–41.

Forer, S. K. (1985, October). *Functional assessment and evaluation systems in medical rehabilitation.* Paper presented at the meeting of the New England Society of Physical Medicine and Rehabilitation, Newport, RI.

Forer, S. K., Granger, C. U., Hamilton, B., Harvey, R., Keith, R. A., Mackey, F., Miller, L. S., Swope, M., Melvin, J., Gordon, W., Warren, C., & Johnston, M. (1984, October). *Functional assessment and evaluation in medical rehabilitation: A uniform national data system.* Forum presentation at the American Congress of Rehabilitation Medicine, Boston, MA.

Forer, S. K., & Magnuson, R. I. (1984). Feedback reporting. In C. Granger & G. Gresham (Eds.), *Functional assessment in rehabilitation medicine* (pp. 171–193). Baltimore: Williams & Wilkins.

Forer, S. K., & Miller, L. S. (1980a). Rehabilitation outcome: Comparative analysis of different patient types. *Archives of Physical Medicine and Rehabilitation, 61*, 359–365.

Forer, S. K., & Miller, L. S. (1980b). Paraprofessional volunteers and the collection of program evaluation data (Abstract). *Archives of Physical Medicine and Rehabilitation, 61*, 490.

Forer, S. K., & Miller, L. S. (1983). Cost effectiveness arguments for comprehensive medical rehabilitation: A literature review. *Journal of the Organization of Rehabilitation Evaluators, 3*, 38–44.

Franklin, J. L., & Thrasher, J. H. (1976). *An introduction to program evaluation.* New York: John Wiley & Sons.

Gabow, P. A., Hutt, D. M., Baker, S., Craig, S. R., Gordon, J. B., & Lezotte, D. C. (1985). Comparison of hospitalization between nursing home and community residents. *Journal of the American Geriatrics Society, 33*, 524–529.

Gilchrist, E., & Wilkinson, M. (1979). Some factors determining prognosis in young people with severe head injuries. *Archives of Neurology, 36*, 355–359.

Granger, C. V., Albrecht, G. L., & Hamilton, B. (1979). Outcome of comprehensive medical rehabilitation: Measurement of PULSES profile and Barthel. *Archives of Physical Medicine and Rehabilitation, 60*, 145–154.

Granger, C. V., & Gresham, G. (Eds.). (1984). *Functional assessment in rehabilitation medicine.* Baltimore: Williams & Wilkins.

Granger, C. V., Hamilton, B., & Forer, S. (1985). Development of a uniform national data system for medical rehabilitation (Abstract). *Archives of Physical Medicine and Rehabilitation, 66*, 538–539.

Guy, M. E., & Moore, L. S. (1982, June). The goal attainment scale for psychiatric inpatients. *Quality Review Bulletin,* 19–29.

Harasymiw, S. J., & Stahl, P. L. (1979). Rehabilitation information system (REHABIS): Computer based medical and demographic statistics at a comprehensive rehabilitation center over an eleven year span. *Official program of the American Congress of Rehabilitation Medicine, 56th Annual Session,* 21.

Harvey, R. F., & Jellinek, H. M. (1981). Functional performance assessment: A program approach. *Archives of Physical Medicine and Rehabilitation, 62*, 456–461.

Harvey, R. F., & Jellinek, H. M. (1983). Patient profiles: Utilization in functional performance assessment. *Archives of Physical Medicine and Rehabilitation, 64*, 268–271.

Hemenway, D. (1983). Quality assessment from an economic perspective: A taxonomy of approaches with applications to nursing home care. *Evaluation and Health Professions, 6*, 379–396.

Hertan, U. J., Dernopoulos, J., Yang, W., Calhoun, W., & Feningstein, H. (1984). Stroke rehabilitation: Correlation and prognostic value of computerized tomography and sequential functional assessment. *Archives of Physical Medicine and Rehabilitation, 65*, 505–508.

Hertan, J., & Yang, W. (1980). Correlation and prognostic value of CT scan and Barthel Index in stroke rehabilitation. *Official Program of the American Academy of Physical Medicine and Rehabilitation, 42nd Annual Assembly,* 103.

Hinnant, H. (1983). Monthly performance reports: Management's tools for control. *Journal of Long Term Care, 11*, 11–21.

Hospital Utilization Project of Pennsylvania. (1974). *Rehabilitation facility program procedure manual.* Pittsburgh: Author.

Howe, M. J., Coulton, J. R., Almon, G., & Sandrick, K. M. (1980, March). Developing scaled outcome criteria for a target patient population. *Quality Review Bulletin,* 17–23.

Iverson, I., Silberberg, N., Stever, R., & Schoening, H. (1973). *The revised Kenny self care evaluation.* Minneapolis: Sister Kenny Institute.

Ives, W. R., Lounsbury, J. W., & Tornatzky, L. G. (1976). An experimental comparison of two community-based drug abuse treatment programs. *Journal of Community Psychology, 4*, 253–258.

Jellinek, H. M., Torkelson, R., & Harvey, R. (1982). Functional abilities and distress levels in brain injured patients at long term follow-up. *Archives of Physical Medicine and Rehabilitation, 63*, 160–162.

Jennette, B., & Bond, M. (1975). Assessment of outcome after severe brain damage: A practical scale. *Lancet, 1*, 480–484.

Jette, A. M. (1980). Functional status index: Reliability of a chronic disease evaluation instrument. *Archives of Physical Medicine and Rehabilitation, 61*, 395–401.

Johnston, M. V., & Keister, M. (1984). Early rehabilitation for stroke patients: A new look. *Archives of Physical Medicine and Rehabilitation, 65*, 437–441.

Kane, R., Melvin, J., Hosek, S., Carney, M., Hartman, J., Roboussin, D., & Serrato, C. (1986). *Changes and out-*

comes for rehabilitative care: Implications for the prospective payment system (Grant No. R–3424–HCFA). Report prepared for the Health Care Financing Administration. Santa Monica, CA: RAND Corp.

Katz, S., Ford, A., Moskowitz, R., Jackson, B., & Jaffe, M. (1963). Studies of illness in aged; index of ADL: Standardized measure of biological and psychosocial function. *Journal of the American Medical Association, 185*, 914–919.

Kaufert, J. M. (1983) Functional ability indices: Measurement problems in assessing their validity. *Archives of Physical Medicine and Rehabilitation, 64*, 260–267.

Keith, R. A. (1984). Functional assessment measures in medical rehabilitation: Current status. *Archives of Physical Medicine and Rehabilitation, 65*, 74–78.

Keith, R. A., & Breckenridge, K. (1985). Characteristics of patients from the Hospital Utilization Project data system: 1980–1982. *Archives of Physical Medicine and Rehabilitation, 66*, 768–772.

King, R. D., Hougland, J. G., Shepard, J. M., & Gallagher, E. B. (1980). Organizational effects on mentally retarded adults: A longitudinal analysis. *Evaluation of the Health Professions, 3*, 85–101.

Lehmann, J. F., Delateur, B. J., Fowler, R. S., Jr., Warren, C. G., Arnhold, R., Schertzer, G., Hurka, R., Whitmore, J. S., Masock, A. J., & Chambers, K. H. (1977). Stroke: Does rehabilitation affect outcome? *Archives of Physical Medicine and Rehabilitation, 56*, 375–382.

Linn, M. W., Gurel, L., & Linn, B. S. (1977). Patient outcome as a measure of quality of nursing home care. *American Journal of Public Health, 67*, 337–344.

Lorber, C., & Lundstrom, J. S. (1981). Managing staff resistance to program evaluation. *Journal of the Organization of Rehabilitation Evaluators, 1*, 19–33.

Mahoney, F., & Barthel, D. W. (1965). Functional assessment, the Barthel Index. *Maryland State Medical Journal, 14*, 61–65.

Mattes, J. A., Klein, D. F., Millan, D., & Rosen, B. (1979). Comparison of the clinical effectiveness of "short" versus "long" stay psychiatric hospitalization. *The Journal of Nervous and Mental Disease, 167*, 175–181.

McGinnis, G. E., Seward, M. L., DeJong, G., & Osberg, S. (1986). Program evaluation of physical medicine and rehabilitation departments using self-report Barthel. *Archives of Physical Medicine and Rehabilitation, 67*, 123–125.

Miller, L. S., & Forer, S. K. (1983). Mortality among stroke patients following rehabilitation (Abstract). *Archives of Physical Medicine and Rehabilitation, 64*, 505.

Miller, L. S., & Johnston, M. V. (1985). One hundred point scale in functional assessment (Abstract). *Archives of Physical Medicine and Rehabilitation, 66*, 556.

Miller, L. S., & Miyamoto, A. T. (1979). Computer tomography: Its potential as a predictor of functional recovery following a stroke. *Archives of Physical Medicine and Rehabilitation, 60*, 108–109.

Miller, L. S., Miyamoto, A. T., & Forer, S. K. (1980, October). *The significance of carotid artery occlusion and stroke outcome*. Poster presented at the American Academy of Physical Medicine and Rehabilitation, Washington, DC.

Mor, V., Granger, C. V., & Sherwood, C. (1983). Discharged rehabilitation patients: Impact of follow-up surveillance by a friendly visitor. *Archives of Physical Medicine and Rehabilitation, 64*, 346–353.

Mullner, R., Nuzum, F. J., & Matthews, D. (1983). Inpatient medical rehabilitation: Results of the 1981 survey of hospitals and units. *Archives of Physical Medicine and Rehabilitation, 64*, 354–358.

National Association of Rehabilitation Facilities (1985). NARF position paper on a prospective payment system for inpatient medical rehabilitation services and a study regarding a prospective payment system for inpatient medical rehabilitation services: Final report. Washington, DC: Author.

Powell, J. W., & Scott, R. (1983). The role of computers in managing patient care. *Journal of American Health Care Association, 9*, 4–8.

Rao, N., Jellinek, H., Harvey, R., & Flynn, M. (1984). Computerized tomography head scans as predictors of rehabilitation outcome. *Archives of Physical Medicine and Rehabilitation, 65*, 18–20.

Rao, N., Jellinek, H. M., & Woolston, D. C. (1985). Agitation in closed head injury: Haloperidol effects on rehabilitation outcome. *Archives of Physical Medicine and Rehabilitation, 66*, 30–34.

Rappaport, M., Hall, K., Hopkins, K., & Belleza, T. (1981). Evoked potential and head injury: Clinical complications. *Clinical Electro Encephalography, 12*, 167–176.

Rappaport, M., Hall, K., Hopkins, K., Teodoro, B., & Cope, N. (1982). Disability rating scale for severe head trauma: Coma to community. *Archives of Physical Medicine and Rehabilitation, 63*, 118–123.

Reihman, J., Wolford, K., Knapp, W., MacCallum, J., & Murray, N. (1983). Treatment outcomes in a day treatment program. *International Journal of Partial Hospitalization, 2*, 18–31.

Reyes, R., & Heller, D. (1981) Traumatic head injury: Restlessness and agitation as prognosticators of physical and psychologic improvement in patients. *Archives of Physical Medicine and Rehabilitation, 62*, 20–23.

Robinson, R., Bolduc, P., Kubos, K., Starr, L., & Price, T. (1985). Social functioning assessment in stroke patients. *Archives of Physical Medicine and Rehabilitation, 66*, 496–500.

Romaniuk, J., & Blanks, E. (1984). Assessing automated information requirements in long-term care: Some general considerations. *Journal of Long Term Care Administration, 12*, 11–14.

Sarno, J., Sarno, M., & Levita, E. (1973). Functional life scale. *Archives of Physical Medicine and Rehabilitation, 54*, 214–220.

Schroder, P., & Washington, W. (1982). Administrative decision making: Staff patient ratios: A patient classification system for a psychiatric setting. *Perspectives in Psychiatric Care, 20*, 111–123.

Scranton, J., Fogel, M., & Edman, W. (1975). Evaluation of functional levels of patients during and following rehabilitation. *Archives of Physical Medicine and Rehabilitation, 56*, 375–382.

Susset, V., Vobecky, J., & Balck, R. (1979). Disability outcomes and self assessment of disabled persons: An analysis of 506 cases. *Archives of Physical Medicine and Rehabilitation, 60*, 50–56.

Teasdale, G., & Jennette, B. (1975). Assessment of coma and impaired consciousness: A practical scale. *Lancet, 1*, 480–484.

Timming, R., Orrison, W., & Mikula, J. (1982). Computerized tomograph and rehabilitation outcomes after severe head trama. *Archives of Physical Medicine and Rehabilitation, 63*, 154–159.

Udin, H., & May, B. (1982, November). *Rehabilitation: National norms and regional patterns of payment source and length of stay.* Poster presented at American Congress of Rehabilitation Medicine, 59th Annual Session, Houston.

Vaillant, G. (1966). Twelve year follow-up of New York narcotic addicts: I. Relation of treatment to outcome. *American Journal of Psychiatry, 122*, 727–737.

Van Ryswyk, C., Churchill, M., Velasquez, J., & McGuire, R. (1981–1982). Effectiveness of halfway house placement for alcohol and drug abuse. *American Journal of Drug and Alcohol Abuse, 8*, 494–512.

Wachtel, T., Derby, C., Fulton, J. (1984). Predicting the outcome of hospitalization for elderly persons: Home versus nursing home. *Southern Medical Journal, 77*, 1283–1286.

Watson, G., Daly, W., & Zimmerman, A. (1980). Staff attitudes and treatment effectiveness. *Journal of Clinical Psychology, 36*, 601–605.

Weddell, R., Oddy, M., & Jenkins, D. (1980). Social adjustment after rehabilitation: A two year follow-up of patients with severe head injury. *Psychosocial Medicine, 10*, 257–263.

Weiss, C. (1972). *Evaluation research: Methods for assessing program effectiveness.* Englewood Cliffs, NJ: Prentice-Hall.

Weissert, W., & Scanlon, W. (1985). Determinants of nursing home discharge status. *Medical Care, 23*, 333–343.

Wellington, S., Benditsky, H., Taintor, Z., & McCleery, G. (1985). So you have had a management information system: What's next? *Topics in Health Record Management, 5*, 53–63.

Williamson, J. (1971). Evaluating quality of patient care: Strategy relating outcome and process assessment. *Journal of the American Medical Association, 218*, 564–569.

Zahn, M., & Ball, J. (1972). Factors related to the cure of opiate addiction among Puerto Rican adults. *International Journal of Addictions, 7*, 237–245.

Chapter 10

A Uniform National Data System for Medical Rehabilitation

Byron B. Hamilton, Carl V. Granger,
Frances S. Sherwin, Maria Zielezny, and John S. Tashman

Medical rehabilitation did not begin to come of age until during and after World War II (1939–1945), as hundreds of thousands of disabled servicemen returned home. Their survival stimulated the medical and allied health professions to organize resources and develop better methods for restoring function of disabled individuals. The demands on rehabilitation proliferated as civilian acute care medicine continued to save more lives and as an increasing proportion of the population lived longer.

In the intervening years, significant changes have occurred: physicians and allied health professionals have turned their attention to the problems of rehabilitation in increasing numbers; the rehabilitation disciplines have organized into specialties, subspecialties, and group practices. For the most part third-party payors have covered the costs of rehabilitation services, and costs of providing service have increased . . . substantially!

Congress and the federal government attempted to control the rapidly rising costs of medical care (including medical rehabilitation) for Medicare-supported patients with the passage of the Social Security Amendments of 1983 (Public Law 98-21), which mandated prospective payment for services instead of reimbursement for "reasonable costs." Acute care hospitals were to be paid a predetermined amount for all patients with the same admitting diagnosis, based on the diagnostic related group (DRG), despite what

their care may have actually cost (Eisenberg, 1984).

Patients admitted for medical rehabilitation, however, are not treated on the basis of diagnosis, but rather on the basis of disability. Furthermore, the resources and time required to achieve the goals of rehabilitation are substantially different from those required for stabilizing the patient's medical condition during acute care. For example, the acute care of the spinal cord–injured paraplegic requires about 28 days, whereas the rehabilitation of that same patient requires about 60 days (Stover, Fine, & McEachren, 1982).

In attempting to set rehabilitation prospective payment criteria, the Health Care Financing Administration (HCFA) recognized the absence of a uniform way to measure medical rehabilitation interventions or outcomes. Also inadequate was documentation of a consistent relationship between patients' functional gains or benefits during rehabilitation, the services provided, and the costs incurred. Accordingly, HCFA recommended to Congress in 1983 that medical rehabilitation facilities be exempted from the Medicare prospective payment system until documentation could be provided in a uniform and reliable way. A time extension was requested by HCFA in 1985 after several studies could not resolve the issues. The National Association of Rehabilitation Facilities (NARF) recommended "A patient classification system, coding system, and uniform patient assessment instrument need to be developed

Supported by a grant from the National Institute of Handicapped Research (No. G008435062).

for inpatients of rehabilitation hospitals so that the industry's 'products' can be defined accurately." (NARF, 1985).

Meanwhile, at an October 1983 annual meeting forum concerning assessment of functional outcome, conducted by the American Congress of Rehabilitation Medicine (ACRM) and the American Academy of Physical Medicine and Rehabilitation (AAPMR), it was recommended that the two organizations establish a task force to develop a uniform national data system for medical rehabilitation. In the spring of 1984, the board of governors of each organization endorsed applying for a grant from the National Institute of Handicapped Research (NIHR) to support the task force in developing a data set that would document the outcomes and costs of medical rehabilitation. The need for such a data set was recognized throughout the rehabilitation industry and by those who regulate it. Twelve national organizations have either sponsored, endorsed, or actively cooperated in the development of a uniform medical rehabilitation data system.[1]

CONCEPTUAL FRAMEWORK OF REHABILITATION

The purpose of medical rehabilitation is to decrease disability and handicap of physically impaired individuals and to minimize the extent of impairment. The terms *impairment, disability,* and *handicap* are defined by the World Health Organization (WHO, 1980), and explained in greater detail in Chapter 1 of this text.

"Impairment" is any loss or abnormality of psychological, physiological, or anatomical *structure* or *function.* It pertains to organ systems. "Disability" is any restriction or lack of ability, resulting from an impairment, to perform an everyday *activity* in the manner or within the range considered normal for a person of the same age, culture, and education. "Handicap" is a dis-

advantage for a given individual, resulting from an impairment or a disability that limits or prevents the fulfillment of a *role* that is normal, depending on age, sex, and social and cultural factors, for the individual (WHO, 1980).

The activities and roles referred to here may be combined, for purposes of discussion, and called "life functions." The onset of a disabling impairment diminishes a person's life functions, often catastrophically. Over time, the natural healing process may restore some life functions. Comprehensive medical rehabilitation intervention is believed to augment restoration substantially. Figure 1 illustrates the expected impact of rehabilitation on the return of life functions.

Following a relatively short period of acute care, in which organ system functions are stabilized, the longer rehabilitation process begins. During rehabilitation (time period *a* in Figure 1), increase in life functions (*b* in Figure 1) attributed primarily to rehabilitation occurs. This increase is considered to be a primary outcome of the process. Furthermore, the extent to which life functions increase may reflect effectiveness of rehabilitation.

During rehabilitation, the time, resources, and money used reflect effort or energy expended. Efficiency (cost efficiency) of the rehabilitation process can be estimated by dividing the increase in life function *b* by the costs incurred during time *a*.

If changes in life function and service effort can be measured in a reliable manner, it follows that rehabilitation care providers would have a powerful tool to demonstrate the effectiveness and efficiency of services, thereby facilitating the management of resources. Reliable measures would also permit us to assess the influence on outcome of innovative care (that is, new or alternative programs, procedures, and devices developed through research). These measures of effectiveness and efficiency are consistent with the concept of the Joint Commission on Accredita-

---

[1]Sponsors of the Task Force to Develop a Uniform National Data System for Medical Rehabilitation: American Congress of Rehabilitation Medicine and American Academy of Physical Medicine and Rehabilitation. Endorsing organizations: National Association of Rehabilitation Facilities; Commission on Accreditation of Rehabilitation Facilities; American Hospital Association—Section for Rehabilitation Hospitals and Programs; National Association of Rehabilitation Research and Training Centers; American Spinal Injury Association; National Head Injury Foundation; and National Easter Seal Society. Cooperating Organizations: American Physical Therapy Association; American Occupational Therapy Association; American Speech, Language and Hearing Association; and Association of Rehabilitation Nurses.

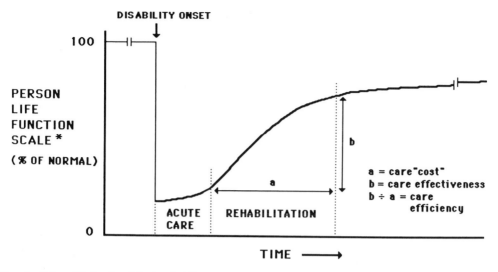

Figure 1.   Return of life functions following disability onset: expected impact of the rehabilitation process. Functions include self-care, mobility, communication, and other person *activities* related to disability; and vocation/education, independent living, and other *roles* related to handicap (WHO, 1980).

tion of Hospitals (JCAH) to demonstrate quality assurance in the delivery of rehabilitation services.

Another outcome attributable to the rehabilitation process concerns function after discharge from rehabilitation. The influence of rehabilitation is not expected to stop at discharge. Measures of postdischarge outcome should account for the extent and duration of gains accomplished during rehabilitation that an individual maintains or increases over time. The Commission on Accreditation of Rehabilitation Facilities (CARF) recognizes, in its requirements for program evaluation and follow-up, that the long-term benefits of rehabilitation are the payoff for society and the disabled individual.

If the means to measure life functions and the accompanying economic consequences of disability are available for the long term, determining cost–benefits and cost-effectiveness of the rehabilitation investment is feasible. The health and economic policy implications of such information, if uniformly and reliably reported, are considerable.

This conceptual framework, which defines and characterizes the rehabilitation process, serves as the basis for development of the uniform data system for medical rehabilitation.

DATA SYSTEM REQUIREMENTS AND DESIGN

A conventional systems description of the rehabilitation process is diagramed in Figure 2. It identifies and characterizes the input (patient attributes), process (rehabilitation provider programs, procedures and devices, as well as the research and training activities that sustain the process), output (patient attributes enhanced by the process), and cost to operate the process (third-party payors). Figure 2 also identifies the data system that interdigitates with and facilitates the care process. This section summarizes a data system design that enables the effectiveness, efficiency, and other outcomes of the rehabilitation process to be determined and then provided to multiple potential users.

The Data System and Data Set

Above the data system bar in Figure 2 are six numbered arrows, which indicate the types and sources of information for the data system.

1. Input Patient Data Accession   These data come from the patient and patient medical record on admission to medical rehabilitation. They characterize the patient and document baseline life functions, and include:

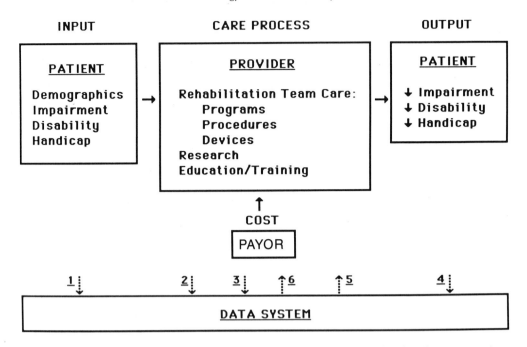

Figure 2.   The rehabilitation process. Elements in the data system are as follows: 1) input patient data, 2) care process data, 3) cost data, 4) output patient data, 5) process management report, and 6) third-party report.

Demographics—birth date, sex, race, English language competence, marital status, with whom living, zip code, and site from which the patient was admitted.

Impairment—impairment group, principal diagnosis, and date of onset of disabling impairment.

Disability—level on admission of independent function in the life activities of self-care, sphincter control, mobility, locomotion, communication, and social cognition. (The scale used to assess disability, the Functional Independence Measure [FIM], is described later in this chapter.)

Handicap—social role function as exemplified by employment and/or educational status prior to admission.

2. Care Process Data Accession   These data come primarily from patient medical records and include: facility code, patient number, admission date, admission class (initial rehabilitation, evaluation only, or readmission), number and duration of care program interruptions, and discharge date. Type and frequency of services provided, which would be derived from patient

financial and service department records, are not included in the initial version of the Uniform Data Set.

3. "Cost" Data Accession   These data come from hospital and physician financial records and include the total inpatient service charges. A surrogate cost estimate is length of stay.

4. Output Patient Data Accession

Impairment—includes medical complications during inpatient admission and at follow-up.

Disability—level at discharge and at follow-up, using the FIM.

Handicap—assessed by independent living and employment and/or educational status at discharge and at follow-up.

5. Process Management Report   These data are generated from the data base, accessed as noted above, and provided to administrative and clinical management of the hospital. Any data may be reported at specified frequencies.

6. Third-Party Report   These data are generated from the data base and would be provided on a restricted basis to "need to know" third parties for purposes of accountability and research. Individual hospital data would remain confidential except as required by law. Aggregate hospital data would be available for regulatory requirements and research.

The critical elements by which the rehabilitation care process may be assessed are derived from this data set. Such important elements as case mix; effectiveness, cost, and efficiency of care; short- and long-term outcome; accountability; and other measures of quality of care, resource utilization, and management may be evaluated. In addition, these data will facilitate research that would be used, in turn, to improve the care process. The documentation derived from this data set can better prepare new generations of clinicians, teachers, and researchers for their roles.

ASSESSMENT INSTRUMENT

The principal measure of human performance ability relevant to medical rehabilitation is disability, that is, the activities of everyday life (WHO, 1980). The instrument within the uniform data set designed to assess these activities is called the Functional Independence Measure (FIM).

Conceptual Basis of the FIM

The underlying conceptual basis of the FIM is the burden of care (type and amount of assistance) required for a disabled individual to perform basic life activities effectively. This burden of care, in turn, should translate into consumption of social and economic resources. Hence, the FIM is expected to reflect the *cost of disability* in social and economic terms.

The FIM does not measure all basic life activities. Rather, it measures a selected *minimum number* of key activities (see chapter Appendix A) intended to be necessary and sufficient (i.e., valid) indicators of level or cost of disability. A more diverse set of human activities is ordinarily assessed and monitored during the rehabilitation clinical care process. The FIM samples some of the more critical ones.

The FIM should measure level of disability regardless of the nature or extent of the underlying pathology or impairment. Hence, the degree of burden of care may be determined for a person with a stroke, cancer, or spinal cord injury as well as for the diverse secondary complications associated with these primary impairments. The FIM has not been specifically designed for use with individuals who have mental impairment only, although it does access certain important cognitive and behavioral activities.

Furthermore, the FIM is expected to be a reliable measure of severity of disability, regardless of the clinical training of the accessor. Its use is appropriate with medical and allied health professionals, as well as nonclinicians, family members, and patients when they have had sufficient orientation.

Finally, the FIM can be used in multiple settings, including a hospital, clinic, nursing home, or individual's home. Also, it should be useful throughout the lifespan, from childhood to old age.

How does the FIM reflect burden of care or cost of disability? Appendix B shows the specific definition of levels and Appendix A the function items included in the FIM. The four levels of the FIM are divided into two categories: "Independent" and "Dependent."

Levels 4 and 3—Independence, complete or modified, means the individual consistently performs the designated activity without the assistance of another person. The implication is that the individual does not incur the social or economic cost of another person in carrying out this necessary life activity.

Levels 2 and 1—Dependence, modified or complete, means the individual consistently performs the designated activity only with the presence or direct assistance of another person. A social (another person's effort) and/or economic cost is incurred by the disabled individual in carrying out a necessary life activity.

There are two levels within independence: at level 4, complete independence, the individual is performing at essentially a normal level. However, at level 3, modified independence, the activity is performed but with some delay, safety risk, or use of an assistive device. Although the assistance of another person is not required at level 3, the individual functions at a less efficient level than normal (a small but real cost to the person, household, work, or society) or he or she requires an assistive device, which must be purchased and maintained.

An important implication of the need for an assistive device is not so much the cost of the device, but the consequence of losing the device or not having it available when needed to perform the designated activity. If that happens, the individual will probably become much less efficient or may even need the assistance of another person. The temporary loss or breakdown of a wheelchair, prosthesis, crutch, or even reading glasses should illustrate the presence of a cost for the assistance provided by the device, or its unavailability.

The heavy cost of disability is reflected within dependence levels 2 and 1, where personal assistance is required. The difference between level 2, modified dependence, and level 1, complete dependence, is the extent (time and effort) to which another person is necessary in order to complete the designated activity. The differentiation of the two is whether the helper provides less than half the effort required to complete the task (modified dependence, level 2) or more than half (complete dependence, level 1). Although exactly how much "half" the effort comprises may sometimes seem unclear, it is obvious that an individual who needs almost total help is in a different category from the one who needs supervision only (level 2a) or touching only (level 2b, minimal assistance). Clinical judgment must be exercised in differentiating level 2c, moderate assistance, from level 1a, maximal assistance. Maximal assistance means the helper makes more than half of the effort to complete the task, while moderate assistance means the subject makes half or more of the effort. Finally, total assistance (level 1b) means the subject makes less than one-fourth of the effort, or none at all.

The helper cost is measured in hours or energy consumed (e.g., heavy lifting), stress of concern or responsibility for the individual's safety (e.g., falling), and the frustration of being on call constantly. The burden on unpaid family and friends is possibly greater than the cost of paid attendants, since the family may spend more total time with the disabled individual, perhaps losing income or the opportunity for recreation themselves.

In one setting, the cost of disability is rather clear. In nursing homes in which Resource Utilization Group (RUG) studies have been conducted, there is a direct and statistically supported relationship between level of patient activities of daily living (ADL) and hours of nursing staff time consumed (Fries & Cooney, 1985). Such a relationship has yet to be established for any functional measure in rehabilitation, including the FIM.

The issue of what would be considered "normal" assistance must also be addressed. We occasionally help another person in the course of normal daily life activities, whether he or she is disabled or not. That is, although a person *can* perform an activity he or she may *choose not to* do it, instead paying someone else to do it or using an assistive device. For example, hair may be washed at the barber shop or beauty salon or an elevator taken up one flight instead of using the stairs. The distinction between "normal" assistance and abnormal assistance is whether the person has a real choice to exercise the alternative. If one has the choice, that is, "can do" but "does not do," then "normal" assistance is employed.

However, it is not uncommon for disabled persons to have substantial assistance from family or friends when having assistance is *easier* than performing the tasks themselves (i.e., the person "can do" but "does not do"). This situation has several implications that challenge the conceptual basis as well as the validity and reliability of the FIM in assessing the cost of disability. For instance, if functional independence of the disabled individual was asssessed at home and numerous "can do" but "does not do" activities were found, how would the real level or cost of disability be determined? The "does not do" activities are performed by someone at some cost.

When using the FIM to assess the fundamental activities of daily living that the disabled individual *should* perform, rating what the person actually *does do* is necessary. The individual should consistently perform all the FIM items without assistance, except in those few situations that "normal" choice can be exercised, as described above. When having assistance with an activity is easier for a disabled individual, the activity is probably difficult for him or her to do independently and consistently, which, in turn, translates to a greater degree of disability. When a well-intentioned "helper" assists an otherwise independent disabled person with many self-care or mobility activities, the assistance, if consistently given, will likely contribute to muscle atrophy and loss of endurance and skill from disuse, which promotes further disability.

Technical Requirements

Validity Validating a functional assessment instrument with rigor is difficult. There are no "gold standards." At the outset, content validation of the FIM is being limited to face validity. That is, expert clinicians and researchers in the field exercise judgment as to whether the measure represents the universe of content and is applied appropriately to assess disability. Particularly necessary is determining whether the FIM is an adequate measure of disability. The method of assessing face validity relies on consensus of experienced clinicians in the field using the instrument under prospective trial conditions. The details of this assessment are discussed later in the section containing trial phase results.

Concurrent validity should be establishable because numerous relevant functional assessment instruments currently in clinical use can be compared to the FIM. Correlational techniques are the principal methods used to draw comparison conclusions. Factor analysis also will aid in establishing the validity of the FIM (Armitage, 1971).

According to Donabedian (1969), "outcomes . . . remain the ultimate validation of the effectiveness and quality of medical care" (p.168). Establishing concurrent predictive validity of the FIM should be possible when the criterion is rehabilitation outcome(s), which presumably can be measured. However, a method to assess predictive validity is not addressed at this time.

Reliability Interrater agreement using the FIM is crucial because any number of clinicians and even nonclinicians could be involved in as-

sessing patient function. The principal evaluators are expected to be physicians, nurses, and physical and occupational therapists.

Test–retest reliability and internal consistency are less important, given the intended use of the instrument (essentially program evaluation), the nature of subjects (known to exhibit slow change on key variables), and the number of items (relatively few items included in the instrument).

Precision Precision of a measure is the degree of change detectable by it, and requirements should be determined by the intended use of the measure. In the design of the FIM, a balance was struck among precision sufficient to determine meaningful change in level of function, adequate reliability, and simplicity of administration. To achieve this balance, the FIM has been designed to discriminate four basic and seven refined levels of functional independence.

A four-level scale with sublevels as described for each item on the FIM is expected to be precise enough to detect change in level of disability from admission to discharge for most patients whom rehabilitation services would expect to benefit. Likewise, follow-up changes, although often small, should still be detectable when item scores are summed.

Assessment of precision adequacy of the FIM has been empirically based through the trial phase. Clinicians have indicated when a four-level FIM was not sufficient for measuring change. Later, a statistical assessment of adequacy of precision will be made.

Instrument Development

The Uniform Data Set is being developed using an iterative process consisting of four phases spanning 3 years: pilot, trial, implementation, and revision. The tasks for the four phases, beginning January, 1985, are:

Pilot Phase (completed April, 1985)—The specific purposes were to determine initial face validity of the data set, identify problems clinicians had in learning how to use the instrument, and estimate time to learn and to administer the instrument. The results are described in the progress section of this chapter.

Trial Phase (completed April, 1986)—The specific purposes were to reassess face validity, determine interrater reliability, gauge level of precision, and reassess time to learn and to administer.

Implementation Phase—With this phase, the system becomes operational. The revised data set is introduced to a number of hospitals. The dissemination (marketing and training) and utilization (data management service and software release) tasks are added to the instrument refinement tasks. Validity and reliability are reassessed. This phase began in the fall of 1986, with a reliability check carried out shortly therafter. The dissemination and utilization tasks are described in greater detail below.

Revision Phase—Every ongoing data system requires periodic assessment for continued validity and reliability. Revisions may be introduced if changing requirements dictate.

DISSEMINATION AND UTILIZATION

Critical aspects of developing a uniform national data system are dissemination and utilization of the system components: the data set, data management service, and computer software. Without sufficient utilization, such a system has little meaning.

To facilitate national use of the data set, a two-path strategy has been proposed. Path A is directed toward developing a centralized data management service into which data collected by rehabilitation hospitals are merged, stored, and reported to data users. Path B is directed toward individual hospital processing of data on that hospital's own mini- or microcomputer using a Uniform Rehabilitation Data Set software package developed specifically for this purpose. This computer program would permit a hospital to collect and maintain its own patient data base for management and research. The program would also permit hospital data to be transmitted easily to a central data management service by disk mailing or telephone modem. In addition, the hospital using the software package could retrieve central data, subject to certain restrictions.

Although the initial development costs of both data management service and software are borne by the project grant, maintenance of the service and initial purchase of the run-time program for the data management software will be the responsibility of participating hospitals. These costs are expected to be quite modest. Both the data management service and software implementation have been targeted for fall of 1986, as part of the implementation phase.

PILOT AND TRIAL PHASE ASSESSMENT

Assessment of the FIM component of the data set has been conducted first as a pilot phase addressing face validity and precision, and second as a trial phase addressing validity, precision, and reliability. The FIM was modified after each phase, based on clinician responses.

Validity

Face validity was assessed by asking experienced clinicians who administered the FIM four questions:

1. Were there items that were difficult to understand?
2. Were there items that were unnecessary?
3. Were there items that should be added?
4. How would you rate the FIM as a measure of severity of disability on a 1 to 5 scale, with 1 = poor, 3 = OK, and 5 = excellent? (Granger, Hamilton, Keith, Zielezny, & Sherwin, 1986).

During the pilot phase, 114 clinicians from 11 medical rehabilitation inpatient facilities assessed 110 patients. The average number of years of clinical rehabilitation experience was 5.8. The clinical disciplines included physical therapy (24%), occupational therapy (20%), nursing (18%), medicine (17%), psychology (8%), speech-language pathology (7%), recreational therapy (4%), and social work (3%).

During the trial phase, 891 clinician assessments were performed at 25 facilities on 250 patients. The average number of years of rehabilitation experience was 6.8. The clinical disciplines included occupational therapy (28%), physical therapy (28%), nursing (27%), and medicine (17%).

The responses to the four validity assessment questions are indicated in Table 1. Face validity appears to be good.

The major revision of the FIM after the pilot and trial phases was addition of subcategories to the "Modified Dependence" and "Complete Dependence" categories. This change, as well as other refinements, improved the overall face validity rating and diminished the frequency of "Add items?" responses.

Precision

The ability of the FIM to detect change in functional level was the most frequently mentioned concern of clinicians in their open-ended written comments during the pilot phase. This concern was also reflected in the high frequency (31%) of "Add items?" responses during the pilot phase. The suggestion to add items decreased to 17% during the trial phase, presumably as a result of elaboration of the "Dependence" levels. Precision will be assessed more rigorously measuring significance of change in the FIM over time for specific patient impairment groups from admission to rehabilitation discharge, and from discharge to follow-up.

Reliability

Interrater reliability based on the sum of all FIM items at four levels of precision appears to be consistent and acceptably high at this point in development. One-way analysis of variance was used to assess 303 pairs of clinicians administering the FIM to patients at admission and 184 pairs at discharge. The intraclass correlation was .86 on admission and .88 at discharge, indicating good agreement between observers.

An alternative means of assessing interrater reliability for each of the single items constituting the FIM was the intraclass correlation, κ (*Kappa*), which adjusts for agreement due to chance (Fleiss, 1981). The average κ for each of

the 18 items comprising the FIM was .54. A κ of .40 to .75 is considered fair to good agreement beyond chance. No single item fell below .43. Therefore, average FIM single-item interrater reliability at this phase of development appears to be fairly good.

We anticipate that refinement of several items and structured training of clinicians in the use of the FIM will result in good to excellent reliability. Pilot and trial phase training was limited to learning from unrefined written material without benefit of feedback. These changes will be assessed during the implementation phase.

The time required to collect the demographic data from the medical and financial records was on average less than 10 minutes per record. The average time required initially to learn to administer the FIM was 41 miniutes and, once learned, 32 minutes per patient to assess and record the data.

Finally, with regard to the other key components of the data system, a second-generation software program and a prototype data management service have been developed by the project staff and consultants. These will be usable in the field on a developmental basis beginning in the fall of 1986.

POTENTIAL USES FOR A UNIFORM DATA SET AND SYSTEM

In conclusion, a uniform data set and system should provide the following information:

1. Uniform language, definitions, and measurements that describe disability and the rehabilitation process.
2. Normative and variability data about impairment, level of disability and handicap, outcomes of care, duration, and costs of (charges for) care.
3. A basis for determining cost–benefits and cost-effectiveness of rehabilitation care.
4. A basis for predicting rehabilitation outcome, which has implications for establishing criteria for admission, discharge, and referral to alternate appropriate and possibly less costly services.

Table 1. Responses to validity assessment

	Pilot	Trial
"Items difficult?"	12%	12%
"Items unnecessary?"	1%	3%
"Add items?"	31%	17%
"Overall rating?" (1–5)	2.98	3.44

5. A basis for justifying payment for services (Medicare—HCFA). The FIM or a derivative of the FIM could be used to establish a prospective payment system for rehabilitation services, provided that the economic basis of the measure is substantiated in quantitative terms.
6. A basis for determining and monitoring quality of care (JCAH), evaluating programs (CARF), and justifying accreditation.
7. Feedback information to care providers, which can facilitate clinical and administrative decision making.
8. A basis for development of policies and planning that will improve the rehabilitation process.
9. A basis for facilitating and evaluating innovative or research interventions.

We expect that many, if not most, of these needs can be satisfied by the data set and system currently under development and described here as the Uniform National Data System for Medical Rehabilitation.

APPENDIX A: FIM ITEMS

Self-Care

Feeding—includes all aspects of eating and drinking, such as opening containers, pouring liquids, cutting meat, and buttering bread, chewing, and swallowing.

Grooming—includes oral care, hair grooming, washing hands and face, shaving, and applying make-up.

Bathing—includes bathing the entire body from the neck down (tub, shower, or bed bath).

Dressing: Upper Body—includes dressing above the waist as well as donning and removing prosthesis or orthosis when applicable.

Dressing: Lower Body—includes dressing from the waist down as well as donning or removing prosthesis or orthosis when applicable.

Toileting—includes maintaining perineal hygiene and adjusting clothing after toileting.

Sphincter Control

Bladder Management—includes complete intentional control of urinary bladder and management of equipment necessary for emptying.

Bowel Management—includes complete intentional control of bowel movement and use of laxatives, suppositories, and manual evacuation.

Mobility

Transfers: Bed, Chair, Wheelchair—includes management of all aspects of transferring to and from bed, chair, or wheelchair, or coming to a standing position, if walking is the typical mode of locomotion.

Transfer: Toilet—includes getting on and off toilet.

Transfers: Tub or Shower—includes getting into and out of a tub or shower stall.

Locomotion

Walking or Using Wheelchair—includes walking, or using wheelchair, once in a seated position, indoors.

Stairs—includes going up and down 12–14 stairs (one flight).

Communication

Comprehension—includes clear comprehension of either auditory or visual communication.

Expression—includes clear expression of either verbal or nonverbal language.

Social Cognition

Social Interaction—includes skills related to getting along and participating with others in therapeutic and social situations.

Problem Solving—includes skills related to using previously learned information to solve problems of daily living.

Memory—includes skills related to awareness in performing daily activities in an institutional or community setting.

APPENDIX B: FIM DESCRIPTION OF GENERAL LEVELS OF FUNCTION

Independent—Another person is not required for the activity (NO HELPER).

4. **Complete Independence**—all of the tasks described as making up the activity are typically performed safely without modification, assistive devices, or aids, and within a reasonable time.

3. **Modified Independence**—Activity requires any one or more than one of the following: an assistive device, more than reasonable time, or safety (risk) considerations.

Dependent—Another person is required for either supervision or physical assistance in order for the activity to be performed, or it is not performed (REQUIRES HELPER).

2. **Modified Dependence**—The subject expends half (50%) or more of the effort. The levels of assistance required are:
   a. Supervision—subject requires no more help than cuing or coaxing, without physical contact
   b. Minimal assistance—subject requires no more help than touching, or subject expends 75% or more of the effort.
   c. Moderate assistance—subject requires more help than touching, or expends half (50%) or more (up to 75%) of the effort.

1. **Complete Dependence**—subject expends less than half (less than 50%) of the effort. Maximal or total assistance is required, or the activity is not performed. The levels of assistance required are: 1a) maximal assistance—subject expends less than 50% of the effort, but at least 25%; 1b) total assistance—subject expends less than 25% of the effort.

REFERENCES

Armitage, P. (1971). *Statistical methods in medical research.* London: Blackwell Scientific.

Donabedian, A. (1969). *A guide to medical care administration. Vol. II. Medical care appraisal: Quality and utilization* (p.168). Washington, DC: The American Public Health Association.

Eisenberg, B. S. (1984). Diagnosis related groups, severity of illness, and equitable reimbursement under Medicare. *Journal of the American Medical Association, 251,* 645–646.

Fleiss, J. L. (1981). *Statistical methods for rates and proportions* (2nd ed.). New York: John Wiley & Sons.

Fries, B. E., & Cooney, L. M. (1985). Resource utilization groups: A patient classification system for long-term care. *Medical Care, 23,* 110–132.

Granger, C. V., Hamilton, B. B., Keith, R. A., Zielezny, M., & Sherwin, F. S. (1986). Advances in functional assessment for medical rehabilitation. *Topics in Geriatric Rehabilitation, 1*(3), 59–74.

National Association of Rehabilitation Facilities. (1985). *NARF position paper on a prospective payment system for inpatient medical rehabilitation services and a study regarding a prospective payment system for inpatient medical rehabilitation services: Final report.* Washington, DC: Author.

Stover, S. L., Fine, P. R., & McEachran, A. B. (1982). *Final report of the UAB spinal cord injury care system.* Birmingham: University of Alabama.

World Health Organization. (1980). *International classification of impairments, disabilities, and handicaps.* Geneva: Author.

SECTION III

Applications to
Rehabilitation Target Groups

Chapter 11

Analyzing Outcomes in the Care of Persons with Multiple Sclerosis

Nicholas G. LaRocca

Functional assessment represents the evaluation of an individual's level of performance, whereas outcome analysis emphasizes the measurement of change in those areas amenable to intervention (Brown, Gordon, & Diller, 1983). Outcome assessment encompasses a wide range of functions along with mediating forces and the social context of the individual. In this chapter, functional assessment in multiple sclerosis (MS) is discussed within the broader perspective of evaluating rehabilitation outcome. The framework of the World Health Organization (WHO, 1980) *International Classification of Impairments, Disabilities, and Handicaps* (ICIDH) will be used. A brief description of MS is followed by some of the early history of assessment in MS. Next is a discussion of the special assessment needs of this illness. The bulk of the chapter describes the Minimal Record of Disability (MRD), a core assessment instrument resulting from international consensus and incorporating the expanded perspective necessary in the evaluation of rehabilitation outcome. Finally, other assessment methods with special application to MS are described.

THE NATURE OF MULTIPLE SCLEROSIS

Etiology and Pathogenesis

Multiple sclerosis is a disease of the brain and spinal cord with onset typically during the adult years. In MS, myelin is destroyed in widely distributed areas of the central nervous system (CNS). Myelin is a multilayered coating of fat and protein produced by oligodendrocytes and wrapped around the axons of nerve cells. Since myelin acts as an insulating sheath for the nerves, its destruction and replacement by sclerotic plaques result in loss of nerve conduction. Signals that ordinarily move rapidly through the CNS are slowed or completely blocked.

The etiology of MS is unknown. Although theories abound, the two most prominent are the autoimmune theory and the viral theory. The autoimmune theory postulates that MS arises from some immunoregulatory deficit, causing the immune system to attack the body's own tissue, perhaps in response to an antigen of myelin or of the oligodendrocytes themselves. The viral theory holds that MS is caused by a latent virus acquired early in life, probably before age 15. It remains dormant until reactivated by unknown means.

Clinical Features

Once MS is contracted, no known treatment can cure the disease or arrest its progress. In a lucky few, the disease remains stable after the initial attack. More commonly, several attacks occur, each followed by a period of partial or total recovery. In some cases, symptoms get progressively worse with no clearly defined attacks or remis-

Preparation of this chapter was supported in part by grants from the National Institute of Handicapped Research (#G008200046) and the National Multiple Sclerosis Society (RG 1459-A-7).

sions. Although unpredictable, the course of MS is generally characterized by slow worsening of symptoms with new symptoms occasionally appearing.

Since any of the myelinated areas, that is, the white matter, of the CNS may be affected, the list of possible symptoms is long. Typically, MS is a disorder of gait accompanied by sensory changes, visual disturbances, and bladder dysfunction. Symptom patterns vary considerably and may also include fatigue, spasticity, intention tremor, nystagmus, bowel problems, dysarthria, sexual difficulties, intellectual decline, emotional lability, and dizziness.

Social and Personal Impact

For the individual, the symptoms of MS generally have a significant negative impact on everyday life. Restricted mobility and reduced independence in activities of daily living (ADL) are perhaps the most important. Ability to work is usually affected; more than 75% of persons with MS are unemployed (Kornblith, LaRocca, & Baum, 1986). Social and recreational activities may be reduced and financial resources stretched to their limit. As a result, psychological distress and family upheaval can ensue.

The impact of MS is particularly acute because it strikes during the peak years of family and career formation. The average age of onset is 34, and 58% of cases begin between the ages of 20 and 50 (Baum & Rothschild, 1981). In 1976, the latest year for which figures are available, the average person with MS lost $4,855 in earnings and spent $1,672 on medical costs annually (Inman, 1984). Since the normal life expectancy is reduced little if at all in MS (Kurzke et al., 1970), the cumulative impact on the individual, the family, and society may be staggering.

The Rehabilitation of Persons with MS

Despite many sobering statistics concerning MS, other aspects are more encouraging. In a national survey of persons with MS, 40% of the respondents reported no mobility restrictions (Baum & Rothschild, 1983). Advances in the management of bladder dysfunction (Blaivas et al., 1984) and in vocational rehabilitation have helped to im-

prove the quality of life for many persons with MS.

The improving situation in MS is in part the result of a shift in emphasis over the last 30 years. Since there is no known way to alter the natural history of the disease, clinical management has moved more in the direction of preventing and minimizing complications while assisting patients and families in adapting to the disease (Scheinberg, Holland, Kirschenbaum, Oaklander, & Geronemus, 1981). The comprehensive model of care (Scheinberg, Giesser, & Slater, 1983), incorporating psychosocial and vocational interventions (Marsh, Ellison, & Strite, 1983), is now widely accepted. As the care of the person with MS has evolved toward a rehabilitative model, interest in functional assessment has grown. Although functional assessment instruments abound, most were developed for use in other conditions and have limited applicability to MS. The extensive involvement of community organizations in planning and providing services for the person with MS has also fostered the search for better ways to assess functional status (Slater, LaRocca, & Scheinberg, 1984).

HISTORY OF ASSESSMENT IN MULTIPLE SCLEROSIS

Early Developments

Despite the critical role of rehabilitation in MS, most assessment methods have originated in neurology. Early efforts were geared toward the evaluation of therapeutic trials (Kurtzke & Berlin, 1954) or the identification of prognostic indicators (Hyllested, 1961). Nevertheless, functional disability has been addressed in virtually every assessment system developed for use in MS.

The diversity of symptoms in MS renders assessment a formidable task. Workers in MS have long recognized the distinction between neurological signs and symptoms and functional disability (Alexander, 1951). Substantial changes in function may accompany small changes in signs and symptoms. It is thus not surprising that several attempts have been made to develop a method for globally rating functional disability in MS. MacLean and Berkson (1951) classified patients as "incapacitated" or "not incapacitated." Later, somewhat more sophisticated systems were proposed, including Thygesen's (1953) 5-point scale, McAlpine, Compston, and Lumsden's (1955) 6-point scale, and Hyllested's (1961) 6-point scale. These early rating scales primarily reflect mobility and independence in everyday activities. They resemble the Kurtzke (1955) Disability Status Scale (DSS), the current standard, which is described below.

Several other detailed MS assessment methods that have been developed focus primarily on neurological impairment. Alexander (1951) devised a complex system of weighted scores in 30 areas, with composite scores ranging from 0 (normal) to -500 (totally disabled). One of the 30 areas rated was mobility, much like the global scales. Fog (1965) proposed a four-part system, including cranial nerves, upper and lower extremities, and the sensory system. Again, ability to walk was incorporated. Pedersen (1965) developed a method for rating patients in six areas. He included not only walking, but also "personal efficiency," that is, independence in everyday activities. These methods resemble the Kurtzke Functional Systems (FS), which, together with the Kurtzke DSS, constitute the most widely used of the several MS impairment/disability systems.

The Kurtzke System

The name John Kurtzke is practically synonymous with assessment in MS. In fact, the most widely used system for grading severity in MS is usually termed the "Kurtzke." This system originally consisted of the Disability Status Scale (DSS), an 11-step ordinal scale ranging from "0" (normal) to "10" (death due to MS). (Kurtzke, 1955). The ratings were based on the results of the neurological examination, but with the greatest weight given to ambulation. Unfortunately, the DDS lacked a standardized method for grading impairment in the various neurological systems. Kurtzke (1961, 1965, 1970) later provided such a method in the form of seven ordinal rating scales known as the Functional Systems (FS). The DSS was then based on the results of the FS but still heavily weighted toward ambulation.

A major limitation of the Kurtzke system has been its lack of a numerical algorithm for deriving the DSS from the FS. Instead, the DSS uses an informal, descriptive combination of the FS and mobility. In addition, many users of the DSS have found that an 11-point scale is not sensitive enough to detect subtle changes in clinical status. Kurtzke (1983) attempted to answer some of these criticisms with a revised version of the FS and an Expanded DSS (EDSS). The new EDSS still ranges from 0 to 10, but in half-point increments, allowing for more precision in evaluating disease severity. Unfortunately, the descriptive method of arriving at the EDSS using the FS was retained. In addition the different grades are not always mutually exclusive. Moreover, patients with a very high rating on only one of the FS (e.g., legally blind but with normal gait) are difficult to rate meaningfully on the EDSS.

Despite these limitations, most patients can be rated quickly and easily. Whereas the FS rate neurological impairments that are little affected by rehabilitation, the emphasis of the EDSS on mobility makes it potentially useful as a very general outcome measure in rehabilitation. The DSS and EDSS provide a common language for clinicians and researchers, and almost every clinical study of MS during the past few years has used the DSS as a measure of severity. Since the FS and DSS form a major component of the MRD, additional characteristics of these instruments are described in detail below.

DEVELOPMENT OF THE MINIMAL RECORD OF DISABILITY

Background and Purpose

Notwithstanding widespread acceptance of the Kurtzke system (1955, 1961, 1970, 1983), the FS and EDSS are primarily measures of neurological impairment revealing little about functional disability. Only fragmentary data have been available concerning the independence, self-care, service needs, and social role performance of persons with MS. Building on a suggestion made in 1972 by Tore Broman, Slater proposed in 1979 that the International Federation of Multiple Sclerosis Societies (IFMSS) create a standardized minimal record of functional status for MS (Slater, 1981). Thereafter, work began on developing the MRD for MS (Slater, Fog & Bergmann, 1981), and has continued since its publication (Haber & LaRocca, 1985; Slater, 1984; Slater & Raun, 1984).

The MRD was designed to be implemented in a variety of settings for the purposes of:

1. Providing an internationally comparable core of information
2. Aiding in planning individual, community, and national services
3. Complementing neurological examinations and other measures in clinical trials
4. Evaluating outcomes of medical, social, and rehabilitative interventions
5. Researching the individual, familial, social, and economic ramifications of MS
6. Serving as a quantitative indicator of functional status in clinical settings.

Criteria

Taking into account the intended uses of the MRD and the special requirements of MS, this new instrument was designed to fulfill the following criteria (Haber & LaRocca, 1985):

1. The MRD should include the least information required for practical assessment of the individual's functional capabilities and needs.
2. The descriptors used for various functions must be compatible with the terminology used by the various professions (e.g., neurology, rehabilitation, nursing, and social work) which participate in the medical and social care of patients with MS.
3. The MRD must comprise questions that are adequately inclusive and clearly descriptive of functional disabilities so as to be meaningful when translated into different languages.
4. Existing record systems for MS in different centers should be compatible with the MRD, so that the individual MRD items can be readily correlated with methods of assessment already in use.
5. Sufficient measures of performance should be included, despite possible redundancy, to

assure usefulness to community health professionals for planning services.
6. The MRD should be constructed in such a way that it can be administered either by health professionals or by volunteers trained and supervised by professionals.
7. The design of the MRD should follow as closely as possible the WHO *Classification of Impairments, Disabilities, and Handicaps*.

The MRD was thus seen as the minimal core data set that would facilitate interinstitutional and international communication. It was not assumed that the MRD alone would satisfy all the information needs of a given user. Instead, each user would add to the MRD those measures needed to round out the assessment.

CONTENT OF THE MRD

The MRD has five sections and is organized around the three-tier classification of dysfunction developed by the WHO (1980). Scores for all of the items on the MRD may be recorded on a single two-sided page.

During the course of its development, the MRD has periodically been revised and updated. The latest version as of this writing (Haber & LaRocca, 1985) is available from the National Multiple Sclerosis Society. Data from both the current and previous versions are presented.

Demographic Information

Twelve questions cover identifying information, date of onset and diagnosis of the illness, birthdate, education, marital status, household composition, and vocational data. Questions on topics that are very specific to each country are not included. Instead, users employ their own questions, thus better reflecting local needs. Ethnicity is one such topic. Administered as an interview, this section can be performed by a supervised nonprofessional, and requires less than 5 minutes to complete.

Functional Systems

The first of two measures of neurological impairment, the FS consists of nine single-item scales designed to quantify the results of the neurological examination. John Kurtzke (1961, 1965, 1970, 1983) developed the FS. Functions assessed include pyramidal, cerebellar, brainstem, sensory, bowel/bladder, visual, cerebral (mental), spasticity, and "other." These ordinal rating scales use a 0 and 1, 0 to 3, 0 to 5, or 0 to 6 format. They can be rated only by a physician or other professional competent in performing a neurological examination. The FS are rated after such an examination has been completed. Although the FS require less than 5 minutes to complete, the length of the neurological examination depends upon the thoroughness of the examiner. The FS were not designed to be summed into a composite score, but instead are used descriptively along with other factors to arrive at an overall rating of disease severity.

Disability Status Scale

The DSS (Kurtzke, 1955, 1961, 1965, 1970) and EDSS (Kurtzke, 1983) constitute the second measure of neurological impairment in the MRD. Both are ordinal rating scales that may approach an interval level of measurement. Both range from 0 (normal neurological) to 10 (death due to MS), but the DSS has 11 steps, whereas the EDSS has 20. The EDSS was designed to replace the DSS with a grading scheme more sensitive to change. Ratings are based upon the FS and on the patient's ability to walk. The rater should be a neurologist or other professional competent in performing the neurological examination. Although rating the DSS or EDSS takes just a few seconds, completing the neurological examination and FS adds to the time needed to arrive at a score.

Despite its more than 30-year history, there are suprisingly few published data on the measurement properties of the FS and DSS. Both are clearly ordinal scales, although Kurtzke (1955, 1965, 1983) has pointed out that the bell-shaped distribution usually found with the DSS suggests that its steps may approach an equal interval scale. The reliability of the system was investigated in connection with the cooperative study of adrenocorticotropic hormone (ACTH) (Kuzma et al., 1969). Using an incomplete Latin-square design, both the FS and the DSS were found to be stable across raters and administrations, that

is, in almost all cases, mean differences were not significant. In a study at the Albert Einstein College of Medicine, this author found an intraclass correlation coefficient of .98 between DSS scores on 20 patients obtained independently by two neurologists. The FS were designed to measure nonredundant factors. Supporting this notion, a recent study found intercorrelations of the FS to be modest, ranging from .10 to .57 with a mean of .33 (LaRocca, Scheinberg, & Slater, 1984). In support of the use of the FS and DSS as indicators of change, Kurtzke (1961, 1983) has shown how scores vary between hospital admission and discharge. As would be expected, the vast majority either remain the same (61%) or improve (16%). In the ACTH study (Rose et al., 1970), correlations between the number of items improved on the FS/DSS and the number of items improved on the standard neurological exam (SNE) and Quantitative Examination of Neurologic Functions ranged from .45 to .61. The same study provided further evidence for the validity of the FS/DSS system. Correlations with the SNE were .81 for the DSS and .79 for a composite of the FS.

Incapacity Status Scale

The Incapacity Status Scale (ISS) is a 16-item inventory of functional disability based in large part on the PULSES Profile (Moskowitz & McCann, 1957) and the Barthel Index (Mahoney & Barthel, 1965) with additions to better cover the disabilities seen in MS, such as fatigue. It was assembled by John Kurtzke (1981) and Carl Granger (1981) in collaboration with members of the IFMSS. Each of the 16 items is rated on a 0 to 4 ordinal scale. In addition, there is a 13-item sexual concern inquiry, which is not used in arriving at an overall score. The ratings for each item may be used singly or a composite score may be obtained by summing scores on the 16 items. The ISS can be employed in one of two ways. A structured interview can be administered to the patient, whose responses then form the basis of the ratings. As an alternative, some of the items can be used to rate the results of actual testing of functions, such as ambulation, transfers, and grooming. Thus the ISS may be scored either as a "can do" or a "does do" measure. The interview takes approximately 20 minutes to complete and may be performed by a trained and supervised nonprofessional.

Due in large part to the IFMSS field testing, a large number of data have been gathered concerning the two new components of the MRD, the ISS and the Environmental Status Scale (ESS). Both the North American (LaRocca et al., 1984) and Danish (Fog et al., 1984) studies addressed the question of reliability (internal consistency) of the composite ISS score. The results, summarized in Table 1, are pertinent to the issue of reliability and cross-national validity of the ISS. Although the Danish sample was slightly more disabled than the North American, the Cronbach's alphas were identical (.93) and the patterns of corrected item-total correlations were nearly the same. Despite the high alphas, it is difficult to state what is measured by a score containing items as diverse as vision and sexual function. Both sets of item-total correlations suggest that mobility and self-care constitute the major dimensions underlying ISS scores. Indeed, items unrelated to mobility and self-care have lower item-total correlations.

This issue was illuminated by three factor-analytical studies, the two previously mentioned and one conducted in the Netherlands (Minderhoud,

Dassel, & Prange, 1984). The North American study used principal factoring, the Danish study alpha factoring, and all three employed varimax rotation. Table 2 provides a simplified summary of the results. In all three studies, the greatest proportion of variance is accounted for by an ambulation/self-care factor. Although there are slight differences among the three in the items loading on this factor, the similarities are striking. In contrast, the second and third factors differ markedly among the three studies. These results suggest that composite ISS scores should be used with caution. The ISS is heterogeneous in content and total scores mainly reflect global disability in mobility and self-care, with some important problems not well represented. A weighted ISS composite consisting only of ambulation and self-care items might be preferable to a simple summing of all 16 items. Moreover, at present, the cross-national validity of the ISS is confined to this global indication of disability.

Table 1. Item analysis of the Incapacity Status Scale

	Corrected item-total correlations	
	North America	Denmark
Item		
Transfers	.86	.87
Bathing	.85	.89
Dressing	.84	.86
Ambulation	.83	.86
Stair climbing	.82	.83
Grooming	.73	.71
Societal role	.72	.80
Feeding	.68	.72
Bladder function	.62	.61
Fatigability	.56	.30
Sexual function	.53	.57
Bowel function	.52	.64
Vision	.47	.43
Speech/hearing	.43	.36
Psychic function	.41	.33
Physical problems	.25	.27
Summary statistics		
Total: Mean	17.9	23.0
S.D.	12.5	14.5
Cronbach's alpha	.93	.93

Table 2. Comparison of factor-analytical studies of the Incapacity Status Scale*

North America	Denmark	The Netherlands
Factor #1:		
Stair climbing	Stair climbing	Stair climbing
Ambulation	Ambulation	Ambulation
Transfers	Transfers	Transfers
Bladder		
Bathing	Bathing	Bathing
Dressing	Dressing	Dressing
	Grooming	Grooming
	Feeding	Feeding
		Physical problems
Societal Role		Societal role
Factor #2:		
	Bowel	
	Bladder	
Grooming		
Feeding		
Vision		Vision
		Speech
	Fatigability	
	Psychic function	Psychic function
	Sexual function	
Factor #3:		
		Bowel
		Bladder
	Physical problems	
Fatigability		
		Sexual function

*(items with factor loadings of .50 or higher)

Composite scores for the ISS appear to have good reproducibility. With two independent physician raters, LaRocca et al. (1984) obtained an intraclass correlation coefficient of .94. Using a Pearson correlation coefficient, Johnson, Lambie, Peace, and Thompson (1984) found a somewhat lower level of covariation, .78. However, when only those items that best predict the socioeconomic consequences of MS were used, the correlation coefficient rose to .88. The later study also examined agreement on individual ISS items, finding that fatigue, psychic function, vision, and bladder function had the lowest correlation, all with r values below .50. Similarly, LaRocca et al. (1984) found that the four worst items were fatigue, physical problems, bladder function, and psychic function. Other items showed adequate levels of agreement.

The ISS was designed to measure functional disability. Evidence for the validity of the measure comes from several different sources. First, the ISS is based on widely recognized measures of functional status, the PULSES Profile and the Barthel Index. Scores from the ISS correlate highly with an accepted measure of severity in MS, the DSS. LaRocca et al. (1984) found an r of .81, and Fog et al. (1984) obtained a Spearman ρ of .87. An early study comparing Granger's Long Range Evaluation System and the ISS reported a correlation of .87 (Kurtzke, 1981). Among patients undergoing inpatient treatment at the Burke Rehabilitation Center, this author found a correlation of .74 between ISS scores and the number of hours of home assistance needed.

Environmental Status Scale

Developed by a committee of the IFMSS (Mellerup et al., 1981), the ESS provides an assessment of social handicap resulting from chronic illness. Seven items pertaining to work, finances, home, personal assistance, transportation, community assistance, and social activity are each rated on an ordinal scale ranging from 0 to 5. Although a composite score can be obtained by summing the seven ratings, the heterogeneity of the items favors using them individually. As with the ISS, a structured interview is used to gather information from the patient and arrive at the ratings. Alternatively, the items may

be rated on the basis of records or other knowledge of the patient's situation. The ESS takes about 10 minutes to complete and can be administered by a trained and supervised nonprofessional.

The ESS has been the subject of similar studies in North America (LaRocca et al., 1984) and Denmark (Fog et al., 1984). Considering a composite score, Table 3 shows that both studies found nearly identical patterns of item-total correlations and comparably high alphas. In a factor-analytical study, Minderhoud et al. (1984) found two relatively weak factors. Although the numerical internal consistency of the ESS supports the use of a composite score, the heterogeneity of its content discourages it. It is difficult to state what a score drawn from such diverse items represents. This score could be regarded as a global measure of social handicap resulting from the disease, but such a concept needs to be developed further to achieve respectability. Continued research on a composite ESS score seems warranted, but in service settings it is recommended that ESS items be used as individual indicators.

Both the ESS composite and the individual items appear to have good reproducibility, with an intraclass correlation coefficient of .97 and no item singled out as problematic.

Like the ISS, the ESS correlated highly with Kurtzke's DSS in both North American (r = .76; LaRocca et al., 1984) and Danish samples (Spearman ρ = .74; Fog et al., 1984). Kuroiwa, Itoyama, Shibasaki, Tobimatsu, and Igata (1984)

Table 3. Item analysis of the Environmental Status Scale

Corrected item-total correlations		
	North America	Denmark
Item		
Transportation	.73	.75
Personal assistance	.71	.75
Financial/economic status	.62	.69
Actual work status	.59	.69
Personal residence/home	.59	.24
Community services	.52	.47
Summary statistics		
Total: Mean	8.5	13.6
S.D.	7.5	7.4
Cronbach's alpha	.83	.82

reported high (in excess of .75) correlations between individual ESS items and the DSS. Thus both composite ESS scores and specific items appear to reflect the severity of the illness in a variety of samples.

Applications of the MRD

In developing the MRD, the IFMSS envisioned broad applicability in medical, community, and research settings. Many of these applications, such as formulation of national policy, are beyond the scope of this chapter. The focus therefore will be on those uses of the MRD most germane to rehabilitation.

Clinical Care

Customary medical management of MS patients assumes the character of rehabilitation as neurological specialists assign increasingly high priority to long-term care and restoration of function. Assessment of functional status consequently assumes greater importance. Ordinarily, one product of clinical assessment is semi-legible free text. Conversely, research assessments generally provide standardized quantitative information while lacking mechanisms for recording qualitative data. The MRD has been used to merge the two styles of data recording. A universal progress note, developed at Albert Einstein College of Medicine, serves as the routine clinical progress note for each patient visit and also as a data sheet for research projects. Similar forms are in use at other centers (LaRocca et al., 1984). In addition to spaces for identifying information, MRD scores, and computer field designations, ample space is provided for free text. With a physician's signature at the bottom, no other written or dictated progress note is needed. On subsequent visits, clinicians can refer to both the free text notes and the quantitative ratings of neurological status, ADL, and social handicap. As a result, patient progress can be monitored more effectively and emergent problems pinpointed. The ready availability of comprehensive information on functional status encourages a rehabilitative orientation toward patient care.

Biomedical Research

Poser (1978) pointed out that the earliest standardization of data collection methods in MS was undertaken within clinical trials; these standards focused on functional disability rather than neurological impairment. The heterogeneity of MS symptoms apparently encouraged the use of such disability measures. Neurological signs and symptoms vary so greatly from patient to patient that a common denominator based on functional status was needed.

Modern therapeutic trials in MS demonstrate even greater use of functional status measures. In a large multicenter trial of cyclosporine (Sandoz Pharmaceuticals, 1984), several such measures are used. First, as part of the Quantitative Examination of Neurologic Functions (Potvin & Tourtellotte, 1985), simulated ADL such as putting on a shirt and cutting with a knife are assessed. Second, patients are assessed using the Ambulation Index (Weiner & Ellison, 1983). Third, the FS, EDSS, and ISS portions of the MRD are completed. Such therapeutic trials are generally regarded as part of clinical neurology rather than rehabilitation. Nevertheless, many of the outcome variables used to evaluate therapeutic efficacy are identical to those used as outcome measures in rehabilitation. Thus, therapeutic trials in MS include both neurological impairment and functional disability as significant indicators of outcome.

Rehabilitation

Published studies of rehabilitation in MS are rare. Feigenson et al. (1981) reported a study of costs and benefits of inpatient rehabilitation, but the MRD had not yet been developed. In a study still underway (Francabandera, Reding, LaRocca, Scheinberg, & McDowell, 1986), severely disabled MS patients are being randomly assigned to either inpatient or outpatient rehabilitation and followed for 2 years after treatment. The MRD and health-related expenditures constitute the major outcome parameters. Within each treatment setting, however, more intensive evaluations take place, yielding details not available with the MRD.

OTHER INSTRUMENTS

The major focus of this chapter has been the MRD, the most widely recognized assessment system for MS. However, in recent years, a number of other assessment approaches have been applied to MS. Space only permits a discussion of instruments developed specifically for MS or extensively used with MS patients. Therefore, the description of instruments that follows includes only published methods and lays no claim to being exhaustive.

The Neurological Rating Scale

"Standardized" versions of the neurological examination are proposed from time to time for use in MS. One recent example is the Neurological Rating Scale (NRS) (Sipe et al., 1984). This instrument covers the areas generally regarded as important in MS. It assesses neurological impairment only, and is not designed to assess functional disability or social handicap. What distinguishes the NRS is the use of composite subscales using weighted scores and an overall score to reflect neurological impairment.

In its present form, the NRS poses several problems. When it was published, the authors provided no data to support the summing of items into composite scales. In addition, items were weighted on a theoretical basis that, although reasonable, was not supported by data. The weighting scheme was thus arbitrary. Rudimentary findings were presented on only five patients. Until additional data are presented, the NRS remains a technique of unknown properties.

The Quantitative Examination of Neurologic Functions

Before the advent of sophisticated neuroimaging, electrodiagnostic methods, and physiological techniques, the diagnosis of neurological disorders relied upon the trained hand and eye of the neurologist. Unfortunately, the ordinal grading system used in the neurological examination (e.g., mild, moderate, severe) remains somewhat indeterminate, even with the best of verbal definitions.

One of the more objective approaches to neurological testing in MS and other conditions is the Quantitative Examination of Neurologic Functions (QENF). Most of the major neurological tests, such as strength, sensation, coordination,

and gait, are administered using standardized procedures and materials (Kuzma, Tourtellotte, & Remington, 1965; Potvin & Tourtellotte, 1985; Tourtellotte, Haerer, Simpson, Kuzma, & Sikorski, 1965). Each test assesses an objective parameter such as pounds or seconds. The same approach is used to evaluate ADL. Raw scores can be converted to "percent of normal function" using age- and sex-appropriate norms. The result is a comprehensive and standardized assessment of neurological impairment and disability. Normative data are available for a number of disorders. Despite its many advantages, this technique has not been widely used in MS outside of major clinical trials (Rose et al., 1970; Sandoz Pharmaceuticals, 1984). Its length and need for special equipment appear to have discouraged use. Work underway to implement many of the tests on personal computers may increase the utilization of this and other quantitative methods.

Documentation Sheet for Multiple Sclerosis

Sigrid Poser (1978) developed one of the most extensive and carefully designed of all record systems for MS in conjunction with an epidemiological study in West Germany. Machine-readable optical scanning sheets were used to record information concerning background, demography, neurological impairment, diagnostic testing, disease characteristics, disabilities in ADL, and handicap in social roles. The emphasis, however, was upon neurological impairment with only brief coverage of disability and handicap.

The MS Functional Profile

As part of their previously mentioned study of cost-effectiveness of rehabilitation in MS, Feigenson et al. (1981) developed a 76-item MS Functional Profile (FP). This instrument was based upon one that had been used with stroke patients for some time (Feigenson, Polkow, Meikle, & Ferguson, 1979). The areas assessed include psychological status, sensation, muscle strength, spasticity, coordination, balance, self-care, mobility, and real-life activities. Each item is rated by a medical professional on an ordinal scale ranging from 1 to 3, 4, 5, or 7, depending upon the item. Eighteen subscales have been constructed on the basis of the 76 items. The internal consistency of these subscales is generally good, with only three having a coefficient lambda (Hull & Nie, 1979) of less than .70.

Despite many good features, this instrument appears to have been used very little. A shortcoming of the FP is the tendency to mix neurological impairment (e.g., spasticity) and functional disability (e.g., wheelchair transfers). Some of the items require very fine discriminations or assume that the patient is in a training environment. In addition, some areas are not well covered (e.g., bladder dysfunction). For users who have need for more detail in the assessment of the MS patient, the FP provides a viable if imperfect alternative.

The Ambulation Index

Difficulties in using the DSS led in part to the development of the Ambulation Index (AI) (Weiner & Ellison, 1983). The AI is an ordinal rating scale ranging from 0 (asymptomatic; fully active) to 9 (restricted to wheelchair; unable to transfer independently). Whereas the DSS is heavily weighted toward ambulation, the AI focuses on ambulation exclusively. Many of the grades use objective parameters such as distance walked and time elapsed. Since the construct being measured in the AI is simpler than that in the DSS, interpretation of scores on the AI is more straightforward. The correlation between the DSS and the AI is substantial, however, with a Spearman ρ of .81 (W. Mietlowski, personal communication, 1986). Additional research is needed to determine how much information the AI yields beyond that provided by other instruments.

The Illness Severity Score

The Illness Severity Score (Mickey, Ellison, & Myers, 1984) represents a unique attempt to improve upon existing assessment methods without adding to them. Using 100 random pairings of MS patients, clinicians rated which of the pair was more severely affected. Using nonlinear regression methods, a weighted sum of several variables was developed that most accurately reproduced the clinicians' discriminations. The items utilized were the FS, the DSS, a rating of clinical activity, and course (relapsing, relapsing and progressive, or progressive). The Illness Severity Score was concordant with clinician ratings in 86% of cases. The correlation between scores obtained by two independent examiners was .93.

Although statistically sound and theoretically elegant, the Illness Severity Score may have limited usefulness in rehabilitation. The items constituting the score primarily represent neurological impairment, that is, parameters that are not thought to change with rehabilitation. As a result, this measure would be useful primarily in clinical neurology and therapeutic trials.

The Postal Diary and Standard Day Interview

Lawson, Robinson, and Bakes (1985) reported two methods for evaluating the impact of MS. One is a diary mailed to patients and filled out on a daily basis. The second is the Standard Day Interview, a detailed, tape-recorded, face-to-face interview widely used in Great Britain. Both techniques are primarily designed to yield data concerning the amount of time patients engage in various everyday activities such as sleeping, eating, shopping, and working. These methods seem most suitable for descriptive research and individual case studies.

CONCLUSIONS

Functional assessment in MS remains an ever-changing field. In the past, instruments used in MS generally fell into one of two categories: either they were developed for use in other conditions and were poorly suited to MS, or they were primarily measures of neurological impairment. With the introduction of the MRD, MS now has a brief but reasonably comprehensive instrument that assesses all three areas in the *International Classification of Impairments, Disabilities, and Handicaps* (WHO, 1980). The product of international and multidisciplinary research and consensus, the MRD forms a core data set to which users can add their own more detailed instruments. Although initial studies confirm that the MRD has many sound properties, research leading to improvements in the MRD, as well as to the development of new and better assessment techniques for use in MS, must continue.

REFERENCES

Alexander, L. (1951). New concept of critical steps in course of chronic debilitating neurologic disease in evaluation of therapeutic response: Longitudinal study of multiple sclerosis by quantitative evaluation of neurologic involvement and disability. *Archives of Neurology and Psychiatry, 66*, 253–271.

Baum, H. M., & Rothschild, B. B. (1981). The incidence and prevalence of reported multiple sclerosis. *Annals of Neurology, 10*, 420–428.

Baum, H. M., & Rothschild, B. B. (1983). Multiple sclerosis and mobility restriction. *Archives of Physical Medicine and Rehabilitation, 64*, 591–596.

Blaivas, J., Holland, N., Giesser, B., LaRocca, N., Madonna, M., & Scheinberg, L. (1984). Multiple sclerosis bladder: Studies and care. *Annals of the New York Academy of Sciences, 436*, 328–346.

Brown, M., Gordon, W., & Diller, L. (1983). Functional assessment and outcome assessment: An integrative review. *Annual Review of Rehabilitation, 3*, 93–120.

Feigenson, J., Polkow, L., Meikle, R., & Ferguson, W. (1979). Burke stroke time-oriented profile (BUSTOP): an overview of patient function *Archives of Physical Medicine and Rehabilitation, 60*, 508–511.

Feigenson, J., Scheinberg, L., Catalano, M., Polkow, L., Mantegazza, P., Feigenson, W., & LaRocca, N. (1981). The cost-effectiveness of multiple sclerosis rehabilitation: A model. *Neurology, 31*, 1316–1322.

Fog, T. (1965). A scoring system for neurological impairment in multiple sclerosis. *Acta Neurologica Scandanavica, 41* (Suppl. 13), 551–555.

Fog, T., Heltberg, A., Kyhn, K., Mellerup, E., Raun, N., & Zeeberg, I. (1984). Evaluation of disability, incapacity and environmental status scales in multiple sclerosis. *Acta Neurologica Scandanavica, 70*(Suppl. 101), 77–86.

Francabandera, F., Reding, M., LaRocca, N., Scheinberg, L., & McDowell, F. (1986, April). Rehabilitation options in multiple sclerosis. Poster presented at the annual meeting of the American Academy of Neurology, New Orleans.

Granger, C. (1981). Assessment of functional status: A model for multiple sclerosis. *Acta Neurologica Scandanavica, 64* (Suppl. 87), 40–47.

Haber, A., & LaRocca, N. (Eds.), (1985). *Minimal record of disability for multiple sclerosis*. New York: The National Multiple Sclerosis Society.

Hull, C., & Nie, N. (1979). *SPSS update: New procedures and facilities for Releases 7 and 8*. New York: McGraw-Hill.

Hyllested, K. (1961). Lethality, duration, and mortality of disseminated sclerosis in Denmark. *Acta Psychiatrica Scandinavica, 36*, 553–564.

Inman, R. (1984). Disability indices, the economic costs of illness, and social insurance: The case of multiple sclerosis. *Acta Neurologica Scandanavica, 70*(Suppl. 101), 46–55.

Johnson, R., Lambie, D., Peace, K., & Thompson, G. (1984). Disability in multiple sclerosis and the provision of social and medical services: Findings in Wellington, New Zealand. *Acta Neurologica Scandanavica, 70*(Suppl 101), 105–112.

Kornblith, A., LaRocca, N., & Baum, H. (1986). Employment in individuals with multiple sclerosis. *International Journal of Rehabilitation Research, 9*, 155–165.

Kuroiwa, Y., Itoyama, Y., Shibasaki, H., Tobimatsu, S., & Igata, A. (1984). Minimal Record of Disability in multiple sclerosis—application to Japanese patients. *Acta Neurologica Scandanavica, 70*(Suppl. 101), 100–104.

Kurtzke, J. (1955). A new scale for evaluating disability in multiple sclerosis. *Neurology, 5*, 580–583.

Kurtzke, J. (1961). On the evaluation of disability in multiple sclerosis. *Neurology, 11*, 686–694.

Kurtzke, J. (1965). Further notes on disability evaluation in multiple sclerosis, with scale modifications. *Neurology, 15*, 654–661.

Kurtzke, J. (1970). Neurologic impairment in multiple sclerosis and the Disability Status Scale. *Acta Neurologica Scandanavica, 46*, 493–512.

Kurtzke, J. (1981). A proposal for a uniform minimal record of disability in multiple sclerosis. *Acta Neurologica Scandanavica, 64*(Suppl 87), 110–129.

Kurtzke, J. (1983). Rating neurologic impairment in multiple sclerosis: An Expanded Disability Status Scale (EDSS). *Neurology, 33*, 1444–1452.

Kurtzke, J. Beebe, G., Nagler, B., Nefzger, M., Auth, T., & Kurland, L. (1970). Studies on the natural history of multiple sclerosis. *Archives of Neurology, 22*, 215–225.

Kurtzke, J., & Berlin, L. (1954). The effects of isoniazid on patients with multiple sclerosis: A preliminary report. *American Review of Tuberculosis, 70*, 577–592.

Kuzma, J., Namerow, N., Tourtellotte, W., Sibley, W., Kurtzke, J., Rose, A., & Dixon, W. (1969). An assessment of the reliability of three methods used in evaluating the status of multiple sclerosis patients. *Journal of Chronic Diseases, 21*, 803–814.

Kuzma, J., Tourtellotte, W., & Remington, R. (1965). Quantitative clinical neurological testing—II. Some statistical considerations of a battery of tests. *Journal of Chronic Diseases, 18*, 303–311.

LaRocca, N., Scheinberg, L., & Slater, R. (1984). Field testing of a minimal record of disability in multiple sclerosis: The United States and Canada. *Acta Neurologica Scandanavica, 70*(Suppl. 101), 126–138.

Lawson, A., Robinson, I., & Bakes, C. (1985). Problems in evaluating the consequences of disabling illness: The case of multiple sclerosis. *Psychological Medicine, 15*, 555–579.

MacLean, A., & Berkson, J. (1951). Mortality and disability in multiple sclerosis: A statistical estimate of progress. *Journal of the American Medical Association, 146*, 1367–1369.

Mahoney, F., & Barthel, D. (1965). Functional evaluation: The Barthel Index. *Maryland State Medical Journal, 14*, 61–65.

Marsh, G., Ellison, G., & Strite, C. (1983). Psychosocial and vocational rehabilitation approaches to multiple sclerosis. *Annual Review of Rehabilitation, 3*, 242–267.

McAlpine, D., Compston, N., & Lumsden, C. (1955). *Multiple sclerosis*. Edinburgh: E. & S. Livingstone, Ltd.

Mellerup, E., Fog, T., Raun, N., Colville, P., de Rham, B., Hannah, B., & Kurtzke, J. (1981). The socio-economic scale. *Acta Neurologica Scandanavica, 64* (Suppl. 87), 130–138.

Mickey, M., Ellison, G., & Myers, L. (1984). An illness severity score for multiple sclerosis. *Neurology, 34*, 1343–1347.

Minderhoud, J., Dassel, H., & Prange, A. (1984). Proposal for summing the incapacity status or environmental status scores. *Acta Neurologica Scandanavica, 70*(Suppl. 101), 87–91.

Moskowitz, E., & McCann, C. (1957). Classification of disability in the chronically ill and aging. *Journal of Chronic Diseases, 5*, 342–346.

Pedersen, E. (1965). A rating system for neurological impairment in multiple sclerosis. *Acta Neurologica Scandinavica, 41*(Suppl. 13), 557–558.

Poser, S. (1978). *An analysis of 812 cases by means of electronic data processing.* Berlin: Springer-Verlag.

Potvin, A., & Tourtellotte, W. (1985). *Quantitative examination of neurologic functions I: Scientific basis and design of instrumented tests.* Boca Raton, FL: CRC Press.

Rose, A., Kuzma, J., Kurtzke, J., Namerow, N., Sibley, W., & Tourtellotte, W. (1970). Cooperative study in the evaluation of therapy in multiple sclerosis: ACTH vs. placebo. *Neurology, 20*(#5, Part 2), 1–59.

Sandoz Pharmaceuticals. (1984). *Protocol for a double-blind multicenter trial to assess the safety and efficacy of cyclosporine in the treatment of multiple sclerosis.* East Hanover, NJ: Sandoz Research Institute.

Scheinberg, L., Giesser, B., & Slater, R. (1983). Management of the chronic MS patient. *Neurology and Neurosurgery Update Series, 4(21)*, 1–8.

Scheinberg, L., Holland, N., Kirschenbaum, M., Oaklander, A., & Geronemus, D. (1981). Comprehensive long-term care of patients with multiple sclerosis. *Neurology, 31*, 1121–1123.

Sipe, J., Knobler, R., Braheny, S., Rice, G., Panitch, H., & Oldstone, M. (1984). A neurologic rating scale (NRS) for use in multiple sclerosis. *Neurology, 34*, 1368–1372.

Slater, R. (1981). Functional disability ratings: Medical, social, and economic implications. *Acta Neurologica Scandanavica, 64*(Suppl. 87), 3–4.

Slater, R. (1984). Criteria and uses of the Minimal Record of Disability in multiple sclerosis. *Acta Neurologica Scandanavica, 70*(Suppl. 101), 16–20.

Slater, R., Fog, T., & Bergmann, L. (Eds.). (1981). Symposium on multiple sclerosis services—Functional disability ratings: Medical, Social and economic implications. *Acta Neurologica Scandanavica, 64*(Suppl. 87), 1–138.

Slater, R., LaRocca, N., & Scheinberg, L. (1984). Development and testing of a Minimal Record of Disability in multiple sclerosis. *Annals of the New York Academy of Sciences, 436*, 453–471.

Slater, R., & Raun, N. (Eds.). (1984). Symposium on a Minimal Record of Disability for multiple sclerosis. *Acta Neurologica Scandanavica, 70*(Suppl. 101), 1–217.

Thygesen, P. (1953). *The course of disseminated sclerosis: A close-up of 105 attacks.* Copenhagen: Rosenkilde & Bagger.

Tourtellotte, W., Haerer, A., Simpson, J., Kuzma, J., & Sikorski, J. (1965). Quantitative clinical neurological testing. I. A study of a battery of tests designed to evaluate in part the neurological function of patients with multiple sclerosis and its use in a therapeutic trial. *Annals of the New York Academy of Sciences, 122*, 480–505.

Weiner, H., & Ellison, G. (1983). A working protocol to be used as a guideline for trials in multiple sclerosis. *Archives of Neurology, 40*, 704–710.

World Health Organization. (1980). *International classification of impairments, disabilities, and handicaps.* Geneva: Author.

Chapter 12

Outcome Analysis
in Arthritis Rehabilitation

*Stephen T. Wegener, Carolyn M. Brunner,
and Cynthia A. Stabenow*

The analysis of outcome in arthritis rehabilitation is complicated by the diversity of rheumatic diseases, the unpredictable course of the various disease entities, and the difficulty in making an accurate diagnosis. There are over 100 conditions denoted by the term *arthritis* that may or may not be inflammatory in nature. The more usual adult forms are rheumatoid arthritis (RA), osteoarthritis (OA), ankylosing spondylitis (AS), systemic lupus erythematosus (SLE), scleroderma, and gout. In addition, there are forms of rheumatic disease that affect children. Although OA is the most common form of arthritis, the majority of rehabilitation efforts, measurement studies, and available data have focused on rheumatoid arthritis. This state of affairs is due to the potentially devastating impact of the disease, its prevalence, and its early age of onset. Consequently, the major focus of this chapter is on the population with rheumatoid arthritis. Other diagnostic groups are included where information is available. Measuring the outcome of rehabilitation in arthritis patients as a group is inadequate, because patients with different forms of arthritis may require different outcome measures. Therefore, specifying the type of arthritis under assessment and adopting appropriate outcome measures is essential.

An additional complication in the outcome measurement of arthritis rehabilitation is the un-predictable course of the disease process. Unlike mental retardation or acute spinal cord injury, where the individual's impairment is fixed, rheumatic diseases tend to resemble multiple sclerosis or psychiatric illness, where the impairment may vary over time. In rheumatoid arthritis, some patients experience an unrelenting progression and others have brief attacks interspersed with relative quiescence. In general, longitudinal studies reveal that the number of rheumatoid arthritis patients doing poorly increases with time (Rodnan, Schumacher, & Zvaifler, 1983). This unpredictable course presents problems in measurement frequency, measurement sensitivity, and research design.

In rheumatic disease, outcome must be considered in terms other than the end result of treatment. Figure 1 indicates that end results may not take into account the course of the illness. Wright (1985) describes this well:

> In rheumatoid arthritis, whatever the intervention measures, the ultimate condition of the patient may be similar. However, by the administration of anti-rheumatoid drugs, disability may be reduced for periods, and other outcome measures such as laboratory variables improved. In that case the "area under the curve" is significantly different from those patients who do not receive antirheumatic therapy. This improvement in the quality of life is not to be despised. Therefore, in talking of outcome, we do well to consider immediate improvement, in-

Preparation of this chapter was supported by a National Institute of Handicapped Research Grant (#G008300043). We acknowledge the assistance of Stephanie A. Allen in preparation of the manuscript.

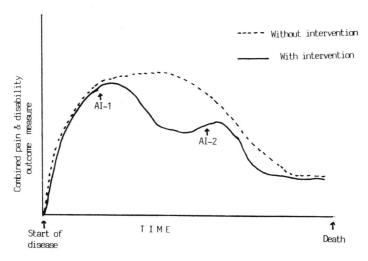

Figure 1.   Curves showing quality of life of patients receiving arthritis interventions (AI) and those who are not. (Adapted from Wright, 1985.)

termediate amelioration, and ultimate prognosis. (p. 986)

Finally, the validity of any outcome measurement is dependent on a number of variables, one of which is the homogeneity of the sample. Several of the rheumatic diseases, including rheumatoid arthritis, are easily diagnosed in the advanced form. In the early stages, however, when some signs may be subclinical or nonspecific, the type of rheumatic disease may be misdiagnosed. Thus, treatment cohorts can be contaminated, leading to erroneous conclusions about treatment efficacy.

With these caveats in mind, this chapter reviews rheumatic disease rehabilitation, provides a model for assessment, reviews specific outcome methods, and describes efforts to improve outcome assessment in rheumatic disease.

Rheumatic Disease Rehabilitation

Rheumatic disease rehabilitation focuses initially on intermediate goals, such as increasing range of motion, decreasing inflammation, and learning new psychological and physical coping skills, with the hope that these gains will translate into long-term improvements in function and quality of life. The roles of the various rheumatic disease rehabilitation team members are diverse, and the treatment methods employed cannot be detailed in this limited space. Interested readers are re-

ferred to volumes by Ehrlich (1986) and Riggs and Gall (1984) for more detailed information.

Because of the lag time between treatment onset and eventual improvement, outcome assessment must encompass measurement of immediate, intermediate, and long-range effects. Potential assessment targets are patient, social, and environmental variables. Measurement tools may assess the entire range from molecular to molar events, from specific joint range of motion to quality of life. A comprehensive outcome assessment program would accommodate both temporal and multimethod considerations.

The Biopsychosocial Model

Adequate efforts to rehabilitate patients with rheumatic disease include diagnosing and treating problems on the biological, psychological, and social levels. The biopsychosocial model (Engel, 1977) encompasses an approach to health care that emphasizes the interdependence of these three systems in determining patient functioning and ultimate disability. This model not only meets the need for an interdisciplinary approach, but also provides guidelines for appropriate assessment procedures. Leigh and Reiser (1980) incorporated the biopsychosocial concept into a Patient Evaluation Grid (PEG; Table 1).

The PEG system encourages clinicians and researchers to consider the interactive nature of the

Table 1. Model to organize assessment information in biological, personal (psychological), and environmental (social) dimensions.

Dimensions	Assessment information		
	Current	Recent	Background
Biological	Symptoms Physical examination Vital signs Status of related organs Medications Disease	Age Recent bodily changes Injuries, operations Disease Drugs	Heredity Early nutrition Constitution Predisposition Early disease
Personal	Chief complaint Mental status Expectations about illness and treatment	Recent illness, occurrence of symptoms Personality change Mood, thinking, behavior Adaptation, defenses	Developmental factors Early experience Personality type Attitude toward illness
Environmental	Immediate physical and in- terpersonal environment Supportive figure, next of kin Effect of help-seeking	Recent physical and inter- personal environmental events Life changes Family, work, others Contact with ill persons Contact with doctor or hospital	Early physical environment Cultural and family environment Early relations Cultural sick role expectation

Adapted from Leigh and Reiser (1980).

illness—health continuum and facilitates comprehensive evaluation. As Schwartz (1982) pointed out, the biopsychosocial model also indicates that treatments will interact and perhaps have synergistic effects. The framework allows theoretical consideration of each treatment's relative contribution to a specific outcome. Furthermore, variables that may have been overlooked are brought to attention. The following review of potential outcome assessment methods is based on this organizational system. It will become apparent that, although biological, and to a lesser extent, psychological measures are becoming established, a great deal of work remains in the development of social-environmental measurement tools.

BIOLOGICAL MEASURES

"Medical" measurements of outcome in rheumatic diseases have been developed mainly for inflammatory types of arthritis, especially rheumatoid arthritis. These measurements have been used to study progression of the disease over years, and are exemplified by the radiographic staging system, or assessment of fluctuations in the activity of the disease. The latter have been refined primarily to be indicators (or endpoints)

used in clinical trials of drug effects in rheumatoid arthritis (Tugwell & Bombardier, 1982). The measures can be divided into those that are 1) "objective"—assessable by the physician, or 2) "subjective"—based on the patient's self-report and the physician's opinion of the patient's condition.

Disease Activity Indicators

For classifying the anatomical staging of rheumatoid arthritis, X-rays provide a readily available, noninvasive, objective measure (Steinbrocker, Traeger, & Battman, 1949). The stages range from grade 1 (no destructive changes, although periarticular osteopenia may be present) to grade 4 (evidence for cartilage and bone destruction, joint deformity, and fibrous or bony ankylosis).

Synovitis, proliferating synovial and inflammatory cells, is associated in the early phases with increased vascularity and loss of calcium from the bone (radiologically, osteopenia). Synovitis later destroys the cartilage, manifested by joint space narrowing, and the subchondral bone. Because synovitis is not limited to the structure within the joints but also involves adjacent structures such as the joint capsule and tendons, persistent synovitis results in tendon laxity and joint instability (subluxation, ulnar deviation).

Various methods have been recommended for measuring the number of painful and/or swollen joints. The Lansbury articular index (Lansbury, 1958) weights involvement of larger joints with a higher score (e.g., knee = 25, wrist = 4) without taking into account severity of joint inflammation. The Ritchie articular index (Ritchie et al., 1968) accounts for a range of joint inflammation (e.g., 0—no tenderness, +1—patient says it is painful; +2—patient says it is very painful). In this index, small joints of the hand and foot are not scored individually, but are grouped in units. In both of these measurements, the observer records a total score.

The time to walk 50 feet is analogous to grip strength of the upper extremities, since it assesses pain in the hip, knee, ankle, tarsal, and metatarsal joints. Test-to-test fluctuations in time may reflect alterations in the activity of the synovitis; fixed times may indicate inactive disease if they are short, irreversible destructive changes in one or more of these joints, *or* significant muscle weakness if they are prolonged (Grace, Gerecz, Kassam, & Buchanan, 1986).

The erythrocyte sedimentation rate (ESR) is a simple, inexpensive laboratory test that measures the rate at which red blood cells (erythrocytes) fall in a vertical cylindrical tube. This fall rate is more rapid in the presence of fibrinogen, which increases with inflammation, and other acute phase proteins. Although inflammation other than rheumatoid synovitis can increase the ESR, the latter has been accepted as a rough (and objective) correlate of disease activity (Dixon, 1982).

Morning stiffness is the duration between awakening and the time of feeling "limber" as reported by the patient. Since the measure is subjective and no means of quantitation is generally available, its continued use is due to its good correlation with other clinical and laboratory parameters and with an easily understood numerical score (e.g., 3 hours).

Finally, subjective impressions of both the observer and the patient about disease activity, and of the patient regarding pain, are frequently incorporated into the overall assessment. These measures may be influenced by factors extraneous to rheumatoid arthritis, and reproducibility is often difficult to achieve (Rind, Bird, & Wright, 1980).

Generally, a single indicator is not used to measure disease activity. Instead, some constellation of the above measures is selected and reported.

Remission Indicators

Because complete remission may occur in rheumatoid arthritis, either spontaneously or with the use of drugs, a committee of the American Rheumatism Association (ARA) was appointed to define such remission. The preliminary report (Pinals, Masi, Larsen, & the Subcommittee for Criteria of Remission, 1981) indicated that a minimum of five of the following requirements must be fulfilled for at least two consecutive months in a patient with "definite or classic RA" (as defined by ARA criteria):

1. Morning stiffness not to exceed 15 minutes
2. No fatigue
3. No joint pain
4. No joint tenderness or pain on motion
5. No soft tissue swelling in joints or tendon sheaths
6. ESR less than 30 mm/hr (females) or 20 mm/hr (males)

In the patient studies described by Pinals and co-workers (1981), there was 100% specificity in discriminating rheumatoid arthritis patients with active disease and 72% sensitivity for clinical remission. The aim was to achieve uniformity in clinical application, using generally acceptable and convenient measurements, rather than to identify an absolute state of remission that could be documented only by extraordinary measures, such as biopsy of synovial tissue or radiological procedures.

Flexibility and Strength

Range of motion (ROM) and grip strength are two clinical assessments routinely done with rheumatic disease patients. Physicians use these indicators to document effects of medications or surgery. Physical and occupational therapists employ these assessments to measure change associated with modalities (e.g., heat, cold, ul-trasound) or splints. Researchers traditionally include a measure of grip strength in drug and other outcome studies (Pincus et al., 1984).

The standard method for measuring joint ROM is based on procedures for measuring and recording adopted by the American Academy of Orthopedic Surgeons (AAOS, 1966). Subsequent studies of interrater reliability of joint ROM illustrate the variable nature of this measurement over time and its questionable use as an outcome measure (R. O. Smith & Benge, 1985).

For patients with rheumatic disease in the hands or wrists, an adapted sphygmomanometer should be used to measure grip strength (Melvin, 1982). A standard dynamometer is not recommended because of inflexibility and hardness, which can produce pain, and because grasping it adequately is difficult for patients with moderate or severe joint deformity. The assessment of hand function includes evaluation of both prehension and nonprehension activities. Prehension involves grasping by either finger–thumb, as in holding a pencil, or full hand, as in holding a glass. Nonprehension involves activities such as pushing, pulling, sorting objects, or applying pressure.

Although ROM and grip assessments provide some information, they do not demonstrate how the patient can use muscular substitutions and adaptive methods to perform a functional task. This outcome is influenced by pain in the wrist and finger joints, presumably related to pain or joint destruction. Outcome is generally correlated with the articular index for the upper extremities (Lee, Baxter, Dick, & Webb, 1974). There are many types of functional hand assessments currently in use, but the standardized tests (Jebsen, 1969; MacBain, 1970; H. Smith, 1973), are preferred for outcome measurement.

PAIN MEASURES

The pain that accompanies rheumatic disease is a multidetermined experience influenced by biological, psychological, and social variables. A separate section is devoted here to pain measurement because studies (Brena, Chapman, Stegall, & Chyatte, 1979; Downie et al., 1978) have indi-cated that, in rheumatic disease, pain plays a prominent role in patient's lives. A recent study by Kazis, Meenan, and Anderson (1983) investigated the importance of pain in explaining the health status and health behavior of persons with arthritis. The Arthritis Impact Measurement Scales (AIMS) was used to measure physical, psychological, and pain variables in a sample of 729 patients. The AIMS is an established measure in arthritis research with acceptable psychometric properties (Meenan, Gertman, Mason, & Dunaif, 1982). The results confirmed the hypothesis that pain makes a highly significant contribution to explaining both physicians' and patients' overall health assessments. Furthermore, pain was the most important of the three health status variables in accounting for medication usage and the variable most associated with subsequent physical disability. Therefore, some measure of pain experience is appropriate for inclusion in rehabilitation outcome studies.

A number of methods have been used to measure pain in scientific studies. These efforts have included psychophysiological approaches, numerical and verbal ratings, and assessment of pain behaviors. Historically, the use of laboratory psychophysiological techniques to produce and measure pain threshhold and tolerance have been confined to nonpatient populations. Only a few studies (e.g., Moldofsky & Chester, 1970; Wolff, 1971) have used these methods with arthritis patients. The use of a pressure dolorimeter to detect joint tenderness and provide a reproducible pain stimulus is a method that has been used with some success (Moldofsky & Chester, 1970) and deserves wider consideration. Although many psychophysiological procedures may not be practical in many investigations, the clinician–researcher may find the precision useful in some outcome studies.

Early outcome studies used crude numerical or verbal ratings of pain intensity. These measures were of questionable value because little consideration was given to the psychometric properties of the scales. More recently, sophisticated scales accounting for the intensity, duration, and trend of the pain have been developed. Many of the functional assessment questionnaires discussed in the subsequent section have subscales measuring pain. A comparison of the major functional assessment questionnaires' pain scales may be derived from a study by Liang, Larson, Cullen, and Schwartz (1985). These authors administered five health status instruments (AIMS, Functional Status Index [FSI], Health Assessment Questionnaire [HAQ], Index of Well Being [IWB], Sickness Impact Profile [SIP]) in random order to 50 arthritis patients before and after total joint arthroplasty. Only the AIMS, FSI, and HAQ can be compared, because the SIP and IWB do not have pain scales. These three instruments all had significantly correlated pain scales and all measured a reduction in pain postoperatively. Although these measures have some different characteristics that should be considered in choosing a pain scale, there are no conclusive data to support one scale over another for pain measurement.

Additional self-report measures of pain include visual analogue scales and questionnaires designed specifically to measure pain. Scott and Huskisson (1976) have described the use of visual analogue scales in chronic pain measurement. Although this type of measurement has a number of problems, including variations in line length as a result of reproduction method and inability of some arthritis patients to grasp the concept of a line representing their pain, this measurement tool is widely accepted and used.

A number of attempts have been made to use verbal pain descriptors to measure acute and chronic pain. The most widely used instrument of this genre is the McGill Pain Questionnaire (MPQ) developed by Melzack (1975). The MPQ measures the temporal, intensity, and qualitative aspects of the pain experience through the use of verbal descriptors. A body of research has accumulated on the MPQ suggesting it has acceptable reliability and face, construct, discriminant, and concurrent validity. This instrument has been used to evaluate the efficacy of psychological interventions upon rheumatoid arthritis patients' self-reports of pain (Bradley, Turner, Young, Agudelo, Anderson, & McDaniel, 1984; Randich, 1982) with success.

A novel approach to pain measurement using a pictorial, nonverbal rating scale has been used by Frank, Moll, and Hart (1982). They compared the use of a visual analogue scale, a verbal descriptor 5-point rating scale, and a series of eight drawings of faces. The faces depicted ranged from extremely sad and painful to happy and pain free. Their results showed moderately high correlations between the three measures. The results indicate that a nonverbal, self-report pain measure may be useful with persons of poor literacy, although more research is needed to establish the psychometric properties of the tool.

Fordyce (1976) emphasized the importance of observable behaviors as the critical outcome measure in the treatment of chronic pain and illness. Recently, there have been some efforts to use the observation of pain behaviors as an outcome measure in arthritis treatment. A system for making reliable and valid observations of pain behaviors was developed by Keefe and Block (1982) for use with chronic low back pain patients. The method uses the analysis of a 10-minute videotape during which the patient is observed performing a standardized set of activities including sitting, standing, and walking. The tape is scored for several classes of pain behaviors such as grimacing and guarding. These authors reported significant correlations with self-report and found the measure was sensitive to treatment changes. Bradley and his colleagues (McDaniel et al., in press) have adapted this system for use with rheumatoid arthritis patients. Their preliminary data indicate patients' pain behaviors are correlated positively with self-report and functional disability. The use of a standardized pain behavior rating measure is a significant and useful development, because all other pain measurement tools rely on self-report of one form or another. The use of this type of approach in conjunction with a self-report measure would provide high-quality outcome data.

PSYCHOLOGICAL MEASURES

The biopsychosocial model alerts the clinician–researcher to the fact that rheumatic disease may affect psychological health as well as the traditionally measured physiological consequences. Several authors (Fries, 1981; Meenan, Yelin, Nevitt, & Epstein, 1981) have suggested that psychological, quality of life, functional abilities, and pain outcomes are extremely important to patients. Although traditional biological measures (e.g., inflammation indexes, ROM) may be useful as process measures to health care professionals, patients are focused on more personal experiences.

To this end, a wide range of measures have been employed to assess psychological status in persons with rheumatic disease. Early reports employed psychiatric interviews and projective psychological tests to investigate the relationship between certain personality variables and disease process. Because these methods have poor psychometric properties, they cannot be recommended for outcome measurement. Recently, efforts have focused on the use of traditional psychological adjustment inventories to measure variables of interest, including depression, anxiety, and global adjustment. Instruments such as the Minnesota Multiphasic Personality Inventory, (MMPI; Hathaway & McKinley, 1967) and the Symptom Checklist-90 (Derogatis, 1977) have been widely used to assess general adjustment and specific psychological states (Nalvan & O'Brien, 1964; Polley, Swenson, & Steinhilber, 1970; Wegener, 1986). Specific scales for depression, including the Beck Depression Inventory (Beck, 1978) and the Zung Self-Rating Depression Scale (Zung, 1965), have been used as well. The majority of studies report higher levels of depression in arthritis patients than controls (Zaphiroporelos & Burry, 1974).

However, these findings and the use of psychological assessment tools developed for psychiatric populations are suspect both intuitively and psychometrically. Patients with physical illness may respond differently to these measures than other patient groups. Many of the items included in depression scales are concerned with somatic symptoms, which may be disturbed by rheumatic disease, thus yielding spurious scores. Green (1982) has argued against the use of traditional psychological tests with medical patients on the grounds that these tests and the related norms were developed using psychiatric populations. Therefore, it is psychometrically unsound to apply these measures to medical patients without additional validity studies.

The current trend in psychological assessment has been the development of specific assessment instruments for rheumatic disease. This development is a result of the recognition of the psychometric considerations outlined above and an increased awareness of the role cognitive factors may play in overall functioning. Two efforts have focused on assessing the patient's attitudes and beliefs regarding their disease.

Wallston, Pincus, Nicassio, Woodward, and Dodd (1983) developed the Arthritis Helplessness Index, which assesses the extent to which patients believe they are responsible for their general health and management of their arthritis symptoms. O'Leary (1985) and her colleagues at the Stanford Arthritis Center have developed a self-efficacy scale to measure a person's belief that he or she is able to make efficacious changes in the process and outcome of the disease. Beliefs and attitudes regarding disease may be important in persons with arthritis because perceived control may prevent the development of learned helplessness and depression, as discussed by Seligman (1975).

SOCIAL FUNCTIONING MEASURES

In addition to experiencing affective changes, pain, and physical disability, persons with arthritis have adjustments to make in their social functioning. Impairments in employment, family functioning, social activities, and quality of life have been reported. Recently, investigators (Burkhardt, 1985; Meenan et al., 1981) have attempted to document these social changes using standardized techniques. Meenan and his group used structured interviews and questionnaires to assess the sociomedical impact of arthritis on 245 persons. The results indicated that major losses in work, finances, and family functioning are very prevalent. Work disability was identified as the most important sociomedical consequence of rheumatoid arthritis because it was linked to income and other psychosocial losses. Burkhardt (1985) investigated the impact of arthritis on the quality of life. She found that the severity of the arthritis-induced impairment indirectly affected overall quality of life through mediating variables. This type of outcome criteria measurement is difficult to undertake because of methodological problems, including a paucity of reliable instruments, difficulty in operationally defining the variables, and the need for longitudinal studies. Overcoming some methodological problems is possible by using more sophisticated techniques, such as those employed in the studies above. Research indicates that these global measures are important in outcome measurement both to patients and policymakers, and therefore need to be pursued.

FUNCTIONAL MEASURES

Functional capacity is, in the final analysis, the major criterion for evaluating the impact of arthritis on an individual's life. The preservation and restoration of function is a primary goal of the interdisciplinary arthritis rehabilitation team. Halpern and Fuhrer (1984) defined functional assessment as the "measurement of purposeful behavior in interaction with the environment" (p. 3). The accurate assessment of this dynamic relationship is critical to the measurement, prediction, and evaluation of a disability or handicap.

The ARA functional classification system divides patients into four groups, ranging from Class I (ability to perform all activities) to Class IV (incapacitation, or confinement to bed or wheelchair use) (Rodnan et al, 1983). The ARA system is found lacking on at least two points. First, the criteria were not sensitive enough to describe or measure the more subtle aspects of patient functioning. Second, the criteria focused primarily on what the person could *not* do as opposed to highlighting areas of competency. Initial efforts to address these issues focused primarily on the assessment of the activities of daily living (ADL). These measurement tools have been expanded in an attempt to measure overall health status and have included a broad range of activities. The major functional status instruments used with arthritis patients are listed in Table 2.

The selection of items for inclusion in these measures is based primarily on their relevance to personal behaviors, social role, or specific impairment expected to arise from a rheumatic disease. Although all of these measures have been used in rheumatic disease studies, most of the instruments are designed for outcome measurement, not diagnosis or treatment planning.

It is impossible to review the psychometric properties and test utility of all 15 instruments listed. Himmel (1984) has indicated three criteria useful in choosing an instrument: psychometric quality, a graded response format, and utility. Of the instruments discussed, reliability and validity criteria have been established for the AIMS, HAQ, FSI, PI, Index of ADL, SIP, and IWB. Other measures should be used with caution until psychometric data are available. Some measures use a performance gradient response, inquiring as to difficulty of the tasks or the degree of restriction. This graded response format is preferable to a dichotomous yes/no response. The inclusion of a response gradient increases sensitivity and enhances clinical relevance.

The issue of test utility has not been sufficiently addressed to date, because few investigations have been done to evaluate the instruments for diverse measurement purposes. One study by Liang and co-workers (1985), described in the previous section on pain measurement, compared five of the major health status instruments. In addition to pain scale comparison, relative efficiency and sensitivity in the measurement of mobility, physical function, social role, social activity, and global health were assessed. In general, the instruments had highly correlated subscales, but the interinstrument correlations were higher for social and global scales than pain or mobility. Liang et al. concluded that no single instrument outperformed the others. Researchers are advised to critically review instruments and choose one that targets the rehabilitation criteria of interest.

CONCLUSION

A recent conference on arthritis rehabilitation sponsored by the National Institute for Disability and Rehabilitation Research, The National Institutes of Health, and the Arthritis Foundation developed consensus statements regarding outcome measurement. The conferees supported the importance of functional status assessment in outcome measurement and encouraged the applica-

Table 2. Functional assessment scales for arthritis patients

Instrument[a]	Type of administration	Major areas assessed
ADL (Katz, Downs, Cash, & Grotz, 1970)	Interview/observation	Only ADL: dressing, bathing, eating, etc.
AIMS (Meenan, Gertman, & Mason, 1980)	Self-report	Mobility, physical activity, dexterity, social role & activity, pain, ADL psychological impact
ARA Classification of Functional Capacity (Steinbrocker et al., 1949)	Interview	Discrete global categories from completely independent to incapacitated
Activity diary (Skevington, 1983)	Self-report	List of 11 activities (e.g., sleep, recreation, passive)
Assessment of Function (Ehrlich, 1973)	Self-report/interview	Homemaking assessment
Brief Objective Evaluation (Swezey, 1978)	Observation/interview	18 functional activities (e.g., butter bread, put on garment)
FSI (Jette, 1980)	Self-report	Mobility, hand activities, personal and home care, interpersonal activities with dependence and pain rating for each
HAQ (Fries, Spitz, Kraines, & Holman, 1980)	Self-report	ADL, mobility, hand activities, sexuality, medical costs, pain
IFI (Lee, Jasani, Dick, & Buchanan, 1973)	Self-report/interview	List of functional activities (e.g., open doors)
IWB (Kaplan, Bush, & Berry, 1976)	Self-report	Mobility, physical activity, social activity
Keitel Functional Test (Eberl, Fasching, Rahlts, Schleyer, & Wolf, 1976)	Observer ratings of exercises	List of functional activities to be performed and observed
MHAQ (Pincus, Summey, Soraci, Wallston, & Hummon, 1983)	Self-report	Shorter HAQ, disability, satisfaction, need for help
PI (Convery, Minteer, Amiel, & Connett, 1977)	Interview	Daily living skills, mobility
Rheumatic Disease Self-Assessment (Swezey, 1978)	Self-report	ADL, mobility, lifting, home activities
SIP (Bergner, Bobbitt, Carter, & Gilson, 1981)	Self-report/interview	Mobility, work and home activities, ADL, social interaction

[a] AIMS = Arthritis Impact Measurement Scales; FSI = Functional Status Index; HAQ = Health Assessment Questionnaire; ADL = Index of Activities of Daily Living; IFI = Index of Functional Impairment; IWB = Index of Well Being; MHAQ = Modified Health Assessment Questionnaire; PI = Polyarticular Index; SIP = Sickness Impact Profile.

tion of these techniques in clinical care. Support was found for the acceptance of self-report in assessing psychological and social areas of functioning. Finally, the use of multiple measures and multiple perspectives on outcome was advocated. This chapter has reviewed a diverse group of measures that fulfill these recommendations.

The authors of this chapter have used an evaluation system that employs input from the patient, the health care professional, and the patient's significant others (Wegener, O'Leary, & Brunner, 1986). The data indicate poor agreement between these various individuals' ratings of patient functioning and rehabilitation outcomes. Although additional research is needed, preliminary conclusions indicate that the answer to the question, "What effects do arthritis rehabilitation interventions have?," may depend on whom is asked.

Outcome measurement in rheumatic disease rehabilitation poses a number of idiosyncratic difficulties; however, progress can be expected as more rehabilitation specialists become aware of the rheumatic diseases as appropriate targets for their efforts. Using the biopsychosocial model as a guiding principle, researchers will avoid the pitfalls that characterize current research. Clinicians and researchers in rheumatic disease rehabilitation must be cognizant of the interaction of multiple organism systems to understand fully the impact of interventions.

REFERENCES

American Academy of Orthopedic Surgeons. (1966). *Joint motion—method of measuring and recording*. Chicago: Author.

Beck, A. T. (1978). *Depression inventory*. Philadelphia: Center for Cognitive Therapy.

Bergner, M., Bobbitt, R. A., Carter, W. B., & Gilson, B. S. (1981). The sickness impact profile: Development and final revision of a health status measure. *Medical Care, 19,* 787–805.

Bradley, L. A., Young, L. D., Anderson, K. O., McDaniel, L. K., Turner, R. A., & Agudelo, C. A. (1984). Psychological approaches to the management of arthritis pain. *Social Science and Medicine, 19,* 1353–1360.

Brena, S. F., Chapman, S. L., Stegall, P. G., & Chyatte, S. B. (1979). Chronic pain states: Their relationship to impairment and disability. *Archives of Physical Medicine and Rehabilitation, 60,* 387–389.

Burkhardt, C. S. (1985). The impact of arthritis on quality of life. *Nursing Research, 34,* 11–16.

Convery, F. R., Minteer, M. A., Amiel, D., & Connett, K. L. (1977). Polyarticular disability: A functional assessment. *Archives of Physical Medicine and Rehabilitation, 58,* 494–499.

Derogatis, L. R. (1977). *SCL-90 R (revised) version manuals*. Baltimore: Johns Hopkins University Press.

Dixon, J. S. (1982). Biochemical and clinical changes in rheumatoid arthritis: Their relation to the action of antirheumatoid drugs. *Seminars in Arthritis and Rheumatism, 12,* 191.

Downie, W. W., Leatham, P. A., Rhind, V. M., Wright, V., Branco, J. A., & Anderson, J. A. (1978). Studies with pain rating scales. *Annals of Rheumatic Disease, 37,* 378–381.

Eberl, D. R., Fasching, V., Schleyer, I., & Wolf, R. (1976). Repeatability and objectivity of various measurements in rheumatoid arthritis: A comparative study. *Arthritis and Rheumatism, 19,* 1278–1286.

Ehrlich, G. E. (1973). *Total management of the arthritis patient*. Philadelphia: Lippincott.

Ehrlich, G. E. (Ed.). (1986). *Rehabilitation management of rheumatic conditions*. Baltimore: Williams & Wilkins.

Engel, G. L. (1977). The need for a new medical model: A challenge for biomedicine. *Science, 196,* 129–136.

Fordyce, W. E. (1976). *Behavioral methods for chronic pain and illness*. St. Louis: Mosby.

Frank, A. J. M., Moll, S. M. H., & Hart, J. F. (1982). A comparison of three ways of measuring pain. *Rheumatology and Rehabilitation, 21,* 211–217.

Fries, J. F. (1981). Toward an understanding of patient outcome measurement. *Arthritis and Rheumatism, 26,* 697–704.

Fries, J. F., Spitz, P., Kraines, R. G., & Holman, H. R. (1980). Measurement of patient outcome in arthritis. *Arthritis and Rheumatism, 23,* 137–145.

Grace, E. M., Gerecz, E., Kassam, Y., & Buchanan, W. W. (1986). Fifty foot walking time: An inappropriate outcome measure. *Arthritis and Rheumatism, 29* (Suppl.), 516.

Green, C. (1982). Psychological assessment in medical settings. In T. H. Millon, C. Green, & R. Meagher (Eds.), *Handbook of clinical health psychology* (pp. 339–376). New York: Plenum Press.

Halpern, A. S., & Fuhrer, M. J. (Eds.). (1984). *Functional assessment in rehabilitation*. Baltimore: Paul H. Brookes Publishing Co.

Hathaway, S. R., & McKinley, J. C. (1967). *The Minnesota Multiphasic Personality Inventory manual (revised)*. New York: The Psychological Corporation.

Himmel, P. B. (1984). Functional assessment strategies in clinical medicine: The care of arthritic patients. In C. V. Granger & C. E. Gresham (Eds.), *Functional assessment in rehabilitative medicine* (pp. 343–363). Baltimore: Williams & Wilkins.

Jebsen, R. H. (1969). An objective and standardized test of hand function. *Archives of Physical Medicine and Rehabilitation, 50,* 311–319.

Jette, A. M. (1980). Functional status index: Reliability of a chronic disease evaluation instrument. *Archives of Physical Medicine and Rehabilitation, 61,* 395–401.

Kaplan, R. M., Bush, J. W., & Berry, C. C. (1976). Health status: Types of validity for an index of well being. *Health Services Research, 11,* 478–507.

Katz, S., Downs, T. D., Cash, H. R., & Grotz, R. C. (1970). Progress in development of the Index of ADL. *Gerontologist, 10,* 20–30.

Kazis, L. E., Meenan, R. E., & Anderson, J. J. (1983). Pain in the rheumatic diseases. *Arthritis and Rheumatism, 26,* 1017–1022.

Keefe, F. J., & Block, A. R. (1982). Development of an observation method for assessing pain behavior in chronic low back pain patients. *Behavior Therapy, 13,* 363–375.

Lansbury, J. (1958). Report of a three year study on the systemic and articular indices in rheumatoid arthritis: Theoretic and clinical considerations. *Arthritis and Rheumatism, 1,* 505–522.

Lee, P., Baxter, A., Dick, W. C., & Webb, J. (1974). An assessment of grip strength measurement in rheumatoid arthritis. *Scandinavian Journal of Rheumatology, 3,* 17–23.

Lee, P., Jasani, M. K., Dick, W. C., & Buchanan, W. W. (1973). Evaluation of a functional index in rheumatoid arthritis. *Scandinavian Journal of Rheumatology, 2,* 71–77.

Leigh, H., & Reiser, M. F., (1980). *The patient: Biological, psychological, and social dimensions of medical practice*. New York: Plenum Press.

Liang, M. H., Larson, M. G., Cullen, K. E., & Schwartz, J. A. (1985). Comparative measure of efficacy and sensitivity of five health status instruments for arthritis research. *Arthritis and Rheumatism, 28,* 542–547.

MacBain, K. P. (1970). Assessment of function in the rheumatoid hand. *Canadian Occupational Therapy Journal, 37,* 95–102.

McDaniel, L. K., Anderson, K. O., Bradley, L. A., Young, L. D., Turner, R., Agudelo, C., & Keefe, F. J. (in press). Development of an observation method for assessing pain behavior in rheumatoid arthritis patients. *Pain*.

Meenan, R. F., Gertman, P. M., & Mason, J. H. (1980). Measuring health status in arthritis: The arthritis impact measurement scales. *Arthritis and Rheumatism, 23*, 146–152.

Meenan, R. F., Gertman, P. M., Mason, J. H., & Dunaif, R. (1982). The arthritis Impact Measurement Scales: Further investigations of a health status measure. *Arthritis and Rheumatism, 25*, 1048–1053.

Meenan, R. F., Yelin, E. M., Nevitt, M., & Epstein, W. V. (1981). The impact of chronic disease. *Arthritis and Rheumatism, 24*, 544–549.

Melvin, J. L. (1982). *Rheumatic disease: Occupational therapy and rehabilitation* (2nd ed.). Philadelphia: Davis.

Melzack, R. (1975). The McGill Pain Questionnaire: Major properties and scoring methods. *Pain, 1*, 277–299.

Moldofsky, H., & Chester, W. J. (1970). Pain and mood patterns in patients with rheumatoid arthritis: A prospective study. *Psychosomatic Medicine, 32*, 309–318.

Nalvan, F., & O'Brien, J. (1964). On the use of the MMPI with rheumatoid arthritis patients. *Arthritis and Rheumatism, 7*, 18–24.

O'Leary, A. (1985). *Psychological factors in rheumatoid arthritis pain and immune function: A self-efficacy approach*. Unpublished doctoral dissertation, Stanford University, Stanford, CA.

Pinals, R. S., Masi, A. T., Larsen, R. A., & The Subcommittee for Criteria of Remission of Rheumatoid Arthritis of the American Rheumatism Association Diagnostic and Therapeutic Criteria Committee. (1981). Preliminary criteria for clinical remission in rheumatoid arthritis. *Arthritis and Rheumatism, 24*, 1308–1315.

Pincus, T., Callahan, L. F., Sale, W. G., Brooks, A. L., Payne, L. E., & Vaughn, W. K. (1984). Severe functional declines, work disability, and increased mortality in seventy-five rheumatoid arthritis patients studied over nine years. *Arthritis and Rheumatism, 27*, 864–872.

Pincus, T., Summey, J. A., Soraci, S. A., Wallston, K. A., & Hummon, N. P. (1983). Assessment of patient satisfaction in activities of daily living using a modified Stanford health assessment questionnaire. *Arthritis and Rheumatism, 26*, 1346–1353.

Polley, H. F., Swenson, W. M., & Steinhilber, R. M. (1970). Personality characteristics of patients with rheumatoid arthritis. *Psychosomatics, 11*, 45–49.

Randich, S. R. (1982). Evaluation of pain management program for rheumatoid arthritis patients (Abstract). *Arthritis and Rheumatism, 25*, S11.

Riggs, G. K., & Gall, E. (1984). *Rheumatic disease rehabilitation and management*. Boston: Butterworth Publishers.

Rind, V. M., Bird, N. A., & Wright, V. (1980). A comparison of clinical assessments of decreased activity in rheumatoid arthritis. *Annals of Rheumatic Disease, 39*, 135–137.

Ritchie, D. M., Boyle, J. A., McInnes, J. M., Jasani, M. K., Dalakos, T. G., Grieveso, P., & Buchanan, W. W. (1968). Clinical studies with an articular index for the assessment of joint tenderness in patients with rheumatoid arthritis. *Quarterly Journal of Medicine, 37*, 393–406.

Rodnan, G. P., Schumacher, H. R., & Zvaifler, N. J. (Eds.). (1983). *Primer on the rheumatic diseases* (8th ed.). Atlanta: Arthritis Foundation.

Schwartz, G. (1982). Testing the biopsychosocial model: The ultimate challenge facing behavioral medicine. *Journal of Consulting and Clinical Psychology, 50*, 1040–1053.

Scott, P. J., & Huskisson, E. C. (1976). Graphic representation of pain. *Pain, 2*, 175–184.

Seligman, M. E. (1975). *Helplessness*. San Francisco: Freeman.

Skevington, S. M. (1983). Activities of illness behavior in chronic pain. *Pain, 15*, 295–307.

Smith, H. (1973). Smith hand function evaluation. *American Journal of Occupational Therapy, 27*, 244–251.

Smith, R. O. & Benge, M. W. (1985). Pinch and grasp strength: Standardization of terminology and protocol. *American Journal of Occupational Therapy, 39*, 531–535.

Steinbrocker, O., Traeger, C. H., & Battman, R. C. (1949). Therapeutic criteria in rheumatoid arthritis. *Journal of the American Medical Association, 140*, 659–662.

Swezey, R. L. (1978). *Arthritis: Rational therapy and rehabilitation*. Philadelphia: Saunders.

Tugwell, P., & Bombardier, C. (1982). A methodologic framework for developing and selecting endpoints in clinical trials. *Journal of Rheumatology, 9*, 758–762.

Wallston, K. A., Pincus, T. P., Nicassio, P., Woodward, N., & Dodd, M. A. (1983, March). *Correlates of functional capacity in patients with rheumatoid arthritis*. Paper presented at·the meeting of the Society of Behavioral Medicine, Baltimore.

Wegener, S. T. (1986). *The prediction of rehabilitation outcome in rheumatoid arthritis patients*. Unpublished manuscript.

Wegener, S. T., O'Leary, A., & Brunner, C. M. (1986, March). *The Tripartite model in arthritis rehabilitation assessment*. Paper presented at the meeting of the Society of Behavioral Medicine, San Francisco, CA.

Wolff, B. B. (1971). Factor analysis of human pain responses: Pain endurance as a specific pain factor. *Journal of Abnormal Psychology, 78*, 292–298.

Wright, V. (1985). Measurement of outcome in rheumatic disease. *Journal of the Royal Society of Medicine, 78*, 985–994.

Zaphiroporelos, G., & Burry, H. C. (1974). Depression in rheumatoid disease. *Annals of Rheumatic Diseases, 33*, 132–135.

Zung, W. (1965). A self-rating depression scale. *Archives of General Psychiatry, 12*, 63–70.

Chapter 13

A Comprehensive Battery for the Measurement of Rehabilitation Outcomes after Major Burns

Kent A. Questad, Michael Boltwood,
Al Alquist, and Barbara J. deLateur

Private and public agencies that pay for most rehabilitation services are demanding an increasingly more accurate description of what they are paying for. From a scientific standpoint, any valid description of a complex process such as rehabilitation after a burn injury requires the measurement of selective factors that describe the process and how these factors relate. Therefore, from a global (interdisciplinary) perspective, the use of multivariate measures and analysis techniques in rehabilitation research and practice is frequently recommended. The purpose of this chapter is to describe the development of a comprehensive, multivariate battery to measure the physical and psychological rehabilitation of patients who have suffered a major burn injury.

WHAT TO MEASURE

When determining what should be measured before assembling a battery, one temptation is to include every measure that might be relevant. Unfortunately, a battery developed by this approach usually produces a great quantity of numbers that are difficult to assemble into a coherent picture of a patient. This is the result of several inherent weaknesses in this approach. First, every measure chosen implies a specific implicit hypothesis, but the various hypotheses are not required to fit into a coherent model of the rehabilitation process or to reflect the patient as a whole. The only way of resolving this problem systematically is to formulate hypotheses overtly that fit into a theoretical model first, then develop a battery that measures only factors that fit into the model. A second implicit assumption is that the measures chosen are valid and reliable. Although this assumption is especially questionable for measures that are developed clinically, even well-standardized and widely accepted measures usually cannot be considered valid or reliable unless data support their use with the specific type of patients evaluated. If such data are not available, the validity of measures should be determined by formulating and testing hypotheses about relationships that should exist among them if they are indeed measuring what they are supposed to be measuring.

DESIGNING THE BATTERY

With the above strategy in mind, the first step was to develop a general structure of hypotheses to test in the battery. Retrospective research and common sense suggest that preinjury factors, the extent and location of the burn, other medical problems, and the nature of treatment would all influence a patient's health status, physiological status, physical function, psychological function, and social function after a burn injury. Research in medical psychology suggests that some secondary characteristics (covariates) might also relate to outcome that are not related to the nature of the injury or treatment. These characteristics involve the degree and quality of social support patients receive (Brian et al., 1985) and the amount of control they feel they have over their health (Achterberg-Lawliss, 1983; Lau, 1982). The overall hypothesis adopted was that patients generally recover completely from their burn injury both physically and psychologically 1 year postburn. A schematic outline of the battery's hypotheses is shown in Figure 1.

The next step was to find measures appropriate for testing the hypotheses. The following rules were used to choose measures. Measures should be well standardized, accepted, understood, and applicable to multiple patient populations. Data should also be available from different populations, including healthy individuals, to provide a context for interpreting what the measures really mean. To meet the criteria of being accepted and understood, measures need to be

tied to an accepted conceptual framework of health and illness. The World Health Organization (WHO, 1980) has developed a taxonomy of terms to describe health status. This system, including definitions of impairment, disability, and handicap, is described in Chapter 1 of this volume.

To measure outcome, there are many excellent, well-standardized questionnaires about health and illness as well as many indices of physical function commonly used in rehabilitation. Recently, several large-scale projects have been directed toward developing standardized measures of self-reported health. The Sickness Impact Profile (SIP) and Rand mental health form are results of such projects (Bergner, 1985; Gilson et al., 1975; Ware, Johnson, Davies-Avery, & Brook, 1979). The SIP, including assessments of patient recovery in degree of independence, physical well-being, and psychosocial status, has proven to be a valid, reliable measure of self-reported health with a variety of patient populations (Bergner, 1985; Deyo, Inui, Leininger, & Overman, 1983; Mclean, Dikmen, Tempkin, Wyler, & Gale, 1984). Because the questions in these scales ask patients to assess the

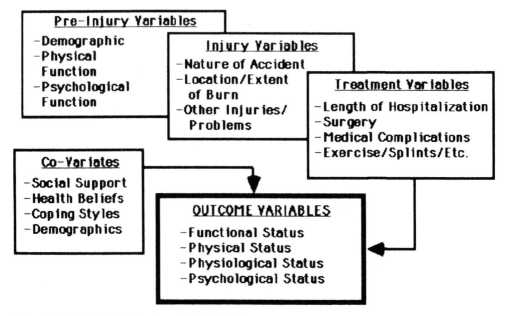

Figure 1.   University of Washington burn rehabilitation study.

impact of a specific impairment, such as that resulting from a burn injury, on many aspects of their lives, they provide information about patients' perceptions of their health in a form that conforms nicely with the WHO definitions. When combined with standard clinical indices of physical function, such as active range of motion (ROM) measurements, they provide a reasonably complete description of both the patient's and the clinician's assessment of the patient's health status.

In some cases, however, a certain amount of creativity was necessary to find measures that met the criteria described above. For example, demographic characteristics such as patients' educational level, age, and type of residence are particularly difficult to quantify in a standard, generally understood fashion. These same factors, however, have been found to be highly related to an individual's full-scale IQ on the Wechsler Adult Intelligence Scale (Revised) (Barona, Reynolds, & Chastain, 1984). Therefore, it is possible to summarize demographic characteristics in the form of an estimated IQ. Along with the person's income, these are used as measures of the influence of demographic factors.

One of the hardest areas for which to develop measures is the seriousness of the burn itself. The most widely recognized measure is the total body surface area burned. Because there are some well-known problems with this measure, and other measures of burn severity are not yet generally accepted, length of hospital stay and the total number of surgical procedures received throughout acute treatment were added as indicators of the general severity of the person's injury. To control or account for the probable effects of burn location, subjects were divided into groups according to whether or not they had burns or grafts to a joint, hand, or cosmetically important area. If they had one or more burned joints they were classified as a "1," and if they had one or more grafted joints they were classified as a "2." A similar strategy has been used with hand burns and burns to cosmetic areas. The classification systems selected and used depend on the clinical question being evaluated. Measures used in the battery are shown in Table 1.

Table 1.   Variables and measurements

Variable	Measurement
1. Self-reported health	Sickness Impact Profile
2. Preinjury health	Rand physical and mental health measures
3. Upper extremity motion	Sum of deviations from normal of range of motion
4. Muscle strength	Cybex testing
5. General stamina	Submaximal oxygen consumption testing
6. Locus of control	Health locus of control scale
7. Social support	Social support questionnaire

THE BATTERY IN DETAIL

Covariates

Data on preinjury health were gathered from the subjects' medical records and from having subjects complete the Rand mental and physical health forms while in acute burn care. To measure two other covariates of burn recovery, questionnaires measuring social support (Schaefer, Coyne, & Lazarus, 1981) and health-specific locus of control (Lau & Ware, 1981) were also administered.

Self-Reported Health Measures

The SIP and the Rand mental health battery were used to obtain these measures. Individual responses on the SIP were scored to provide 12 subscales: ambulation, mobility, body care and movement, social interaction, communication, alertness behavior, emotional behavior, sleep and rest, eating, work, home management, and recreation. These scales were combined together as shown in Table 2 to form composite scales representing levels of self-reported disability, handicap, and emotional impairment.

Table 2.   Sickness Impact Profile scales

Disability scales	Handicap scales	Emotional scales
Body care	Home maintenance	Emotional behavior
Mobility	Social interest	Sleep
Ambulation	Employment	Alertness behavior
Eating	Recreation	

The Rand mental health battery responses were scored to yield five subscales: anxiety, depression, loss of behavioral/emotional control, general positive affect, and emotional ties. Anxiety, depression, and loss of behavioral/emotional control were combined to give a psychological distress score and general positive affect and emotional ties were combined to give a well-being score. A combination of all five basic subscales produced a cumulative mental health index score (Brooks et al., 1979). These scales provide measures of emotional disabilities that may be the result of a burn injury.

Muscle Strength and Endurance Measures

Skeletal muscle strength and endurance variables were measured with a Cybex II isokinetic dynamometer, dual channel recorder, speed selector, and upper body exercise table. The isokinetic (constant rotational velocity) dynamometer accommodates a range of rotational velocities and provides a resistance equal and opposite to the torque output of the working limb throughout the range of motion.

Four large muscle groups responsible for the motion of the two major limb joints were tested for strength and endurance. The isokinetic dynamometer was used to measure the torque output (foot-pounds) of knee and elbow flexors and extensors. The dual-channel recorder simultaneously plotted torque output and position angle. Each muscle group was tested for maximal strength at five velocities: 0 (isometric), 10, 20, 30, and 40 rpms. Reciprocal contractions were conducted so peak extension and flexion torques were obtained in a short, nonfatiguing test. Patients were told to exert maximum force against the input arm throughout the entire ROM for five repetitions. If a decrement in torque was observed in both flexors and extensors by the third or fourth repetition, the patient was told to stop, thus avoiding superfluous work (fatigue). The order of velocity testing was randomized to avoid ordering effects. An endurance test was then administered, which consisted of 20 maximal extensions of the knee and 20 maximal extention/flexion reciprocal contractions of the elbow joint at 20 rpms. A fatigue index was computed for

each muscle group tested by dividing the minimum torque produced over the last five contractions by the maximum produced over the 20 performed.

Kinetic and Respiratory Efficiency

Many patients with major burns cannot comfortably perform traditional maximal exercise testing. A modified oxygen consumption test was developed to collect data from these patients and healthy, unburned subjects for all the tests described below. Oxygen consumption tests were conducted using four modes of exercise: 1) leg cycling on a Monark bicycle ergometer, 2) arm cycling on a Monark arm ergometer, 3) walking on a Quinton Q55 motorized treadmill, and 4) free walking 30.3 meters in a standard tile hallway. The test protocols were tailored for each mode and sex to preclude excessive stress. All tests included similar procedures:

1. The working stages were submaximal.
2. The treadmill, arm, and leg cycling tests consisted of four exercise stages (12 minutes) and were preceded by a resting and followed by a recovery stage.
3. A three-lead electrocardiogram was monitored continually throughout each test.
4. Each stage was 3 minutes in length to theoretically allow subjects to operate at steady state prior to and throughout the third minute (sample minute).
5. Air expired during the last minute of each stage was collected in a Douglas bag and analyzed quantitatively with a gas meter and qualitatively for carbon dioxide and oxygen content with a Perkin–Elmer 1100 mass spectrometer.

The respiratory quotient (McArdle, Katch, & Katch, 1981) was calculated to reveal how efficiently patients transported and metabolized energy stores and the by-products of performing work. The quotient thus represents a measure of patients' general stamina.

Pulse Intensity Calculation

The patient's heart rate was measured at each exercise level and converted to an exercise intensity index. The intensity index (II) is a function of the subject's resting heart rate (RHR), theoretical maximum heart rate (MHR), and the heart rate observed during exercise (EHR). The MHR was determined by the well-established, age-predicted formula MHR = 220 − age (in years). In the II, MHR − RHR represents the theoretical maximum increase in heart rate that could occur as a result of exercise. The value EHR − RHR represents the exercise-induced elevation in heart rate from rest. Dividing EHR − RHR by MHR − RHR provides a measure of the additional exercise-associated stress to the subject that is standardized with respect to age and the general physiological stress the subject is under while resting. Thus the formula for the II is (EHR − RHR)/(MHR − RHR). A standardized measure of heart rate response to exercise, the II is another measure of general stamina.

Upper and Lower Extremity Evaluations

Active and passive ROM were measured by standardized methods for the shoulder, elbow, wrist, and hand. Computation of the indices and scores derived from those measures was accomplished using microcomputer software written by the first author of this chapter.

Active ROM of the lower extremities was measured using the methods outlined by the American Orthopedic Association. Standard tests of lower extremity functions included tests for hip flexion and rectus femoris contractures, as well as contracture of the tensor fasciae latae and/or iliotibial tract. Straight leg raises also were assessed. Other tests were conducted of running, deep knee bends, toe raises, and walking on heels. In addition, gait deformity was assessed.

OTHER MEASUREMENTS

Grip strength, palmar pinch and two-point discrimination (Hunter, 1978) were measured by conventional methods.

Mouth Measurements

Height and width of the mouth were measured for all patients. Both are active measurements.

Neck Measurements

Seven measurements were recorded, six active ROM and one neck circumference. Range of motion was measured with the patient sitting erect in a straight-back chair with head in the neutral position.

Time

Time must also be considered when interpreting all of the measures described above. Referencing events to time since injury rather than to time since discharge is preferable. The reason for this may not be obvious. For clinical purposes, time since discharge from the hospital often serves as a useful gauge for evaluating how well a patient is progressing. For purposes of outcome assessment, however, it is a poor measure because it is related directly to the length of a patient's hospital stay, which in turn is closely related to the severity of the patient's injury. This confounding variable makes comparing different patients' rates of recovery impossible. Using postinjury time, on the other hand, puts all patients on the same time scale, making comparisons of recovery rate possible.

VALIDITY OF THE BATTERY

Criteria

All of the measurement techniques and instruments have been found to be reasonably reliable and valid when used with other patient groups, but their validity for measuring recovery from burn injuries is not well established. The validity of each measure in the battery was assessed by measuring: 1) the degree to which it is related to other measures as hypothesized, 2) the degree to which it detects changes in patients as they recover, and 3) its subjective, clinical validity for adequately representing patients as seen by clinicians.

Impairment Measures

The following are examples of some findings that reflect on the validity of the battery. The first is an example of a general hypothesis developed by the physical and occupational therapists working on the project. Their hypothesis was that all patients would have less than normal grip strength at discharge. From their clinical experience, they had noticed that patients in general seem to be weaker than normal at discharge. The therapists also hypothesized that the patients' grip strengths would be related to the condition of their hands and also to the general severity of their injury.

Patients' grip strengths at discharge were compared with available age- and sex-specific norms (Mathiowetz et al., 1985). The graph in Figure 2 shows that, as hypothesized, all patients had grip strength substantially below normal, regardless of their hand condition, that is, whether the hands were uninjured, burned but not grafted, or burned and grafted. All of the differences from normal levels seen in this figure were found to be statistically significant ($p < .05$). There also was a significant relationship between hand condition and grip strength, as predicted.

The severity of the injury, as measured by surgeries, was also related to grip strength (Figure 2), even though two thirds of the patients had no surgeries to the hand. In addition, all groups were significantly below normal. Since these data support the hypothesis of the study, they also support the validity of grip strength as a measure of an impairment related to burn injuries.

A second impairment study focused on general stamina, as reflected by oxygen consumption and heart rate response to submaximal exercise. Sixty patients with major burns performed graded submaximal exercise on a treadmill, bicycle ergometer, and arm ergometer at 3 months postburn. The same exercise was performed by 50 controls. The two groups had comparable oxygen consumption. For burn subjects, however, the pulse response was greater at any given work load or rate of oxygen consumption. Research data to date suggest that this index may be the most valid measure of the effects of burn injuries on the general stamina and intensity of required effort of burn patients.

Disability and Handicaps

Another preliminary set of findings involved patients' self-reported health measure by the SIP at 3 months postburn (Patterson, Questad, & Boltwood, in press). The general hypothesis was that people on average would report few if any problems on the various scales that are measured by the SIP. This expectation was supported by the finding that, across the 12 scales measured by the SIP, 30 patients reported relatively few problems at the 3-month follow-up.

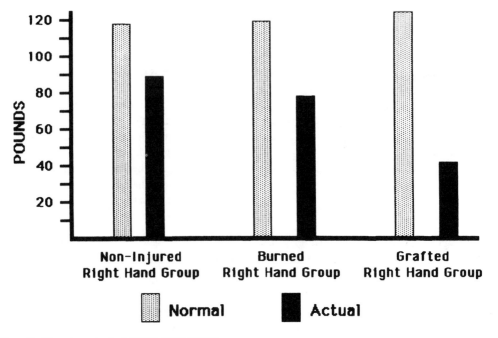

Figure 2.   Normal versus actual right hand grip strength.

It was hypothesized further that significant subgroups would report substantial problems in one or more of the areas measured. Accordingly, the data were subjected to a cluster analysis that divided the 30 patients into groups according to how similar their reports were on the SIP. The analysis produced one group comprising half of the patients who reported less problems than the group as a whole. Two other groups had substantial problems in one area and related elevations on several other SIP scales. The first of these groups contained nine patients. These people reported major vocational problems along with higher levels of emotional and social problems than the patients as a whole. The other major group consisted of five people who reported major levels of emotional problems along with higher elevations of problems on other scales.

A subsequent study (Questad et al., 1986) examined the course of self-reported recovery over the first year postburn. To summarize data, the scales of the SIP were aggregrated into two summary scales, one consisting of scales that measured disabilities and one that measured handicaps. The composition of these scales is shown in Table 2. The hypotheses of this study were: 1) burn patients in general would report fewer disabilities and handicaps as time passed; 2) burn patients in general would not report disabilities or handicaps at 12 months; and 3) the general level and rate of decline of reported handicaps and disabilities would be related to length of hospital stay, preinjury mental health, and postinjury sense of self-control of health. At 3 months, the median score on both the handicap scale and the disability scale were statistically greater than $0 (p < .05)$. By 6 months postburn the median disability score was not statistically different from 0; however, the median handicap score remained greater than 0 until 12 months postburn. Even though the medians were not statistically different from 0, 13% of patients reported that they still had disabilities and 55% that they still had handicaps 12 months postburn. The most frequently reported handicap was a vocational handicap such as no employment or underemployment. A series of multiple regression analyses revealed that preinjury mental health and the self-control scale were not related to either the average level

of the SIP scales over the 12-month period or the rate at which they declined. The length of time the patient had been in the hospital was related to the average level of both of the scales, but not to the rate of decline of either scale.

Total body surface area burned (TBSA) and age are the best established predictors of survival after a burn injury. The purpose of another four studies was to test the relative validity of estimated IQ, income, preinjury mental health, age, and TBSA for predicting self-reported physical and mental health 3 months after a major burn. Subjects were 47 patients who had suffered a major burn injury according to American Burn Association criteria. While in the hospital, subjects completed the Rand mental health form to describe their preinjury mental health, and were interviewed to obtain the approximate income of their household and other demographic variables. Factors such as educational level, sex, and region of residence were used in a previously derived equation to estimate the subject's IQ. Three months after their injury, subjects completed the SIP and Rand mental health form.

A series of multiple regression analyses revealed that preinjury mental health had a strong relationship to all measures of mental and physical health. The exceptions were the SIP scales that measure handicaps; none of the predictors were related significantly to them. Income was also significantly related to all postinjury mental health measures but not to preinjury mental health. Age, TBSA, and IQ were not related to any outcome measures. These results suggest that preinjury mental health and income may be valid, independent predictors of postburn health and that age, TBSA, and demographic factors used to compute an estimated IQ have little predictive validity.

Emotional Impairment

In another study, 55 subjects completed both the SIP and health locus of control scale 3 months after their burn injury. Their responses were analyzed using multiple regression techniques. As in the study described above, the scales of the SIP were reduced to two composite scales, one a summation of scales representing disabilities and the other a summation of scales representing handicaps. Only the handicap scale, the disability scale, and the self-control scale were significantly related to the psychological distress scale of the Rand mental health scale. Similar results were found using the Rand well-being scale. Of the three independent variables, the disabilities scale was most highly related to the Rand scales ($R = .492$ and $R = .522$; $p < .05$) the handicap scale was next ($R = .398$, $R = .454$; $p < .05$), and the self-control scale was least related ($R = .295$, $R = .383$). These results suggest that, when significant disabilities are present, they may be the greatest determining factor of a subject's emotional mental health. Handicaps and perceived self-control of health, however, also may play a significant role in determining psychological adjustment.

CONCLUSIONS

The results presented above suggest that, for patients with major burns, it is generally true that: 1) the level of self-reported disabilities and handicaps, particularly vocational and recreational handicaps, is substantial over a 1-year period postinjury and is related to their length of stay in the hospital; 2) their grip strength is below normal; 3) their response to submaximal exercise is abnormal; and 4) there are significant relationships among measures of disabilities, handicaps, and emotional impairments.

Implications of these studies for the validity of the various elements of the battery are, of course, the most important for this discussion. Most of the hypotheses tested were supported, and thus the general validity of the battery was also supported. What stands out are the few measures that were not related to other measures in the hypothesized manner. First, none of the analyses found that total body surface area burned related significantly to any of the measures of impairment, disability, or handicap. For rehabilitation purposes, length of acute hospital stay and number of surgeries received appear to be more valid indicators of the severity of the injury. Second, estimated IQ has not proven to be a valid indicator of the influence of demographic factors on recovery. However, preinjury income does appear to be a valid predictor of the degree of disability and handicap burned patients report over the course of a year. Finally, although some studies have found that perceived self-control over health is related to some measures of outcome, the relationship has not proven to be as strong or as consistent as originally hypothesized.

Finally, results of these studies have important broader implications for how recovery from burn injuries should be assessed. The effect of a burn injury can be as obvious as facial scarring or amputation of a limb and as subtle as reduced grip strength or reduced recreational activities. When the clinical use of the battery described here is impractical, clinicians must make some sort of comprehensive measurement of burn-related impairments, disabilities, and handicaps to enable a valid assessment of how well patients are recovering from a burn injury.

REFERENCES

Achterberg-Lawliss, J. (1983). Predictive factors of burn rehabilitation. *Journal of Burn Care and Reconstruction, 4,* 437–441.

Barona, A., Reynolds, C. R., & Chastain, R. (1984). A demographically based index of premorbid intelligence for WAIS-R. *Journal of Consulting and Clinical Psychology, 52,* 885–887.

Bergner, M. (1985). A measurement of health status. *Medical Care, 23,* 696–704.

Brian, S., Blanchart, F., Cherrier-Baumann, M., Guenot-Gosse, C., Calles-Blanchard, E., Deschamps, J. P., & Senault, R. (1985). Isolation, social support, life events and health status. *Revue d'Epidemiologie et de Santé Publique, 33,* 48–65.

Brookes, R. H., Ware, J. E., Jr., Davies-Avery, A., Stewart,

A. L., Donald, K. A., Rogers, W. H., Williams, K. N., & Johnson, S. A. (1979). Overview of health status measures fielded in Rand's health insurance study. *Medical Care, 17,*(Suppl.), 1–55.

Deyo, R. A., Inui, T. S. S., Leininger, J. D., & Overman, S. S. (1983). A comparison of traditional scales and a self-administered health status questionnaire in patients with rheumatoid arthritis. *Medical Care, 211,* 180–192.

Gilson, B. S., Gilson, J. S., Bergner, M., Bobbitt, R. A., Kressel, S., Pollard, W. E., & Vesselago, M. (1975). The sickness impact profile: Development of an outcome measure of health care. *American Journal of Public Health, 65,* 1304–1325.

Hunter, S. (1978). *Rehabilitation of the hand.* St. Louis: Mosby.

Lau, R. R. (1982). Origins of health locus of control beliefs. *Journal of Personality and Social Psychology, 42,* 322–334.

Lau, R. R., & Ware, J. E., Jr. (1981). Refinements in the measurement of health-specific locus of control beliefs. *Medical Care, 19,* 1147–1157.

Mathiowetz, V., Kashman, N., Volland, G., Weber, K., Dowe, M., & Rogers, S. (1985). Grip and pinch strength: Normative data for adults. *Archives of Physical Medicine and Rehabilitation, 66,* 69–74.

McArdle, W. D., Katch, F. I., & Katch, V. L. (1981). *Exercise physiology, energy, nutrition, and human performance.* Philadelphia: Lee & Febiger.

McLean, A., Dikmen, S., Tempkin, N., Wyler, A. R., & Gale, J. L. (1984). Psychosocial functioning at one month after head injury. *Neurosurgery, 14,* 393–399.

Patterson, D., Questad, K., & Boltwood, M. (in press). Patient reports about their health and physical functioning three months after a major burn. *Journal of Burn Care and Rehabilitation.*

Questad, K., Boltwood, M., Patterson, D., Covey, M., deLateur, B., Marvin, J., Engrav, L., Dutcher, K., & Heimbach, D. (1986, April). *Self-reported physical health over the course of a year after a major burn: A preliminary analysis.* Paper presented at the annual meeting of the American Burn Association, Chicago, IL.

Schaefer, C., Coyne, J. C., & Lazarus, R. S. (1981). The health-related functions of social support. *Journal of Behavioral Medicine, 4,* 381–406.

Ware, J. E., Johnson, S. A., Davies-Avery, A., & Brook, R. H. (1979). *Conceptualization and measurement of health for adults in the health insurance study: Vol. III. Mental health.* Santa Monica, CA: Rand Corporation.

World Health Organization. (1980). *International classification of impairments, disabilities, and handicaps: A manual of classification relating to the consequences of disease.* Geneva: Author.

Chapter 14

Measuring Rehabilitation Outcomes for Infants and Young Children
A Family Approach

Deborah A. Allen

This chapter is based on the premise that outcome measures in pediatric rehabilitation must consider the entire family. Although a specific intervention may be designed to impact upon the child, the family as a unit will necessarily influence the outcome. After discussing the dynamics of the family approach in rehabilitation outcome analysis, the chapter deals briefly with issues of methodology. Outcome measures are then examined, including selection of outcomes to measure, various categories of outcomes (child, parent, family, costs, and community), and mediating program variables. Finally, a program in Connecticut is evaluated as an illustration.

DEFINING THE POPULATION AND SCOPE OF SERVICE

It is difficult to estimate the number of infants and young children in the United States who could benefit from rehabilitation services. This is due in part to the inability to define the population. The need for services is usually thought to extend to children with diagnoses such as mental retardation, physical-motor disability, emotional disorders, learning disabilities, and serious

chronic illnesses, but there is considerable variance in which diagnoses are included. Moreover, diagnostic categorization is often rendered imprecise by the ever-changing backdrop of human development. Only the minority of children diagnosed as disabled show clearly identifiable impairments at birth. Approximately 160 infants per 100,000 have a serious genetic or central nervous system defect (Hayden & Beck, 1982). A larger number have less severe or less obvious disabilities that may not be detected until after the first year, when developmental milestones fail to appear. Other milder disabilities may be transient or have uncertain prognoses, falling into the grey area that evaluators call "suspect."

Researchers typically separate handicapping conditions of childhood into three broad etiological categories. The first includes infants with known disorders, most often congenital, such as Down's syndrome and spina bifida. The second is the biological risk category. Many of these infants are survivors of neonatal intensive care units and have a range of pre-, peri-, and postnatal complications. The majority are of low birth weight. Although the incidence of low birth weight (less than 2,500 grams) has declined since the mid-1960s (Budetti, Barrand, Mc-

The author is indebted to Glenn Affleck and Suzanne Hudd for their contributions to this chapter and to Sandra Anderson for manuscript preparation. The Family Consultation Project was supported by grants from the Connecticut State Department of Education, National Institute of Mental Health (NIMH), University of Connecticut Research Foundation, and the Research and Training Center for Pediatric Rehabilitation.

Manus, & Heiner, 1981), advances in neonatal medicine have increased the survival rate, particularly for infants of very low birth weight (less than 1,501 grams), who are most likely to show sequelae. The third category is environmental risk. Children in this group are subject to adverse influences on their development such as disadvantaged environments or teenage parents. These infants, apparently healthy at birth, account for the largest number of those eventually requiring services, most often for mild to moderate psycho-educational handicaps.

These three population groupings overlap considerably (Strauss & Brownell, 1985). For example, infants at risk because of a disadvantaged environment are also more likely to experience biological risk from low birth weight or prematurity. Likewise, the distinction between biological risk and known disorders may be blurred by limitations in diagnosis for some conditions (e.g., ventricular bleeds, cerebral palsy).

For young children subject to multiple risks, there are further ambiguities in defining "rehabilitation." A process that occurs over time, rehabilitation traditionally refers to restoring function. For the child, restoration of *original* function is irrelevant since developmental change and rehabilitation are concurrent. Pediatric rehabilitation calls for bringing function to a level expected at a given point in time and hoping that the gains will sustain continued development. This framework also applies to the family, since families change over time in response to the child's changing capacities and demands.

Thus, the concepts of habilitation and rehabilitation merge toward one another when referring to very young children. Services for this population may target preventing future disability, eliminating the possibility of secondary effects from an existing disability, or maximizing developmental potential within the limitations imposed by a disability. Since these goals may assume different degrees of importance over time, the term "early intervention" will be adopted to cover a range of habilitative, rehabilitative, and preventive services. Early intervention programs that primarily focus on compensatory education for economically disadvantaged preschoolers (e.g.,

Head Start) are not covered in this review because they have been analyzed extensively in other sources.

THE FAMILY APPROACH

When measuring rehabilitation outcomes for any individual, considering the entire family is always important. The case for doing so is especially strong where infants and young children are concerned. The family is the filter through which most of the baby's experience is channeled. It provides the earliest social relationships and the nutrients for developmental progress. If quality of life is defined from an ecological perspective as "the reciprocal relationships between persons and their environments" (Alexander & Willems, 1981), then the family and caretaking milieu are the major determinants of quality of life for the infant. It is therefore not surprising that interventions that include parents are more effective (Bronfenbrenner, 1975). Likewise, gains from intervention are typically short-lived when they lack carryover into the child's home environment.

Until recently, most intervention studies have focused exclusively on mothers. The maternal emphasis has also predominated in clinical practice. In the past decade, the roles of fathers (Cummings, 1976; Field, 1981; Marton, Minde, & Perrotta, 1981; Stoneman, Brody, & Abbott, 1983) and siblings (Powell & Ogle, 1985; Skrtic, Summers, Brotherson, & Turnbull, 1984) have gained increasing attention. It is to be hoped that a true family-centered approach is on the horizon. In such an approach, the family is not viewed as a collection of individual members, but rather as a unit comprised of interwoven subsystems (e.g., the marital relationship, sibling relationships, parent–child relationships).

Farber (1960) was the first to bring attention to the impact of the handicapped child on the family. Following his work were investigations of various effects on family integrity such as divorce, stress, lowered earning potential, and social isolation (Price-Bonham & Addison, 1978). Today, advances in family theories of normal human development (Belsky, 1981) and family systems theory (McCubbin, Sussman, & Patterson, 1983) offer useful models for conceptualizing family influences on the handicapped child.

The child, of course, also influences the family in bidirectional, reciprocal fashion (Bell, 1979). For example, many disabled and biologically at-risk infants are less responsive than healthy infants. They may smile less or give less distinctive cues to caregivers, who in turn may reduce their efforts to elicit infants' social behaviors because those efforts are not rewarded. Similarly, the parent who is emotionally depleted by stresses or the demands of the infant's condition may be less likely to give appropriate stimulation to the child.

GENERAL METHODOLOGICAL CONSIDERATIONS

Evaluation of early intervention is plagued by a host of methodological problems. Methodological concerns have figured prominently in reviews of the effectiveness of early intervention for handicapped and biologically at-risk infants (Bricker, 1985; Halpern, 1984; Marfo & Kysela, 1985; Simeonsson, Cooper, & Scheiner, 1982). Lack of methodologic rigor impedes the evaluation of global interventions as well as therapies for specific disabilities, such as physical therapies for children with cerebral palsy (Parette & Hourcade, 1984). Early intervention research is beset by extraordinary heterogeneity in its samples, barriers to sound study design, and confusion about the best measurement strategy. Yet the effects expected from early intervention are generally small, requiring the most sensitive designs and instruments to detect them (Sheehan & Keogh, 1981).

The Sample

Programs usually serve children with a range of handicapping conditions of varying severity. A noncategorical view of child health and health problems (Stein & Jessop, 1982) may facilitate evaluation to the extent that all children and families involved in chronic health crises encounter common life experiences (Pless & Pinkerton,

1975). Despite recent attempts to develop noncategorical measures of children's functional status (Stein & Jessop, 1982), sample heterogeneity is a serious problem for the interpretation of most measures currently in use.

Not only do children have a broad range of disabilities, but the typically small sample sizes make comparisons among children with similar disabilities even more problematic. One way to reduce these effects is through the implementation of collaborative, multisite studies. Another is to devise a means for describing children's progress along some common yardstick such as Simeonsson and Wiegerink's (1975) "index of efficiency." A sort of sliding z score, this index is calculated from the amount of progress expected, the amount of progress made, and the child's relative abilities at the start of the program.

Study Design

For ethical and practical reasons, experimental and even quasi-experimental designs are not always possible in evaluating programs for children with disabilities. Pre- versus postprogram comparisons are the most popular method, but are subject to the ususal methodological criticisms. Another potentially powerful option is the comparison of different treatment variations. Where experimental designs can be employed, there is much debate about whether samples should be matched according to infants' chronological or gestational ages or, for older children, according to chronological age, mental age, or some behavioral criterion. When children are severely delayed, the choice of a comparison group can make a considerable difference in the conclusions drawn about program effeetiveness. In a cogent discussion of this issue, Stoneman and Brody (1984) concluded that the choice should be dictated by theoretical rationale and not by mere convenience, as is usually the case.

Studies are commonly designed to address the question "Is early intervention effective?" Unfortunately, this question is so general as to be almost meaningless (Bricker, Seibert, & Casuso, 1980; Gray & Wandersman, 1980). Rather, researchers should be asking, "For whom do which interventions produce what effects?" Corresponding sophistication in research design is required. Reliance on a single cause–single effect model must yield to multivariate analyses in which interaction terms are considered. Simple main effects have accounted for very little variance in early intervention. To be used appropriately, multivariate techniques will demand the development of casual models that are presently lacking in the field of early childhood development (Halpern, 1984).

Longitudinal follow-up is another important design feature that is too often missing in the study of outcomes for children with disabilities. Since few tests can be used across a very wide age span, longitudinal research with children typically requires the use of different measures for the same construct as the child ages. This problem compounds the usual impediments conducting longitudinal research.

Measurement Strategy

In deciding upon a measurement strategy, the researcher faces a number of options. The strengths and weaknesses of self-report versus observational measures have been reviewed (Eyberg, 1985; Stoneman & Brody, 1984). Self-reports can be obtained through interviews or questionnaires. They may not correspond to actual behavior, but are useful indicators that can be strengthened by obtaining reports from multiple family members.

Traditional observational measures have been unidirectional, capturing only the infant's or the caretaker's behavior in isolation from each other. Although unidirectional measures do provide worthwhile information, dyadic and systems measures are needed to deal with reciprocal relationships. Measures of this type may ask questions about contingent responsiveness, that is, the probability that one family member will make a particular response following the action of another family member. Streams of behavior can be analyzed from a continuous record of interactions (Stoneman & Brody, 1984). The intensive labor involved in these analyses is a drawback, and some people believe that the result fails to capture qualitative aspects of the interaction

(Bakeman & Brown, 1977). Where resources permit, much can be gained from the complementary use of multiple measurement strategies.

OUTCOME MEASURES

Selecting Outcomes to Measure

By far the most common, and often the only, index of intervention effectiveness has been the child's cognitive development as quantified by the intelligence quotient (IQ) or developmental quotient (DQ). This point was illustrated in Marfo and Kysela's (1985) review of 20 early intervention programs in five countries conducted during the last 10 years. In 70% of these programs, child developmental progress was the sole outcome measured.

The overreliance on IQ/DQ has been criticized (Zigler & Trickett, 1978). Even when a child's cognitive development has not improved, benefits from other aspects of the child's life and development may be overlooked. In some cases, change may not be a reasonable goal and intervention success may mean maintenance of existing function. The intervention might also improve parental coping, parent–child interaction, or family status and can have an impact on the community.

Since many interventions work with parents and families to effect and sustain change in the child, evaluating the program's impact on these agents of change makes sense. Yet this does not usually happen. In the Marfo and Kysela (1985) review, parents were trained to teach their children at home in 90% of the programs, but the instructional competence of parents was measured in only one study. In addition, only two of the seven programs that provided parental support measured its effects on parents.

These findings suggest the need for early intervention outcome measures that are more closely related to the program goals. In cases where a goal is considered instrumental to effecting some indirect, ultimate outcome (e.g., improving parental teaching skills to enhance child development), the immediate program impact is more likely to be on the mediator variables than on the child variables. Furthermore, one can argue that positive effects on the change agents, in this case, the parents, are valuable goals in their own right. The desirability of benefiting families *as families* and not just as conduits of intervention therapies for the child is consistent with a growing concern about family burdens and stresses (Gallagher & Vietze, 1986; Turnbull & Winton, 1984).

Child Outcomes

Despite the fact that developmental status is the most frequently measured outcome, the many difficulties in assessing disabled infants and young children produce results that are often unsatisfactory. There are reliability and validity problems with tests that yield global scores as well as with those that are limited to a specific behavioral domain, such as pediatric motor scales (Berk & DeGangi, 1979).

Most existing developmental scales have been standardized on normal children, and the variety of handicapping conditions has worked against the development of test norms for handicapped children. Instead of a norm-referenced test, the choice may be a criterion-referenced test that evaluates the child's performance with respect to defined behaviors as opposed to the performance of a comparison group of children. This approach is supported by those who point out that the question is not how the disabled child should be functioning if he or she were normal but rather what pattern exists in the individual child's development (Simeonsson & Wiegerink, 1975). Such an ideographic approach, however, can pose difficulties as results are interpreted.

Simeonsson and Wiegerink (1975) recommended adapting standardized scales, carefully detailing the adaptations required for various disabilities, then systematically applying the adaptations. Some tests that have been developed recently follow their advice. One example is the Battelle Development Inventory (Newborg, Stock, Wnek, Guidubaldi, & Svinicki, 1984). It was standardized on a large sample of nonhandicapped children, but provides general and specific modifications for testing children with various disabilities. Accompanying individual

test items are pertinent suggestions for positioning, alternate test materials, and so forth.

Most infant tests rely heavily on motor behaviors that can discriminate against motor-handicapped infants (Kearsley, 1981). Abnormal muscle tone and persistence of primitive reflexes also impede testing. Indeed, prevailing models of infant development tend to rely on the Piagetian concept of a sensorimotor period, which inadequately describes the course of development for infants with sensory or motor impairments. Fraiberg's (1970) work with blind infants shows how blindness can delay the formation of object constancy, affect the onset of self-initiated mobility and midline hand activity, prolong separation anxiety, and influence language acquisition.

The presence of severe handicapping conditions may make the assessment process so difficult that the examiner concludes the child is "untestable" (Alpern, 1976). This situation is unfortunate and often avoidable. Ulrey and Rogers (1982) offered comprehensive guidelines for testing "untestable" children and stressed the importance of a well-trained examiner who is not only familiar with the assessment of disabled children, but also prepared to perform follow-ups and re-evaluations. Scores from IQ/DQ tests can be clinically useful and, if the tests are properly administered, give a good indication of current functioning. However, keep in mind that they do have limited predictive ability, at least for the majority of infants whose impairments are not severe (McCall, 1981). The chain of self-fulfilling prophecy that the premature labeling of children can initiate demands caution in test interpretation.

Other aspects of child functioning have received greater attention lately as outcome measures (Halpern, 1984). These include socio-emotional development, medical management (medication status, seizure control), behavior patterns (crying, sleeping), independence (self-feeding, toileting), and physical growth. Sometimes gross indicators are used (e.g., number of hospitalizations). In other instances, the measures are relatively sophisticated, as, for example, the Vineland Adaptive Behavior Scales (Sparrow, Balla, & Cicchetti, 1984). By and large, there is little agreement as to what aggregate of outcomes constitutes an adequate assessment of the whole child, and further work is needed in this area.

Parent Outcomes

The birth of a disabled or seriously ill infant is a profound crisis for the parents (Waisbren, 1980), and their distress can be lifelong (Wikler, Wasow, & Hatfield, 1981). Most theories postulate orderly stages of parental grieving, as reviewed by Blacher (1984). However, empirical support for stage theories is scant; instead, remarkable variability in parents' responses has been observed (Allen & Affleck, 1985). Program evaluations rarely incorporate any parent outcomes beyond parents' satisfaction with services. On the other hand, researchers trying to uncover reasons for variability in parental adaptation have begun developing some promising measurement approaches.

Although parents' psychological status is of interest as an outcome, most clinical scales that measure psychological status have been designed to discriminate psychopathologies. However, parents' responses seldom fall within the pathological range. Instruments that reflect the more normal range of disturbances are preferable, for example, Lorr and McNair's (1982) Profile of Mood States. Measures of parenting stress and resources (Holroyd, 1974) and subjective stress in response to tragic life events (Horowitz, Wilner, & Alvarez, 1979) have also proven useful.

Coping is a complex theoretical construct (Lazarus, 1981) that encompasses cognitive adaptations as well as affective response. Several cognitive adaptations have been related to parents' reactions to the birth of a disabled child. For instance, parents' attributions as to the cause of their infant's condition have been shown to affect their adjustment (Affleck, Allen, McGrade, & McQueeney, 1982). Other cognitive factors that influence coping with disabled infants include parents' perceptions of personal control and ability to derive personal meaning from an otherwise unanticipated, tragic event (Affleck, Tennen, & Gersham, 1985).

Parental knowledge and competencies have been addressed in some programs. Knowledge of the specific training content of a particular program, as well as knowledge of child development and attitudes toward child rearing (e.g., Field, Widmayer, Stringer, & Ignatoff, 1980), have been assessed. Bromwich (1983) has developed the Parent Behavior Progression to measure the evolution of parenting competencies, a tool with both clinical and evaluative applications.

Parent-Child and Family Outcomes

Parents' views of their child are based on the child's actual behavior and on the parents' expectations. It is well known that expectations can strongly affect the disabled child's subsequent development (Lavelle & Keogh, 1980). For this reason, parent perceptions of caretaking difficulties (Broussard, 1976), infant temperament (Bates, Freedland, & Lounsbury, 1979; Pedersen, Anderson, & Cain, 1976), and child progress are valuable indicators of intervention outcome.

Parents' interactions with their disabled children have been studied in terms of objective units of behavior such as smiling, looking, touching, and vocalizing. Parent–child interactions have also been evaluated in terms of subjective judgments in areas such as physical closeness, contingency of maternal response, or sociability (Yarrow et al., 1976). Some measures assess the parent–child interaction as well as the home environment in which it occurs, usually through a combination of objective and subjective indices. Perhaps the most popular instrument of this type, backed by considerable literature, is the Home Observation for Measurement of the Environment Inventory (Caldwell & Bradley, 1978). It assesses the quality and quantity of developmental supports in the child's environment through information obtained from direct observation and parental report.

Recently, there have been some encouraging attempts to apply family systems methodologies to the study of families with severely disabled children (Stoneman & Brody, 1984). Barnard and her colleagues (Barnard, Snyder, & Spietz, 1984) have developed an approach to the assessment of infants and families with physical, health, and social-environmental risks that provides nurses with a tool to evaluate infant and family needs, plan intervention strategies, and monitor progress. At the level of programming for the individual child, family goals, expectations, and constraints may be included in the individualized educational program (IEP). Finally, social support (Crnic, Greenberg, Ragozin, Robinson, & Basham, 1983) and cultural factors play an important role in family adaptation to a disabled child.

Costs and Community Impact There are two outcomes of early intervention for children with disabilities that have received virtually no consideration: costs and impact on the community. In studies of the cost-effectiveness of programs for economically disadvantaged preschoolers, early intervention has been found to be cost-effective in terms of dollars saved on remedial education, social services, and correctional services (e.g., Schweinhart & Weikart, 1980). These data are used to justify the existence of the programs to policymakers. Comparable analyses of programs for handicapped youngsters have not been conducted, perhaps because services for handicapped children are less likely to be considered a luxury. Even for services that are mandated, however, comparing the costs of alternate, equally effective treatment strategies for handicapped children would be useful.

The impact of rehabilitation programs on the community has been addressed almost exclusively in relation to handicapped adults, for whom deinstitutionalization and the establishment of community residences have forced study of the issue. Researchers seem to be operating under the doubtful assumption that programs for young children lack appreciable community impact since children are typically constrained to the immediate caretaking environment. However, increasing calls to remedy shortages of day care, respite care, and case coordination and referral systems for handicapped youngsters have made early intervention a community issue. Public awareness has increased with the recent publicity given to cases involving the withholding of medical treatment for handicapped newborns. Unfortunately, methods for measuring community outcomes are lacking, and community assessment entails a number of political and methodological dilemmas described elsewhere (Allen, in press). Nevertheless, neglect of this area should not be allowed to continue.

Program Variables Few studies of intervention programs for disabled infants and toddlers document how the intervention is actually accomplished. Only 10% of the studies included in the Marfo and Kysela (1985) review showed any concern for the collection of process data. This omission is particularly distressing in light of the emphasis on program flexibility. Intervention activities depend upon the individual family's needs, preferences, and resources as well as the nature of the child's problems. Moreover, the nature of the relationship between the intervenor and the parent is rarely described, although it is the proposed catalyst for change in most programs.

When the intervention is documented, it is normally done by intervenor report. In only a few studies is the intervention itself actually observed (Gray & Wandersman, 1980). Gray and Ruttle (1980) found that reports by home visitors of their activities in the Family-oriented Home Visiting Program contradicted an observer's analysis of those visitors' actual activities. Although the home visitors were convinced that they were working with the mother, the analysis revealed that they were spending considerably more time with the child.

Documenting program variables allows replication of the program and accounts for some variability in program outcome. Children and families who profit less from the intervention may in fact have received qualitatively or quantitatively different services. Intervention should be considered not an all-or-nothing event, but a continuum of services to be documented and treated as an independent variable in analyzing outcomes.

INTERPRETING INTERVENTION OUTCOMES

If an intervention designed to promote cognitive gains in children fails to do so but does improve parents' coping, is it successful or unsuccessful? Since it is unlikely that all outcomes measured will be intercorrelated, how can a verdict be delivered? Ultimately, certain value judgments are involved, and different people diverge in valuing various outcomes. The administrator may give priority to cost-effectiveness, the early childhood educator may value cognitive gains, and the psychologist may stress parental adjustment. Parents themselves differ as to how they evaluate the success of a program. This point was illustrated by a study of parents of handicapped preschool children enrolled in an intervention program in England (Sandow, Clarke, Cox, & Stewart 1981). Parents whose children were moderately handicapped considered program success in terms of their children's intellectual and social gains, whereas parents whose children were profoundly handicapped judged success in terms of emotional and informational support.

For many outcome measures, the superiority of one score over another is by no means clear (Holmes, 1985). The "sooner is better" assumption, which values accelerated attainment of developmental milestones, is not always justified for improving future development. Nor is it always true that "you can't have too much of a good thing" where children's development is concerned. For example, it was once erroneously assumed that infants who cried louder when approached by strangers were more attached to their caregivers and would hence develop better. Qualitative measures that categorize children according to characteristic response patterns would seem to avoid such value judgments. However, when qualitative measures are used for program evaluation, judgments tend to be placed on the inherent worth of certain categories (e.g., "secure" attachment) without empirical justification that one behavior pattern is necessarily better than another for improving future outcome (Holmes, 1985).

THE FAMILY CONSULTATION PROJECT: AN ILLUSTRATION

From 1979 through 1984, the author and her colleagues carried out and evaluated the effects of a family-oriented, home-based early intervention program called the Family Consultation Project, which enrolled over 100 handicapped and biologically at-risk infants. The program structure and philosophy are described elsewhere (Affleck, McGrade, McQueeney, & Allen, 1982). Several notable features of the program evaluation are outlined below.

Method

First, information was derived from multiple sources: neonatal nurses, follow-up clinic physicians, the intervention workers, independent researchers, and the parents themselves. Second, multiple assessments took place. Most data came from researchers' home visits after the infant's birth and at 9, 18, and 40 months, but additional data were collected during interim periods. Third, the intervention was documented, not only in terms of the amount of intervention but also by monthly activities reports of the intervenors and parental reports of what had transpired. Although treatment and comparison groups were randomly assigned, ethical considerations dictated that many comparison infants be enrolled in other existing services. The nature of these services and parental perceptions of these other services were documented as well. Fourth, multiple forms of measurement were used: qualitative and quantitative measures and standardized and nonstandardized assessment tools from among those described earlier in this review. Efforts were made to establish the reliability and validity of each measure. Fifth, the variables measured included a wide variety of indicators of child status, parental perceptions and adjustment, parent–child interactions, and home circumstances. Many measures addressed parental coping in some fashion because this was the primary focus of the supportive intervention.

Results

Program participants as a group showed short-term gains in the quality of the parent–child relationship and home environment and long-term advantages for mothers' emotional and cognitive adaptation. Relative gains in these areas were particularly evident in families whose children were exhibiting poorer development. With the exception of the child's social-emotional status at 40 months of age, effects of the program were not seen in objectively measured child outcomes. Within certain family subgroups (e.g., with infants of very low birth weight, teenaged mothers), the children who received the intervention program exhibited more positive social and emotional characteristics (e.g., cooperativeness, sociability) and/or fewer negative emotional characteristics. The absence of effects on the children's 40-month IQ or social maturity quotient may have been due to the extremely wide variability on these measures.

Within several categories of familial risk (lower social class, single-parent families, teenage mothers, preintervention coping difficulties, poorer infant development), effects of program participation were seen in the mothers' longer term adaptation. Mothers from these families appeared to benefit by developing more positive attitudes toward their children's development, resolving the emotional turmoil associated with the early crisis, showing less distress, and holding more positive expectations for the future.

Conclusion

Was the Family Consultation Project effective? Not in the way that effectiveness is usually defined. Had the evaluation concentrated on children's cognitive development and not distinguished family subgroupings, the results would not have been nearly so encouraging. As it was, the broad family-oriented view of outcome adopted suggested that the intervention did indeed yield certain benefits. More importantly, the specificity in outcome measurement allowed for refinement in the intervention strategy for second-generation programs.

REFERENCES

Affleck, G., Allen, D. A., McGrade, B. J., & McQueeney, M. (1982). Maternal causal attributions at hospital discharge of high risk infants. *American Journal of Mental Deficiency, 86,* 575–580.

Affleck, G., McGrade, B. J., McQueeney, M., & Allen, D. (1982). Promise of relationship-focused early intervention in developmental disabilities. *Journal of Special Education, 16,* 413–430.

Affleck, G., Tennen, H., & Gersham, K. (1985). Cognitive adaptations to high-risk infants: The search for mastery, meaning, and protection from future harm. *American Journal of Mental Deficiency, 89,* 653–656.

Alexander, J. L., & Willems, E. P. (1981). Quality of life: Some measurement requirements. *Archives of Physical Medicine and Rehabilitation, 62,* 261–265.

Allen, D. A. (in press). The identity crisis in community research. In J. A. Mulik & R. F. Antonak (Eds.), *Transitions in mental retardation: Vol. 3. The community imperative: A comprehensive review.* Norwood, NJ: Ablex.

Allen, D. A., & Affleck, G. (1985). Are we stereotyping parents? A postscript to Blacher. *Mental Retardation, 23,* 200–202.

Alpern, G. D. (1976). Measurement of "untestable" autistic children. *Abnormal Psychology, 72,* 478–486.

Bakeman, R., & Brown, J. V. (1977). Behavioral dialogues: An approach to the assessment of mother–infant interaction. *Child Development, 48,* 195–203.

Barnard, K. E., Snyder, C., & Spietz, A. (1984). Supportive measures for high-risk infants and families. *Journal of Birth Defects, 20,* 291–329.

Bates, J., Freedland, C., & Lounsbury, M. (1979). Measurement of infant difficultness. *Child Development, 50,* 794–803.

Bell, R. Q. (1979). Parent, child and reciprocal influences. *American Psychologist, 34,* 821–826.

Belsky, J. (1981). Early human experience: A family perspective. *Developmental Psychology, 17,* 3–23.

Berk, R. A., & DeGangi, G. A. (1979). Technical considerations in evaluation of pediatric motor scales. *The American Journal of Occupational Therapy, 33,* 240–244.

Blacher, J. (1984). Sequential stages of parental adjustment to the birth of a child with handicaps: Fact or artifact? *Mental Retardation, 22,* 55–68.

Bricker, D. (1985). The effectiveness of early intervention with handicapped and medically at-risk infants. In M. Frank (Ed.), *Infant intervention programs: Truths and untruths* (pp. 51–65). New York: The Haworth Press.

Bricker, D., Seibert, J. M., & Casuso, V. (1980). Early intervention. In J. Hogg & P. J. Mittler (Eds.), *Advances in mental handicap research: Vol. 1* (pp. 225–266). New York: Wiley.

Bromwich, R. M. (1983). *Manual for the Parent Behavior Progression (PBP).* Northridge, CA: The Center for Research, Development and Services, Department of Educational Psychology, California State University.

Bronfenbrenner, U. (1975). Is early intervention effective? In M. Guttentag & E. Streuning (Eds.), *Handbook of evaluation research: Vol. 2* (pp. 519–603). Beverly Hills: Sage Publications.

Broussard, E. R. (1976). Neonatal prediction and outcome at 10/11 years. *Child Psychiatry and Human Development, 7,* 85–93.

Budetti, P., Barrand, N., McManus, P., & Heiner, L. (1981). *The implications of cost-effectiveness analysis of medical technology* (Library of Congress Catalog No. 80-600161). Washington, DC: U. S. Government Printing Office.

Caldwell, B. M., & Bradley, R. H. (1978). *Home observation for measurement of the environment.* Little Rock: The Center for Child Development and Education, University of Arkansas at Little Rock.

Crnic, K. A., Greenberg, M. T., Ragozin, A. S., Robinson, N. M., & Basham, R. B. (1983). Effects of stress and social support on mothers and premature and full-term infants. *Child Development, 54,* 209–217.

Cummings, S. T. (1976). The impact of the child's deficiency on the father: A study of fathers of mentally retarded and of chronically ill children. *American Journal of Orthopsychiatry, 46,* 246–255.

Eyberg, S. M. (1985). Behavioral assessment: Advancing methodology in pediatric psychology. *Journal of Pediatric Psychology, 10,* 123–137.

Farber, B. (1960). Family organization and crisis: Maintenance of integration in families with a severely mentally retarded child. *Monographs of the Society for Research in Child Development, 25*(1).

Field, T. (1981). Fathers' interactions with their high-risk infants. *Infant Mental Health Journal, 2,* 249–256.

Field, T. M., Widmayer, S. M., Stringer, S., & Ignatoff, E. (1980). Teenage, lower-class, black mothers and their preterm infants: An intervention and developmental follow-up. *Child Development, 51,* 426–436.

Fraiberg, S. (1970). Intervention in infancy: A program for blind infants. *Journal of the American Academy of Child Psychiatry, 10,* 381–405.

Gallagher, J., & Vietze, P. (1986). *Families of handicapped persons: Research, programs and policy issues.* Baltimore: Paul H. Brookes Publishing Co.

Gray, S. W., & Ruttle, K. (1980). The Family-oriented Home Visiting Program: A longitudinal study. *Genetic Psychology Monographs, 102,* 299–316.

Gray, S. W., & Wandersman, L. P. (1980). The methodology of home-based intervention studies: Problems and promising strategies. *Child Development, 51,* 993–1009.

Halpern, R. (1984). Lack of effects for home-based early intervention? Some possible explanations. *American Journal of Orthopsychiatry, 54,* 33–42.

Hayden, A., & Beck, G. (1982). The epidemiology of high-risk and handicapped infants. In C. Ramey & P. Trohanis (Eds.), *Finding and educating high-risk and handicapped infants* (pp. 19–51). Baltimore, MD: University Park Press.

Holmes, D. L. (1985, April). *Value judgments and descriptive categories in infant research.* Paper presented at the meetings of the Society for Research in Child Development, Toronto.

Holroyd, J. (1974). The questionnaire on resources and stress: An instrument to measure family response to a handicapped member. *Journal of Community Psychology, 2,* 92–94.

Horowitz, M., Wilner, N., & Alvarez, W. (1979). Impact of event scale: A measure of subjective stress. *Psychosomatic Medicine, 41,* 209–218.

Kearsley, R. (1981). Cognitive assessment of the handicapped infant: The need for an alternative approach. *American Journal of Orthopsychiatry, 51,* 43–53.

Lavelle, N., & Keogh, B. K. (1980). Expectations and attributions of parents of handicapped children. In J. J. Gallagher (Ed.), *New directions for exceptional children, No. 4* (pp. 1–27). San Francisco: Jossey-Bass.

Lazarus, R. S. (1981). The stress and coping paradigm. In C. Eisdorfer, D. Cohen, A. Kleinman, & P. Maxim (Eds.), *Theoretical basis for psychopathology* (pp. 177–214). New York: Spectrum.

Lorr, M., & McNair, D. (1982). *Profile of Mood States-B.* San Diego: Educational and Industrial Testing Service.

Marfo, K., & Kysela, G. M. (1985). Early intervention with mentally handicapped children: A critical appraisal of applied research. *Journal of Pediatric Psychology, 10,* 305–324.

Marton, P., Minde, K., & Perrotta, M. (1981). The role of the father for the infant at risk. *American Journal of Orthopsychiatry, 51,* 672–679.

McCall, R. B. (1981). Predicting developmental outcome: Resume and redirection. In C. C. Brown (Ed.), *Infants at risk: Assessment and intervention* (pp. 57–69). Piscataway, NJ: Johnson and Johnson Pediatric Round-Table Series.

McCubbin, H. I., Sussman, M. B., & Patterson, J. M. (1983). *Social stress and the family: Advances and developments in family stress theory and research. Marriage and Family Review (Vol. 6, Nos. 1–2).* New York: Haworth Press.

Newborg, J., Stock, J. R., Wnek, L., Guidubaldi, J., & Svinicki, J. (1984). *The Battelle Developmental Inventory.* Allen, TX: DLM Teaching Resources.

Parette, H. P., & Hourcade, J. J. (1984). A review of therapeutic intervention research on gross and fine motor progress in young children with cerebral palsy. *The American Journal of Occupational Therapy, 38,* 462–468.

Pederson, F. A., Anderson, B. J., & Cain, R. L. (1976, April). *A methodology for assessing parental perceptions of infant temperament.* Paper presented at the fourth biennial Southeastern Conference on Human Development.

Pless, I. B., & Pinkerton, P. (1975). *Chronic childhood disorder: Promoting patterns of adjustment.* London: Henry Kimpton.

Powell, T. H., & Ogle, P. A. (1985). *Brothers and sisters—a special part of exceptional families.* Baltimore: Paul H. Brookes Publishing Co.

Price-Bonham, S., & Addison, S. (1978). Families and mentally retarded children: Emphasis on the father. *Family Coordinator, 27,* 221–230.

Sandow, S. A., Clarke, A. D. B., Cox, M. V., & Stewart, F. L. (1981). Home intervention with parents of severely subnormal preschool children: A final report. *Child: Care, Health and Development, 7,* 135–144.

Schweinhart, L. J., & Weikart, D. P. (1980). Effects of the Perry Preschool Program on youths through age 15. *Journal of the Division for Early Childhood, 4,* 29–39.

Sheehan, R., & Keough, B. K. (1981). Strategies for documenting progress of handicapped children in early education programs. *Educational Evaluation and Policy Analysis, 3,* 59–67.

Simeonsson, R. J., Cooper, D. H., & Scheiner, A. P. (1982). A review and analysis of the effectiveness of early intervention programs. *Pediatrics, 69,* 635–641.

Simeonsson, R. J., & Wiegerink, R. (1975). Accountability: A dilemma in infant intervention. *Exceptional Children, 41,* 474–481.

Skrtic, T. M., Summers, J. A., Brotherson, M. J., & Turnbull, A. P. (1984). Severely handicapped children and their brothers and sisters. In J. Blacher (Ed.), *Severely handicapped young children and their families: Research in review* (pp. 215–246). New York: Academic Press.

Sparrow, S., Balla, D., & Cicchetti, D. (1984). *Vineland Adaptive Behavior Scales.* Circle Pines, MN: American Guidance Service.

Stein, R. E. K., & Jessop, D. J. (1982). A noncategorical approach to chronic childhood illness. *Public Health Reports, 97,* 354–362.

Stoneman, Z., & Brody, G. H. (1984). Research with families of severely handicapped children: Theoretical and methodological considerations. In J. Blacher (Ed.), *Severely handicapped young children and their families: Re-*

search in review (pp. 179–214). New York: Academic Press.

Stoneman, Z., Brody, G. H., & Abbott, D. (1983). In-home observations of young Down syndrome children with their mothers and fathers. *American Journal of Mental Deficiency, 87,* 591–600.

Strauss, M. S., & Brownell, C. A. (1985). A commentary on infant stimulation and intervention. In M. Frank (Ed.), *Infant intervention programs: Truths and untruths* (pp. 133–139). New York : The Haworth Press.

Turnbull, A. P., & Winton, P. J. (1984). Parent involvement policy and practice: Current research and implications for families of young, severely handicapped children. In J. Blacher (Ed.), *Severely handicapped young children and their families* (pp. 377–397). New York: Academic Press.

Ulrey, G., & Rogers, S. J. (1982). *Psychological assessment of handicapped infants and young children.* New York: Thieme-Stratton.

Waisbren, S. E. (1980). Parents' reactions after the birth of a developmentally disabled child. *American Journal of Mental Deficiency, 84,* 345–351.

Wikler, L., Wasow, M., & Hatfield, E. (1981). Chronic sorrow revisited: Parent vs. professional depiction of the adjustment of parents of mentally retarded children. *American Journal of Orthopsychiatry, 51,* 63–70.

Yarrow, L., Cain, R., Pedersen, F., Rand, C., Fivel, M., & Abramson, A. (1976). *Rating scales of maternal and infant characteristics.* Unpublished document, Social and Behavioral Sciences Branch, NICHHD, Bethesda, MD.

Zigler, E., & Trickett, P. (1978). IQ, social competence, and evaluation of early childhood intervention programs. *American Psychologist, 33,* 789–798.

Chapter 15

Correlates of Employment Outcomes of Blind Clients of State Vocational Rehabilitation Agencies

J. Martin Giesen and William H. Graves

The employment problems of blind people are a central concern of administrators of state rehabilitation agencies as well as other professionals. Reducing the unemployment and underemployment problems of the blind persons served by a rehabilitation agency frequently requires that the agency administrator examine the contribution of the services to the outcome of rehabilitation. Often rehabilitation administrators have lacked sufficient information about the contributions to case outcome of different rehabilitation services to enable allocation or reallocation of agency resources according to their potential for reducing client unemployment.

Administrators of rehabilitation agencies have lacked the necessary information on which to base resource allocation decisions because relatively little outcome research has focused on blind and severely visually impaired clients of state rehabilitation agencies (Giesen & Graves, 1984; Giesen, Graves, Machalow, Schmitt, & Dietz, 1984; Schmitt, 1984). Much of the existing literature deals with nonvocational adjustment to blindness (Ammons, 1978), restricts itself to a population of blind persons in a specific geographic region (Knowles, 1969) or a single state agency (Crouse, 1974), or describes employed blind persons (Bauman & Yoder, 1963, 1964).

Agency administrators have been hampered further in their resource allocation decisions by investigations that examined rehabilitation outcome in the "successful or status 26" versus "unsuccessful or status 28" classification system. As Kirchner and Peterson (1982) illustrated, the successful or status 26 category contains at least three subgroups, that is, persons closed as competitively employed, homemakers, or sheltered workshop employees, each with unique characteristics and case service needs. If the agency's goal is to reduce the underemployment and unemployment of its blind and visually impaired clients through competitive employment closures, the agency administrator will need to know which rehabilitation services contribute to which client outcomes, including those that are not competitive employment closures. Outcomes should therefore be examined in terms of more specific outcome categories, as Dunn (1975) argued, so that more accurate estimations of client benefits from the delivery of rehabilitation services can be made.

Both interpretation and prediction methodology should be practical in the outcome classification system that is employed. Prediction methodology in Dunn's list of functional outcomes (1975) is too extensive to be practical. Additionally, the outcome criteria system should address closure issues of concern to these administrators, such as allocating resources for improving the agency's competitive employment closure rate, identifying service needs of persons

Development of this document was supported by Rehabilitation Research and Training Center Grant G008103981 from the National Institute for Handicapped Research, Department of Education, Washington, D.C. Opinions expressed in this document are not necessarily those of the granting agency.

closed in sheltered employment, and examining service delivery issues and client characteristics of persons closed as homemakers.

SUMMARY OF OUTCOME RESEARCH LITERATURE

An extensive body of literature relates various elements of the rehabilitation process to client outcomes. The purpose of most client outcome studies has been to identify those client characteristics that are related to rehabilitation outcome (Bolton, Butler, & Wright, 1968). Outcome studies have been cited as the first step toward providing individualized service programs (Bolton, 1972b).

Although numerous predictive outcome studies have been conducted over the years, the majority of these studies are difficult to compare because they were carried out in specific geographic locations, focused on selected or mixed disability groups, used different criteria for success, or employed different data collection techniques or statistical procedures. To improve the state of the art of predicting rehabilitation outcomes, Bolton (1979) has recommended that no mixed disability groups be employed in the same study and that multivariate analyses be used in outcome research. The study reported below conforms to these recommendations.

Predictive and Descriptive Outcome Studies Specific to Blindness

Relatively few studies have attempted to predict rehabilitation outcome of legally blind clients of state rehabilitation agencies. Several of these studies have described the personal characteristics of the successful blind rehabilitant. Other studies have dealt with a segment of the blind population, such as those blinded during a war, or predicted nonvocational outcomes such as adjustment to blindness or ability for independent living. These studies have been summarized to identify variables potentially indicative of the employment outcome of blind and severely visually impaired clients.

Bauman and Yoder (1963) surveyed 408 legally blind persons employed in 14 occupations. Over 50% of the subjects were totally blind, and

less than 14% had any useful residual vision. The most common traits possessed by these successful professionals were good mobility skills, above-average written and spoken communication skills, good memory, pleasant appearance, and adequate self-confidence. Bauman and Yoder (1964) also investigated the characteristics of over 700 clerical, industrial, and service employees. The typical blind worker in those occupations was a man between 35 and 45 years of age, who 1) had some travel vision, 2) traveled independently using a cane, 3) had graduated from high school, 4) was married with children, 5) produced on an equal level with sighted workers, 6) obtained employment through a state agency for the blind, 7) was trained on the job by his employer, 8) was satisfied with services received, 9) had no major health problems, and 10) believed that persistance, self-confidence, and hard work were the keys to success.

Scholl, Bauman, and Crissey (1969) also reported factors that contributed to the vocational success of visually handicapped clients. The study used 16 personal variables collected for 644 subjects from five states. Vocational success was defined in terms of three criterion variables: percentage of time worked, income, and a socioeconomic index for occupations. The best predictors for percentage of time worked were IQ, sex, travel ability, educational level, and other disabilities. The best predictor variables for income were IQ, sex, functional vision, marital status, educational level, and other disabilities. For the occupational socioeconomic index, IQ, sex, educational level, money spent, travel ability, and other disabilities were the best predictor variables. Intelligence, sex, education, and disabilities other than blindness were the predictor variables common to all three outcome criteria. Descriptive data also revealed that the clients were employed in a limited range of occupations, with more than 50% of the men employed in 13 occupations and 50% of the women employed in only 9 occupations.

Knowles (1969) employed three levels of inferential statistics to study successful and unsuccessful vocational rehabilitation of 461 legally blind clients. The sample contained 245 successful rehabilitants and 216 clients closed unsuccessfully. The only variables found significant in all three analyses were mobility and orientation training and vocational classification before rehabilitation. Three other highly significant discriminators between the success and nonsuccess groups were age at which blindness occurred, years of blindness, and age at rehabilitation.

Personal and program service characteristics were investigated by Crouse (1974) to determine predictors of rehabilitation outcome for legally blind clients of a state rehabilitation agency. The personal characteristic variables of age, sex, race, marital status, number of dependents, and educational level were not as useful as the program service characteristics in predicting rehabilitation success. Within the group of program service variables, personal adjustment services and physical restoration services proved to be the most useful predictors of successful outcome.

Kirchner and Peterson (1982) described three outcome groups of legally blind and otherwise visually impaired persons closed in the 1980 fiscal year by state-federal vocational rehabilitation agencies. Kirchner and Peterson divided the status 26 closures into competitive employment, sheltered workshop, and homemaker groups. Those clients closed in competitive employment were generally the least severely visually impaired, had no second disabling condition, were slightly more likely to be male, were under 36 years old, were either never married or currently married, had at least a twelfth-grade education, were primarily white, received neither Social Security Insurance (SSI) or Social Security Disability Insurance (SSDI), and were either not working or competitively employed at referral. The vast majority of sheltered workshop closures were the most severely visually impaired, and considerably more than half had a second disabling condition. They were slightly more likely to be male, between 25 and 54 years old, white (over a quarter were black), and never married, with a ninth-grade education or less; three quarters were recipients of SSI, SSDI, or both, and the majority were not working at the time of referral. Half the homemaker closures were legally blind with the other half being visually impaired. Just over half had a second disabling condition and over three quarters of the group were female.

The homemakers were generally over 54 years old, currently married or widowed, white, and either homemakers or not working at the time of referral, with less than a twelfth-grade education. Two thirds received no benefits, and one third were recipients of either SSI or SSDI.

The Kirchner and Peterson (1982) analyses are limited by two major factors. First, their analyses of the R-300 tape were restricted to cases closed in RSA status 26 in a single fiscal year. It must be noted, however, that the analyses subdivide the 26 closure population into three categories and provide a significant and unique analysis of rehabilitation outcome data that addresses issues of considerable interest to the blindness field. Omitting cases closed in status 28 from the analyses, however, does restrict the number of implications that can be drawn by rehabilitation administrators. The second limitation is that the R-300 data base does not contain information that previous research has shown to be related to the outcome of services provided blind persons. For example, Scholl et al. (1969) and Knowles (1969) found that blind persons who received orientation and mobility training were more likely to have successful rehabilitation outcomes. Age at onset of blindness (Knowles, 1969) was reported to be predictive of outcome as well. Neither of these two variables was available to Kirchner and Peterson in their examination of the FY 1980 vocational rehabilitation placements of blind and visually impaired clients.

Additional Potential Predictors of Rehabilitation Outcome

No studies identifying variables related to outcome were found that examined the influence of the labor market, that is, unemployment rate, on employment outcome for blind clients of the state rehabilitation system. Levitan and Taggart (1977) stated that "the disabled are disproportionately affected by labor market changes. . . . In bad times, those who become disabled are the most expendable workers, and disabled job seekers lose out in competition with others who are sounder in mind or body" (p. 23). This study, therefore, examined the contribution of labor market conditions to the prediction of employment outcome, specifically the county or Standard Metropolitan Statistical Area (SMSA) unemployment rate of the client 60 days prior to case closure.

Attempts have not been made to assess the impact of the proximity of rehabilitation facilities, rehabilitation counseling services, and protected employment for blind/severely visually impaired persons on the outcome of the rehabilitation process. Crouse (1974) found the use of a facility in a rehabilitation case to be positively related to a successful closure. However, proximity as such has not been investigated in a systematic manner.

Although the contributions of education to the prediction of rehabilitation outcome (Scholl et al., 1969) have been examined in prior research, the contribution of a closely related factor, the blind client's occupational history, has not been systematically studied. A considerable body of literature (e.g., "New study affirms," 1983) indicates that the briefer the period of unemployment prior to referral for rehabilitation services, the greater the likelihood of competitive employment outcome. Other occupational factors, such as difficulty level of the job held by the blind person prior to the provision of rehabilitation services, have not been investigated.

Other variables not investigated in prior outcome studies include use of optical and nonoptical aids, low vision aid training services, Individualized Written Rehabilitation Plan (IWRP) vocational goal levels, number of changes in IWRP vocational goals, and case services expenditure data.

PURPOSE OF STUDY

The present study was designed to assist vocational rehabilitation agencies serving blind and visually impaired persons to identify client characteristics and agency resources associated with four client employment outcomes. It was also intended to fill gaps in the rehabilitation literature regarding the employment outcomes of rehabilitation for blind clients of state rehabilitation agencies. The four employment outcomes are competitive employment closures, sheltered workshop employment closures, homemaker closures, and nonworking closures. The categories of variables used to predict client employment status outcome

include personal, financial, occupational, rehabilitation process, counselor, and environmental variables.

The study was designed to identify the following variables predicting employment outcome:

1. Those associated with the rehabilitation service delivery system process
2. Those characteristic of the client, including those related to disability and to personal/biographical characteristics
3. Those related to the financial status of the client
4. Those related to the occupational history of the client
5. Those related to the rehabilitation counselor
6. Those related to the environment

METHOD

Subjects

The states of Florida, Kansas, Mississippi, and Ohio were selected to participate in the study. The four states represented a sampling of different geographic locations, agency structures, and urban/rural populations. Case files of individuals closed in rehabilitation status 26 (successful) and status 28 (unsuccessful) during federal fiscal years 1978 through 1980 (October 1, 1977 to September 30, 1980) served as the population from which the cases were selected.

The systematic quota sampling procedure used called for selecting every 17th case file from a master list of all cases closed to ensure that the sampling would be distributed across the client population of each state. This sampling method resulted in each state being represented in proportion to the total served and to the 26/28 closure ratio for each state. All 619 cases selected were persons at least legally blind, having Rehabilitation Services Administration (RSA) disability codes of 100–119.

Data Collection

Based on the literature review, studies of R-300 data, case file previews, and identification of previously unexplored variables, 136 specific variables were abstracted from case files by a team of data collection specialists. Seventy-one "R" variables were obtained from the R-300 form or a modified version of the form used by the state. Case file information provided 32 "C" variables, including specific information on type and number of additional eye disabilities, type and number of other (noneye) disabilities, receipt of mobility training, use of adaptive aids, ability and achievement test scores, occupational history information, job titles, *Dictionary of Occupational Titles* (DOT) codes (U.S. Department of Labor, 1977), locations and addresses of counselor and service facilities, and counselor demographic information, including training and experience. Each job title was coded by its DOT code and assigned a job difficulty index number, the Total Vocational Quotient (TVQ) (McCroskey, 1980). The DOT code was useful for descriptive purposes and the TVQ index permitted inclusion of employment information in quantitative analysis. The third section of the coding form was designed for coding up to 28 case service expenditure ("E") totals.

Predictor Variables

A total of 151 variables were identified from the initial set from the coding form, recoded variables, indicator variables, and special computed indices. All of these variables were quantitative. This set of 151 variables included variables that were "outcome" rather than "predictor" variables, and there were missing data unavailable from the case files on some variables.

In order to address these problems, the list of variables was carefully examined. Variables that themselves could be considered "outcome" variables or that were descriptive of rehabilitation outcome, such as weekly earnings at closure and outcome of extended evaluation or vocational rehabilitation services, were identified. It was deemed inappropriate to employ variables that were unknown until at or near the time of closure to predict outcome. Another restriction for selection of a predictor was that it have little, if any, missing data, because variables with substantial missing data may tend to show relationships that are restricted to particular subsets of the sample. Also, when the selected set of predictor variables was analyzed, the number of cases available for

the variable with the smallest N was used to limit the number of cases on all other variables to this same minimum value. Using the restrictions noted above, a subset of 101 candidate predictors was selected from the initial set of possible predictors. These variables were not outcomes of the process, and were complete for all, or nearly all (99%), of the cases in the sample. Variables recorded in the database and used in data analysis are listed completely in Giesen et al. (1985).

RESULTS AND DISCUSSION

Employment Outcome Groups

Using wages earned and employment setting at case closure as criteria, four employment outcome groups were established: competitive (CPT), sheltered (SHL), homemaker (HMK), and unemployed (UNP). The CPT group consisted of those employment outcomes for which wages were earned in nonsheltered settings. The outcome categories for the CPT group were competitive labor market, state agency–managed Business Enterprise Program (BEP), and self-employed (except BEP). The SHL group were employed in protected work settings. The SHL categories included sheltered workshop and homebound industry closures. The HMK group outcome categories were homemaker and unpaid family worker. The HMK group consisted of status 28 closures with outcome categories of not working–student, not working–other, and trainee or worker (noncompetitive labor market). This classification system is based on the nine-group coding system used in the RSA manual for reporting vocational rehabilitation client work status at closure. Although the nine-group system provides more information about the outcome of the vocational rehabilitation process than the four employment categories system of the present study, it is too cumbersome to facilitate prediction and interpretation of the results. The employment outcome groups were assigned an index of 1 through 4, which reflects the earning potential at closure. This index, therefore, permits quantitative analysis of the dependent variable, employment outcome group at closure. A detailed breakdown of the distribution of cases in each employment group over the

10 RSA work status closures is available in Giesen et al. (1985).

Data collected on large numbers of variables examined in this study yielded information that went well beyond the initial scope of the project but that has value to vocational rehabilitation administrators in planning service delivery for blind and severely visually impaired clients. This information is available in Giesen et al. (1985) and by request from the authors. It includes:

1. R-300 data
2. Specific eye disorder data coded both by the R-300 coding system and by The International Classification of Diseases, 9th Revision, Clinical Modifications (ICD-9; Commission on Professional and Hospital Activities, 1980)
3. Selected case record data not included in the R-300
4. Extensive case service expenditure data
5. Comparisons of visual disorders in this investigation to those provided by the National Society to Prevent Blindness (1980)
6. Data on disabilities present in addition to blindness
7. Extensive descriptive data on the employment outcome groups, including such variables as age at referral, gender, education, earnings at referral and closure, and occupation skill levels at closure
8. Comparison of occupations of successfully rehabilitated blind clients with the U. S. labor force
9. Reasons for unsuccessful closure

Discriminant Function Analysis

Stepwise multiple discriminant analysis was employed to identify specific variables that discrimi-

nate or help classify cases into outcome categories using the information from the independent variable list. The discriminant analysis was performed by the Statistical Package for the Social Sciences (Nie, Hull, Jenkins, Steinbrenner, & Bent, 1975), Release 9.0, using the Wilks' method, prior probabilities determined by group size, and other parameters at default values. The results of the discriminant analyses yielded an eigenvalue and a set of coefficients for each discriminant function, as shown in Table 1. The eigenvalue for canonical function 1 indicates that 58.7% of the "explainable" variance is accounted for by the groups and amounts to a moderate amount of discriminatory power for the first function. Functions 2 (25.8%) and 3 (15.5%) have less discriminatory power. All three functions were significant.

Because this study is an exploratory search for potentially discriminating variables, some of the variables entered into the equation (see Table 2) were weak discriminators as well as intercorrelated, thereby having redundant discriminatory information. In stepwise discriminant analyses, the first variable "entered" into the equation is the single best discriminating variable. The order of entry of the variables can be assumed to reflect the order of importance of the variables in the discrimination process as they enter the equation. Table 3 shows the order of variables selected for entry into the stepwise discriminate equation. The Wilks' lambda value for the collection of variables entered up to step 20 was 0.426, and all lambdas for the discriminating variables were significant from step 1 on. A total of 52 discriminating variables was entered before the stepwise selection ceased. The results discussed are limited to an examination of the first 11 of these variables.

Table 1.   Summary of discriminant functions

Function	Eigenvalue	Canonical correlation	After function	Wilks' lambda	df	Chi square
—	—	—	0	.307	156	681.9*
1	.892	.687	1	.582	102	313.8*
2	.392	.531	2	.809	50	122.4*
3	.235	.437	—	—	—	—

*significant at $p < .001$.

Table 2.   Means and group differences for discriminating variables

Variable	F-ratio[a]	Employment group number[b]			
1. C2—Age at onset of blindness	63.1	2 16.2	1 19.2	4 28.1	3 46.7
2. C11—Occupational goal TVQ at first IWRP	41.4	3 50.5	2 51.0	4 55.6	1 61.2
3. E36—Expenditures for personal adjustment training–vocational adjustment training (PAT/VAT)	15.1	1 587	3 703	4 904	2 2746
4. R9A—Gender	19.4	1 .406	4 .420	2 .460	3 .730
5. R33D—Primary support at referral: other personal sources	11.9	3 .054	4 .100	2 .111	1 .243
6. R26—Highest grade completed	14.9	2 8.17	3 9.58	4 10.5	1 11.2
7. C26—Proximity in miles to VR counselor	5.66	4 13	2 18.1	3 21.1	1 21.2
8. R64A—Received noninstitutional training	6.10	4 .260	3 .348	1 .391	2 .556
9. R60A—Received institutional training	26.4	3 .029	2 .079	4 .213	1 .337
10. R59—Received physical restoration services	7.13	4 .347	2 .365	1 .480	3 .574
11. NDIS—Number of additional disabilities	23.5	1 .738	2 1.10	4 1.24	3 1.38

[a]All significant at the .05 level.

[b]1 = Competitive; 2 = Sheltered; 3 = Homemaker; and 4 = Unemployed. Group subsets with a common underline are not significantly different by the Newman-Keuls Test at the .05 level.

Classification of Cases and Prediction of Employment Outcome

Prediction/classification of the employment status case outcome of blind clients was accomplished through discriminant function analysis with moderate accuracy (see Table 3). Blind persons closed in the HMK group were correctly classified 84% of the time and more often correctly classified than the other work status groups members. With a 78.5% correct classification rate, blind persons closed in the competitive labor market were the second most accurately classified group. Of persons closed as employed in a sheltered workshop setting, 46.7% were correctly classified. Cases closed unemployed were the least successfully classified (41.2% correct).

Table 3.   Classification results of the stepwise discriminant analysis

Actual group	No. of cases	Predicted group membership			
		1	2	3	4
Competitive—1	200	157 (78.5%)	4 (2.0%)	21 (10.5%)	18 (9.0%)
Sheltered—2	60	6 (10.0%)	28 (46.7%)	14 (23.3%)	12 (20.0%)
Homemaker—3	200	8 (4.0%)	4 (2.0%)	168 (84.0%)	20 (10.0%)
Unemployed—4	148	38 (25.7%)	8 (5.4%)	41 (27.7%)	61 (41.2%)
Percent of "grouped" cases correctly classified: 68.09%					

For all groups, an overall correct classification rate of 68% was achieved. This rate is a 272% improvement over the assumed chance rate of 25% correct.

Relationship among the Employment Groups

Table 3 shows a summary of the mean differences between employment groups for the discriminating variables, which are listed in order of entry into the discriminate analysis. *F* ratios are for the one-way analysis of variance for each variable.

Vocational Rehabilitation Process Variables

IWRP Vocational Goal   A major finding of this study is the importance of the job difficulty level of the client's vocational objective. The pattern of the results for the job difficulty index (TVQ) was HMK = SHL < UNP < CPT (see Table 2).

The lack of quantification of occupations and occupational goals in previous research has denied the field a method to assess the contribution of a major variable leading to employment outcome. Because of its importance, the IWRP vocational goal skill level (TVQ) merits the attention of rehabilitation counselors and administrators. McCroskey and Perkins (1981) identified 7573 DOT job titles with TVQ scores (skill levels) equal to or less than that of the competitive group.

Personal-Vocational Adjustment Training (PAT/VAT)   Crouse (1974) has reported that receipt of personal adjustment services was a useful predictor of rehabilitation outcome. In this study, PAT/VAT expenditure was significantly greater for the SHL group than for any other group. The other groups were not significantly different from one another. Large expenditures for these services appear to be associated with sheltered employment outcomes. Rehabilitation administrators, in anticipation of the increasing number of multihandicapped blind persons entering the system, need to allocate additional funds to meet the personal and vocational adjustment training needs of blind multihandicapped persons.

Institutional and Noninstitutional Training   Training has been found to be indicative of successful rehabilitation outcome (Bowman & Micek, 1973). Previous studies, like the Bowman and Micek (1973) study, have not examined the relationship between training category and specific employment outcome, nor were the studies focused on the effect on outcome of the training with blind clients.

Noninstitutional training (on-the-job or vocational training at miscellaneous sites) was more likely to be associated with wage-earning outcomes (CPT, SHL) than with non-wage-earning outcomes (HMK, UNP). Blind persons closed in sheltered employment were more likely to receive noninstitutional training than the other three work status groups. Individuals in the CPT outcome group were more likely to receive noninstitutional training than the UNP group.

A minority (111, or 17.9%) of the cases received institutional training, which includes college or other academic training, business school, or vocational school training. As expected, significantly fewer HMK (2.9%) and SHL closures (7.9%) received institutional training than either the CPT (33.7%) or the UNP (21.3%) outcome groups. Significantly more of the CPT outcome group than of the UNP outcome group received institutional training.

Physical Restoration   The results of this study were consistent with those of Crouse (1974), who found that receipt of physical restoration was related to rehabilitation outcome. The UNP group and the SHL group, less likely to receive physical restoration services, were not significantly different from each other. The CPT and HMK groups were more likely to receive physical restoration services, but were not different from one another. The HMK group was more likely to receive services than either the UNP or SHL groups, and the UNP group was less likely to receive services than either the CPT or HMK groups.

The results suggest that administrators of rehabilitation agencies can anticipate that slightly under half (46.7%) of the cases will require physical restoration. More cases in the CPT and HMK groups were found to have received these kinds of services than in either of the other groups. Because the CPT and SHL groups share an average onset age of blindness during adolescence, further study is needed to determine why there are differences in the rates at which physical restoration was received by the two groups and, more importantly, why receipt of the service was more often associated with a competitive closure than with a sheltered closure.

Personal and Disability-Related Variables

Age at Onset of Blindness Age at onset of blindness was reported by Knowles (1969) to be related to the rehabilitation outcome of blind cases. Earlier onset ages were found to be associated with wage-earner outcomes. The latest age of onset (mean = 46.7) was associated with the HMK group. Between the HMK group and the CPT and SHL groups was the UNP unemployed group, with an average onset age of 28.1 years.

The results suggest that persons whose onset of blindness occurs while the individual is age appropriate for the educational system learn skills that assist them in entering the world of work. Persons who become blind after age 22 and prior to middle age often do not have the opportunity to learn, practice, and acquire proficiency at those skills, taught to blind youth in the educational setting, that have the potential for transfer to the employment setting. Because this group is still young enough to have wage-earner vocational goals, vocational rehabilitation plans or IWRPs are often developed since they appear to be age appropriate and in concert with the goals of the agency and the blind person. Investigations are needed to determine what services are required to assist these individuals in achieving a wage-earning closure.

Gender Prior studies (Bolton, 1972a; Scheinkman, Dunn, Menz, Andrew, & Currie, 1975; Wright & Trotter, 1968) have indicated that successful rehabilitation or status 26 outcomes occurred more often with males than with females. In contrast with the other studies, gender differences were not indicative of closure in status 26 in the present study. There were no differences in the distribution of males and females in CPT, SHL, and UNP categories. The HMK group, traditionally categorized as a 26, con-

tained a higher proportion of females than the other three groups. Because of the prevalence rate of blindness among females (National Society to Prevent Blindness, 1980), additional studies are needed to examine the effects of the rehabilitation service delivery system on the employment outcome of blind women.

Educational Level Educational level was recorded in terms of highest grade completed. All groups were significantly different on this variable. The order of groups from lowest to highest was SHL, HMK, UNP, and CPT. Whereas most previous research (e.g., Berkowitz, Englander, Rubin, & Worrall, 1975) indicates that a higher educational level is associated with successful closure, the present results suggest that the pattern is not consistent across successful closure groups. In the present study, the UNP group (status 28) was found to have an average educational level of 10.5 while the CPT group reported 11.3 years. However, if the categories are collapsed using the traditional 26-28 system, the mean educational level of the 26 group (CPT, SHL, and HMK) was approximately 10.2 whereas the 28 group (UNP) was 10.4 years. These findings could have been interpreted to mean that more education is associated with unemployment among blind persons or that education does not matter. Using the broader dichotomous categories of status 26 and 28 may therefore obscure important subpopulation differences, that is, differences between competitive, sheltered, and homemaker closures, as Dunn (1975) has suggested. Using these categories may then lead to inappropriate conclusions about the effects of various elements of the rehabilitation service delivery system on benefits clients receive from the services. Future research, in order to be viable, must differentiate between the three major closure groups within the successful (status 26) closure category.

Number of Additional Disabilities All cases included in the present study are considered by RSA criteria to be persons with severe disabilities. Consequently, additional disabilities could have significant implications for behavioral functioning. Previous research (Scholl et al., 1969) suggests that additional nonvisual disabilities are associated with lower socioeconomic status, percentage of time worked, and lower income. These results, through identifying secondary and tertiary disabilities, indicate that fewer additional disabilities are associated with CPT outcomes. Conversely, additional disabilities were found to be associated with the other outcome groups.

The HMK group had, on the average, 1.38 additional nonvisual disabilities. Given that this is the oldest group, it is the group most likely to have disabilities associated with aging. The principal secondary and tertiary disabilities—diabetes, hypertension, and cardiovascular disease—are ones associated with the aging process. This group can also be expected to need physical restoration services. Slightly over 57% received some form of physical restoration services, with an average hospital convalescence expenditure of $195.00. The relatively high percentage of cases receiving physical restoration services with a relatively low hospitalization cost suggests that some of these costs were shared by a third party. Administration agencies serving large numbers of persons who are likely to be closed as homemakers can expect that the provision of physical restoration services will be a frequent agency service. It is one, however, where third-party cost sharing can be expected. Counselors serving this type of client need to know how to use third-party sources to reduce the cost of the IWRP for this group of agency clients.

Financial and Disincentive Variables

Client financial resources at referral have been found to be associated with rehabilitation outcome in previous research (Bolton, 1972a; De-Mann, 1963; Scheinkman et al., 1975). Presence of personal income at referral such as current earnings, workman's compensation, and private annuities, rather than transfer payments or funds from family and friends, was associated with competitive closures. Of the CPT group, 24.3% had support from these sources at referral. More than 90% of the other 3 groups relied on non-personal sources of support at referral, such as transfer payments.

Although having personal sources of support at referral was associated with competitive employment outcomes, it should be noted that, in

the rehabilitation of the blind community, over three fourths of the competitive closures group received financial support at referral from non-personal sources. This situation may indicate that financial disincentives favoring noncompetitive employment closures among blind clients are not as strong as previous research has indicated (e.g., Walls & Tseng, 1976).

Geographic and Environmental Variables

Proximity in miles of the rehabilitation counselor's office to the home of the blind client and its relationship to outcome has not been examined in previous research. This variable is important for blindness agencies, given the low prevalence of the disability and the dispersion of clients within the state. "Proximity to VR counselor" showed that clients most likely to be closed in the UNP group were those residing closest to the counselor (mean = 13.0 miles). The SHL group at 18.1 mean miles did not differ significantly from the UNP group. The UNP group did differ significantly from the HMK (mean = 21.1 miles) and the CPT (mean = 21.2 miles) groups. Possible explanations for the finding include: 1) the rural/urban dimension interacts with service delivery and need patterns, 2) case selection by the counselor is more important when greater travel distances are involved, 3) multihandicapped blind persons may be prohibited from access to rehabilitation services when significant travel is involved, and 4) referral systems function differently when the rehabilitation counselor is located in close proximity.

IMPLICATIONS

These results have implications for policies and delivery of services by state rehabilitation agencies affecting the employment and underemployment of blind and visually impaired clients of these agencies.

Policy Issues

1. The research based on the traditional successful (26) versus unsuccessful (28) closure dichotomy obscures important differences among employment outcomes of

blind clients. At a minimum, future researchers must separate outcome categories into competitive, sheltered, homemaker, and nonworking groups to further understand the interplay of factors impacting on employment outcomes of blind clients.

2. The relatively large proportion of cases found with cataracts (22.5%) indicates that physical restoration services, optical aids, and related services can be expected to continue and increase with the aging of the U.S. population as major services of state rehabilitation agencies.

3. Counselors and agencies are very often dealing with cases that are more severely disabled than records indicate. Case management procedures need to be initiated that identify secondary nonvisual disabilities and specify in the development of the employment goals how their impact on role performance will be eliminated or minimized.

4. Policies are needed that assure meeting the total rehabilitation needs of the client. This need is particularly great for cases involving diabetes mellitus, which was found to be the most frequent nonvisual disability of the sample.

5. The mean weekly wage at closure for the competitively employed outcome group, approximately $129, is less than might have been expected. Agency administrators need to be assured that the wages received by the client with a competitively employed closure are comparable to those of nondisabled persons who are employed in similar positions.

6. The importance of age at onset of blindness suggests that it needs to be included in the agency information system for comparison with other information and case outcome.

7. Case management policies are needed that encourage the use of occupational histories in the case management process and that focus the counseling interview on occupationally relevant behaviors.

8. Case loads need to be examined in terms of the zip codes (or another system of geographic location) of the client at referral to determine if there are areas that are underserved.

Practice Issues

1. Rehabilitation professionals need to know the etiology, treatment, associated nonvisual disorders, and availability and use of optical and nonoptical aids in the rehabilitation of persons blinded by cataracts or diabetic retinopathy.

2. Rehabilitation counselors will need to be encouraged to arrange for efficient delivery of physical restoration services to shorten the period between referral and receipt of services.

3. Rehabilitation counselors need to be encouraged to arrange for comprehensive medical diagnostic studies, including dietary counseling, of the diabetic blind referral.

4. Rehabilitation counselors with many homemaker closures can expect to allocate a substantial portion of their case funds for physical restoration services. Their clients will also need the services of rehabilitation teachers and orientation and mobility specialists.

5. Ways in which occupational history information can be used in the vocational counseling process, including vocational goal development, need to be included in both preservice and continuing education programs of rehabilitation professionals.

6. Rehabilitation counselors need to plan more vocational counseling interviews for blind clients who have competitive vocational goals than for those clients whose vocational goals may be classified as homemaker in order to monitor the appropriateness of the IWRP vocational goal.

7. Findings suggest that, when optical aids are purchased for severely visually impaired persons, low vision training should be included.

REFERENCES

Ammons, J. M. (1978). *Benefit category prediction for adjustment of blindness and training at a rehabilitation center.* Unpublished doctoral dissertation, University of South Carolina.

Bauman, M. K., & Yoder, M. (1963). *Placing the blind and visually handicapped in professional occupations.* Philadelphia: Pennsylvania Office for the Blind, Commonwealth of Pennsylvania.

Bauman, M. K., & Yoder, M. (1964). *Placing the blind and visually handicapped in clerical, industrial and service occupations.* Philadelphia: Pennsylvania Office for the Blind, Commonwealth of Pennsylvania.

Berkowitz, M., Englander, V., Rubin, J., & Worrall, J. D. (1975). *An evaluation of policy-related rehabilitation research.* New York: Praeger Publishers.

Bolton, B. (1972a). Predicting client outcome from intake data. *Rehabilitation Research and Practice Review, 4*(1), 23–25.

Bolton, B. (1972b). The prediction of rehabilitation outcomes. *The Journal of Applied Rehabilitation Counseling, 3*(2), 16–24.

Bolton, B. (1979). *Rehabilitation counseling research.* Baltimore: University Park Press.

Bolton, B. F., Butler, A. J., & Wright, G. M. (1968). *Clinical versus statistical prediction of client feasibility* (Monograph No. 7). Madison: Wisconsin Studies in Vocational Rehabilitation, University of Wisconsin, Regional Rehabilitation Research Institute.

Bowman, J. T., & Micek, L. A. (1973). Rehabilitation service components and vocational outcome. *Rehabilitation Counseling Bulletin, 17*, 100–109.

Commission on Professional and Hospital Activities. (1980). *The international classification of diseases, 9th revision, clinical modification* (Vols. 1 and 2). Ann Arbor, MI: Commission of Professional and Hospital Activities.

Crouse, R. J. (1974). Predictors of vocational rehabilitation outcomes for the legally blind. (Doctoral dissertation, University of Northern Colorado, 1974). *Dissertation Abstracts International, 35*(5), 2801A.

DeMann, M. M. (1963). A predictive study of rehabilitation counseling outcomes. *Journal of Counseling Psychology, 10*, 340–343.

Dunn, D. (1975). Vocational evaluation services in the human services delivery system. *Vocational Evaluation and Work Adjustment Bulletin, 8*(Spec. ed.), 7–9.

Giesen, J. M., & Graves, W. (1984, August). *Predicting employment outcomes of blind clients of state rehabilitation agencies.* Paper presented at the meeting of the American Psychological Association, Toronto, Canada.

Giesen, J. M., Graves, W. H., Machalow, S., Schmitt, S., & Dietz, P. (1984, May). *The impact of rehabilitation services on the employment status and job skills of blind clients of four state rehabilitation agencies.* Paper presented at the meeting of the National Association of Rehabilitation Research and Training Centers, Chicago, Illinois.

Giesen, J. M., Graves, W. H., Schmitt, S., Lamb, A. M., Cook, D., Capps, C., & Boyet, K. (1985). *Predicting work status outcomes of blind/severely visually impaired clients of state rehabilitation agencies (Technical Report).* Mississippi State: Mississippi State University, Rehabilitation Research and Training Center on Blindness and Low Vision.

Kirchner, C., & Peterson, R. (1982). Vocational and rehabilitation placements of blind and visually impaired clients: U.S. 1980. *Journal of Visual Impairment and Blindness, 76*, 426–429.

Knowles, L. L. (1969). Successful and unsuccessful vocational rehabilitation of the legally blind: A multi-statistical approach. (Doctoral dissertation, University of Southern California, 1969). *Dissertation Abstracts International, 29*(12), 4326A.

Levitan, S., & Taggart, R. (1977). *Jobs for the disabled.* Baltimore: Johns Hopkins University Press.

McCrosky, B. (1980). *The encyclopedia of job requirements, Vol 1: Jobs by title.* Mississippi State: Mississippi State University.

McCrosky, B. J., & Perkins, E. (1981). *The manual for the McCrosky vocational quotient system.* St. Cloud, MN: Vocationology, Inc.

National Society to Prevent Blindness. (1980). *Vision problems in the U.S.* New York: Author.

New study affirms cost effectiveness of rehabilitation services in Minnesota. (1983). *Rehabilitation Forum, 10*(3), 24–37.

Nie, N. H., Hull, C., Jenkins, J., Steinbrenner, K., & Bent, D. (1975). *SPSS: Statistical package for the social sciences* (2nd ed.). New York: McGraw-Hill.

Scheinkman, M., Dunn, D., Menz, F., Andrew, J., & Currie, L. (1975). *The unsuccessful state vocational rehabilitation client. An analysis research report I: Project overview and description of client sample characteristics* (RT-22). Menomonie: University of Wisconsin–Stout, Research and Training Center, Dept. of Rehabilitation and Manpower Services.

Schmitt, S. A. (1984). *The prediction of work status outcome of blind women.* Unpublished doctoral dissertation, Mississippi State University.

Scholl, G., Bauman, M., & Crissey, M. (1969). *A study of the vocational success of groups of the visually handicapped.* Ann Arbor: The University of Michigan, School of Education.

U.S. Department of Labor, Bureau of Statistics. (1977). *Dictionary of occupational titles.* Washington, DC: U.S. Government Printing Office.

Walls, R., & Tseng, M. (1976). Measurement of client outcomes in rehabilitation. In B. Bolton (Ed.), *Handbook of measurement and evaluation in rehabilitation* (pp. 207–255). Baltimore: University Park Press.

Wright, G., & Trotter, A. (1968). *Rehabilitation research.* Madison: The University of Wisconsin Press.

Chapter 16

Analyzing Rehabilitation Outcomes of Persons with Head Injury

Leonard Diller and Yehuda Ben-Yishay

Outcomes in rehabilitation are in a sense like paintings. They depict aspects of reality that can be portrayed in many ways, viewed from different perspectives, and understood from several frames of references. The consequences of traumatic brain injury (TBI) and the epidemiological constraints under which they take place are complex. Traumatic brain injury, for example, may not be a single entity but an aggregate category, such as cancer, where site, nature, and extent of damage are important in understanding outcome. Furthermore, constellations of sequelae may be difficult to relate to antecedent pathology. Sequelae may range from circumscribed mental impairment to combinations of physical and mental impairments. Whereas some consequences are apparent at the time of injury, others are more likely to unfold with the passage of time, resulting in outcomes ranging from total recovery to death.

Outcome assessment in the rehabilitation of persons with TBI depends on three considerations: 1) the nature of brain damage and its consequences, 2) the settings in which rehabilitation services are provided, and 3) the language of outcome assessment in relation to TBI. This chapter examines each of these considerations.

THE CONSEQUENCES OF BRAIN DAMAGE

The sequelae of brain damage and the course of natural recovery have been studied from the standpoint of etiology, severity, time frames for recovery, and population characteristics.

Etiology

Three groups have been noted: 1) open head injuries from penetrating objects, 2) closed head injuries from forces applied to a stationary skull, and 3) closed head injury from a rapidly decelerating skull. The location and extent of damage on impact and the secondary effects on the structure and dynamics of the brain all must be considered.

Many of the earlier studies that identified people by locus of lesion either did not consider etiology or, if they did, focused on wartime populations with a higher frequency of open head injuries. Wartimes provide the most TBIs, and outcomes in these populations may differ from those in modern civilian rehabilitation programs.

Severity of Brain Damage

Many indicators of severity have been used, including the presence of focal neurological lesions, loss of consciousness, and posttraumatic amnesia, as well as the presence of epilepsy and depressed skull fracture (Levin, Benton, & Grossman, 1982). It is readily apparent that indices of mental rather than physical impairment may serve both as useful predictors of long-term outcomes and as useful measures of severity of brain damage.

Over the last decade, the Glasgow Coma Scale (GCS; Teasdale & Jennett, 1974) has become

Preparation of this chapter was supported by grant #G0083000039 from the National Institute of Handicapped Research.

widely adopted as a measure of brain damage severity. It is one of the few assessment devices designed specifically for use with TBI patients. The GCS is a simple, 15-point behavioral measure in three dimensions (eye opening, motor responses, and verbal response) that can be used as indicators of emergence from coma. Cutoff scores on this 15-point scale have been used to classify TBIs into mild, moderate, and severe. It should be noted that GCS scores have been devised for use in an acute care neurosurgical setting, where outcome concerns often hover around the prediction of life or death. The widespread use of the GCS is evident in its adoption as a standard of TBI severity in multicenter studies nationally as well as internationally.

Depending on the cutoff score used for the GCS, grossly categorized outcomes are predictable. For example, a cutoff of 8 and below on the GCS predicts death in approximately half of the patients before they leave the hospital (Strub & Block, 1981). Patients with higher GCS scores perform better on outcome measures 1 year later (Levin et al., 1982). In working with less severe cases, Rimel, Giordani, Barth, and Jane (1982) and Rimel and Jane (1983) found that, compared to patients with mild head trauma (GCS scores of 13 +), patients with moderate trauma (GCS scores of 9–12) had a greater incidence of unemployment, changes in activities of daily living, subjective complaints, and neuropsychological impairments. Whereas outcomes in the moderate group were related to characteristics of the brain damage, outcomes in the mild cases were related to premorbid demographic characteristics. Considering this feature of the mild TBI group, research findings by McClean, Temkin, Dikman, and Wyler (1984) are particularly relevant. A control group drawn from friends of persons with TBI showed amounts of subjective anxiety, irritability, temper tantrums, and complaints equal to those of the TBI group. However, the TBI group had more headaches, dizziness, subjective feelings of fatigue, and difficulties in concentration. This suggests that even persons with mild TBI may wind up with permanent residual problems; these problems, however, must be evaluated within their social context.

Time Frames for Recovery

When is the measurement of outcome appropriate? It is difficult to interpret the benefits of interventions that are administered while active recovery is taking place. Consequently, plateaus of recovery have become an important subject of study. Investigators of recovery and those studying rehabilitation seem to view recovery from different vantage points: The former tend to emphasize a prospective view, tracing recovery from the time of injury or emergence from coma, whereas the latter tend to view recovery from the retrospective vantage of a particular facility. Prospective studies encounter the problem of a selective attrition of subjects that is due, for instance, to losing contact with them. Retrospective studies must deal with a loss of subjects resulting from exclusionary criteria specifying who is admitted for rehabilitation.

In a study using the Glasgow Outcome Scale (GOS), Jennett and Bond (1975) chose 1 year as the time period for assessing outcome and observed that most recovery took place within the first 6 months. Tracking recovery from time of onset from a prospective standpoint, they proposed that patients' status on a 5-point scale (death, permanent vegetative state, severely, moderately, and mildly disabled) remains relatively invariant from 6 months on. A parallel finding appears in a prospective follow-up series in New York City of patients with severe head trauma who emerged from a coma (Diller & Ben-Yishay, 1983).

Whereas earlier studies involving neuropsychological measures reported a plateau of recovery in 12 months (Mandelberg, 1975), Dikmen, Reitan, and Temkin (1983) found that patients continued to improve at 18 months. Kay, Ezrachi, and Cavallo (1986) noted that recovery results from groups of patients are generally expressed in terms of mean scores. When the population is divided into subgroups, some patients do indeed plateau; however, some become worse and others continue to improve over time. This is consistent with recent findings using newer brain imaging techniques, which suggest that patients who deteriorate over time may have different patterns of neuropathology (Levin et al., 1986). The findings also help account for reports of patients returning to gainful employment 10 years after severe head injury. There are as yet few long-term, prospective longitudinal studies tracking persons with TBI for a 5- or 10-year period.

Brooks et al. (1984) have posed a number of methodological questions that should be examined in considering outcome studies:

1. What behaviors are being assessed? Verbal intelligence plateaus more rapidly than performance intelligence (Brooks, 1984b), but verbal tests may differ from performance tests on dimensions such as old versus new learning, timed versus untimed tasks, and simple versus complex tasks.

2. Which is the appropriate reference point— the time of injury or the time since emergence from coma? Najenson, Sazhon, Fiselson, Becker, and Schechter (1978) noted that some patients emerge from coma 5 or 6 months after injury. Recovery of abilities in such patients may follow different timetables and yield different results than if one only considered time since onset. Panikoff (1983) working with functional skills and Diller and Ben-Yishay (1983) working with neuropsychological measures found that recovery is lawful in that individuals who are superior within a group of TBI individuals at 2 months will be superior at 12 months.

3. Is there an order of recovery? Meeder (1982), tracking return of skills on a battery of 25 perceptual-motor tasks used in occupational therapy, found an orderliness to recovery. Performance in some tasks (e.g., visual attentiveness) improves more rapidly than performance on others (e.g., figure–ground relations). Najenson et al. (1978) argued that visual and auditory comprehension improve initially, followed by oral expression, reading, and writing.

4. What percent of patients in the original sample are available for follow-up? There appear to be no guidelines as to what is an acceptable attrition rate. The problem has plagued the field from the early work of Conkey (1938), who began with 25 subjects and found that only 4 were available at the end of the study. Attrition is less when subjects receive a service. Thus, the attrition rate for the experimental group is less than for the control group in the study by Prigitano et al. (1986) of an intervention program.

Demographic Characteristics of TBI

Age affects prediction of outcomes in two major ways. First, among adults with increasing age, the chance of recovery decreases. Second, TBI occurs more often in young adult males than in other population groups (Rimel et al., 1982). Although this has obvious consequences for task programming in rehabilitation, it may also have implications for possible differences in the organization of the brain by age and sex. For example, damage to the same area of the brain may have different effects at different ages. Therefore, not only is the kind of injury important, but also the state of the brain that received the trauma. From a societal standpoint, 31% of an adult TBI population in central Virginia had been hospitalized previously for an earlier head injury (Rimel & Jane, 1983). Thus, a number of TBIs may occur among people who already have had brain damage, which in turn may have exposed them to the risk of further brain damage. In a follow-up study of individuals with TBI admitted to municipal hospitals in New York City, a large number had histories of alcoholism, mental illness, or drug abuse (Diller & Ben-Yishay, 1983). Tobis, Puri, and Sheridan (1982) suggested that the reason why so few of their TBI population in a program in southern California returned to work was a history of sociopathic characteristics and depression; these characteristics may have placed them at a risk for an accident. Tobis et al.'s data suggested an additional reason why conclusions based on wartime studies may differ from conclusions based on civilians.

Thus, in considering outcomes, individual differences among persons with TBI may be as important as the severity of brain injury, particularly in the case of mild brain damage. Although one should not infer that persons with TBIs are not necessarily maladjusted, it is nonetheless important to note that demographic considerations color outcomes.

SETTINGS

The *National Directory of Head Injury Rehabilitation Services* (National Head Injury Foundation, 1984) lists more than 200 setting in the United States that offer services to persons with TBI as of 1984. Since each of these settings presumably has treatment objectives and outcome criteria to assess clients' status upon discharge, finding common outcome measures for diverse populations and interventions is important. For example, one study of severe TBIs in an outpatient setting used referral to another agency as a mark of successful outcome (Cole, Cope, & Cervelli, 1985). Others have used reduction of problems (Ben-Yishay, Silver, Piasetsky, & Associates, 1987) or vocational placement. Furthermore, although many settings define criteria for admission in terms of client needs, there is increasing pressure to utilize potential outcomes as a screening measure for service eligibility. Thus, inpatients are admitted and continue in medical rehabilitation settings if progress can be demonstrated. Divisions of vocational rehabilitation operating at the state level specify potential employment as an admission criterion. It is clear that a single set of outcome measures fails to respond to the needs in the field. The Commission on Accreditation of Rehabilitation Facilities (CARF) requires documented program evaluation activity as a criterion for certifying a brain injury program.

In a follow-up study in diverse New York City hospitals of persons with severe TBIs who emerged from coma, Diller and Ben-Yishay (1983) found that at the end of 1 year general medical problems such as fractures, internal organ injuries, or pneumonia had been reduced from an incidence of 75% just prior to discharge to 6%. Neurological residuals such as seizures, paralyses, or aphasia were reduced from 94% to 78%, and cognitive behavioral problems such as depression, sexual dysfunction, memory impairment, impulsivity, affect disturbance, aggression, and apathy rose from 59% to 75%. This

pattern of change parallels a system of settings from emergency and acute medical care through inpatient medical rehabilitation to outpatient services.

Acute Care Programs

The major indices of recovery are: 1) reduction of medical complications, 2) improvement on the GCS, and 3) increase in awareness and orientation. A measure that has been used for assessing awareness and orientation is the Galveston Orientation and Awareness Scale (GOAT; Levin, O'Donnell, & Grossman, 1979). Whereas the GCS can be administered daily or even hourly to track recovery during coma, the GOAT is generally administered daily or weekly. These measures, however, fail to capture many of the conditions treated in rehabilitation settings.

Inpatient Medical Programs

The traditional objectives of inpatient medical programs are to: 1) reduce and prevent medical complications; 2) enhance functional skills, particularly with regard to activities of daily living (ADL); and 3) prepare the patient and family to cope with problems in living with a disability. For TBI, these traditional objectives have to be supplemented in two ways: 1) by reducing cognitive and behavioral dysfunctions, and 2) by facilitating acceptance of problems and strategies for management by patients and families.

Conventional Rehabilitation Outcome Measures Rusk, Block, and Lowman (1969) described outcomes obtained by a conventional multidisciplinary team in terms of ADL and vocational status. A similar approach has been used by Hook (1976) and Najenson et al. (1978), who expanded and refined the metrics for this population. Panikoff (1983) used a modification of conventional ADL scales, supplemented by other measures, to show changes in a TBI population as a result of treatment. Sehgal (1986) has refined this approach in several important ways by: 1) developing uniform scales for the members of a traditional medical rehabilitation team, including physical, speech and occupational therapists as well as nurses, psychologists, and social workers; 2) including measures sensitive to some of the neurobehavioral sequelae of TBI in the cognitive and behavioral domains; and 3) developing the measures in a prospective fashion. Typically, outcome studies had been based on retrospective data.

Specialized Outcome Measures for TBI Neurobehavioral problems are a central feature of TBI that cut across all of the therapies offered in inpatient medical rehabilitation programs. Consequently, a number of investigators have developed measures for classifying patients who cannot be classified by conventional measures because of the need for distinctions on cognitive and behavioral rather than motoric and behavioral bases. Perhaps the most well known is the Rancho Levels of Cognitive Function Scale (LCFS; Hagen, Malkmus, & Durham, 1979), developed in 1972 at Rancho Los Amigos Hospital. Using a global set of descriptors divided into eight levels, the LCFS describes various levels of responsiveness to stimuli in a nontest environment, such as responses to verbal commands, alertness, agitation, purposeful and nonpurposeful behavior, memory, attention span, new learning, and social behavior.

The GOS has been expanded and used in inpatient medical rehabilitation programs (Hall, Cope, & Rappaport, 1985; Najenson et al., 1978; Roberts, 1979; Stover & Zeiger, 1976). The most sophisticated version, the Disability Rating Scale (DRS), has been expanded from 5 to 30 times reflecting different levels of disability (Hall et al., 1985; Rappaport et al., 1982). The DRS has been shown to be reliable and more sensitive to changes in patients than previous measures, and to have both concurrent and predictive validity. The DRS has been used as an outcome measure on followup. This scale, like others, must deal with the following problems:

1. Do the categorical groupings reflect subtle changes?
2. Because the categories combine multiple dimensions of behavior, does change in one dimension correspond to a change in another?
3. What if the behavior does not fall into a single category?

Because persons with TBIs may require interventions that are specific to their special needs, distinctive outcome measures may be necessary.

For example, Corrigan, Arnett, Houcks, and Jackson (1985) assessed reality orientation for an inpatient intervention program designed for patients who were not fully oriented. Braunling-McMorrow, Lloyd, and Fralish (1986) adapted a method for teaching social skills to persons with TBIs and tested for carryover in a natural setting. Nagele (1985) analyzed the task of toothbrushing to assess the cognitive problems and retraining of a TBI person. Although reliability and validity findings are incomplete, these approaches are of interest in that they focus on functional skill content in areas relevant to persons with TBIs. They also imply reanalysis of what is being taught and the purpose for which it is being taught. Part of the problem is that programs with defined missions such as vocational programs often must borrow methods and content from other programs.

From this brief review, two main points are to be noted: 1) few scales have been developed that are sensitive to the specific problems of the TBI patient in inpatient medical rehabilitation programs and; 2) specific scales developed to identify levels of deficit in patients with TBIs and to track improvement in rehabilitation have been used minimally in follow-up studies to assess outcomes.

Outpatient Programs

Because of the size of the TBI population and changes in financing health care, outpatient programs are proliferating rapidly. They differ in terms of the comprehensiveness of services offered, the levels of severity of the populations being served, and their objectives. Program goals might include vocational/educational, cognitive, social, independent living, family relief, or maintenance in the community, singly or in various combinations. Drawing on experiences with other outpatient populations including the developmentally disabled and psychiatric or physically handicapped, a potpourri of TBI programs have been developed that reflect the evolving state of the field. Outpatient programs combining cognitive, social, psychotherapeutic, and prevocational approaches in a holistic way have used psychometric, personality, and job placement criteria singly or in combination (Ben-Yishay et al., 1987; Prigitano et al., 1986; Scherzer, 1986). These programs are noteworthy in that they offer common philosophies of treatment and are beginning to offer different types of evidence to support treatment effectiveness. For example, Ben-Yishay et al. (1987) compared groups that differed in the amount of treatment time devoted to cognitive remediation versus social group processes. Prigitano et al.'s study (1986) compared treated and untreated groups, although subjects were not randomly assigned to the groups. Scherzer (1986) compared successive samples of treated groups to replicate earlier results.

There are many studies that report findings on focused functional goals such as driving, reduction of behavioral disturbances, and enhancement of specific abilities. However, these reports, which are often presented at conferences, have often not been screened for validity and adequacy of measurement.

Many of the "process" issues that are critical for case management may be reflected only indirectly in outcomes. Examples include acceptance by the patient and family of silent impairments (e.g., memory problems), willingness to sustain participation in a program, and ability to internalize the task demands of a program. Although such issues are important in all populations undergoing rehabilitation, they surface as the central problem in persons with TBIs after inpatient rehabilitation has been completed. Furthermore, it might be argued that the true impact of process issues may be better tested several years after the completion of a program.

TBI OUTCOMES AND REHABILITATION

The participants in rehabilitation who are interested in outcome include patients and families, service providers from different professions, administrators, public officials, and third-party payors. The mental set of the participants may lead to observer bias on relevant outcome measures. In psychotherapy studies, for example, outcomes derived from patient self-ratings, therapist ratings, and psychological tests may not agree (Fiske & Shewder, 1966). Differing perspectives guide what to look for and how much

detail to include. Patients and families might focus on relief of complaints. Service providers might focus on changes on standardized tests that are sensitive to the sequelae of TBI. Third-party payors may judge outcomes by changes in economic dependency or reduction of health care costs. Each group, while acknowledging the perspective of other groups, might legitimately focus on more detailed data within the domain of their interest.

Participant bias becomes more striking when one considers the purposes of outcome measures, which are to provide guides for prognosis, case management, allocation of resources, and research. Participants have expectancies around each of these issues. Families and patients may hope for a cure, service providers may be intent on demonstrating usefulness, and the administrator may be determined to balance outcome data against competing demands for resources. Although these expectancies might be exaggerated to different degrees, nonetheless they are built into the situation.

Impairments, Disability, and Handicaps

One logical way of looking at outcomes would be to accept the language of rehabilitation as proposed in the *International Classification of Impairments, Disabilities, and Handicaps* (ICIDH; WHO, 1980). An impairment is a deficit on a measure generally assessed by standard tests. Impairments may be motoric, such as a difficulty in range of motion, or mental, such as a defective score on an intelligence test. A disability is a deficit in a functional skill, that is, a skilled activity that has face validity in daily life. Inability to grasp or release is an impairment in motor function. Inability to hold a cup is a disability. If one fails an intelligence test item, it is not intuitively obvious that failure has a practical consequence. A handicap is a difficulty in carrying out a major role in normal living wherein part of the problem may reside in the environment as well as in the individual. Handicaps generally refer to activities such as employment, living arrangements, and utilization of health care resources. Impairments, disabilities, and handicaps are generally interrelated, although this is not always the case.

Rehabilitation Indicators (Brown, Gordon, & Diller, 1984) use a language that is consonant with the ICIDH system, although with the following modifications pertinent to TBI. Whereas disabilities are behavioral descriptors that are relatively the same in different environments, handicaps are dependent to a greater degree on person–environment interactions. A disability might be viewed as a property of the person, whereas a handicap may be viewed as a property of the environment as much as of the person. Rehabilitation indicators postulate that person–environment behaviors can be divided into two levels. At one level are statuses such as employment and living arrangements, which account for major roles. At the second level are activity patterns, which describe how people use their time. Whereas disabilities are indicators of skills that can be measured against norms, statuses and activity patterns are more value laden and idiosyncratic. In other words, disabilities are indicators of what people can do, and statuses and activity patterns are indicators of what they actually do.

Impairments

The vast majority of outcome studies with TBI populations use batteries of neuropsychological tests adapted from clinical psychology (e.g., the Wechsler Intelligence Scale) or clinical neurology (e.g., the Halstead Reitan battery). A few tests are specifically sensitive to the most critical dimensions of neuropsychological impairments in TBI. These include disturbances in attention/arousal, executive functions (i.e., ability to identify a problem, execute a planned strategy to resolve the problem, monitor the response critically, and change a course of action) and affective awareness/regulation. Newer tests designed to address this problem are being developed, such as tests of problem-solving ability (Hart, Zimmer, Bacley, & Hayden, 1985), executive ability (Lezak, 1983), and new learning (Levin, High, Williams, & Eisenberg, 1985). Because cognitive processes are complex, it is difficult to isolate and pinpoint the source of a breakdown. For example, attention may involve initiation, sustained vigilance, processing multiple sources of information simultaneously, and inhibiting re-

sponse to an inappropriate stimulus. Clinically, one might observe apathy, confusion, perseveration, and impulsiveness as breakdowns in different facets of attention. It is difficult to design tasks that would separate the dimensions of attention disturbance and yet be equally sensitive to the qualities noted in clinical observation.

Neuropsychological tests are designed to be sensitive to behavioral differences between brain-damaged people and others, but not necessarily to differences in functional disability and handicap. There have been recent efforts to correlate neuropsychological impairment measures with functional measures (Hart, Plenger, Helffenstein, & Hayden, 1985; Heaton, Chelune, & Lehman, 1978). At best, these may be indirect markers that only reflect functional outcomes, but are not functional outcome measures in themselves.

In the case of interventions, effects of practice are uncertain, particularly if mildly impaired persons with TBI may profit from practice while the severely impaired may not (Brooks et al., 1984). Although using alternate forms of tests might be one practical approach to the problem, care must be taken that the alternative forms are equally difficult and randomly administered. Brooks et al. (1984) found that the paragraphs used to measure recall on the different forms of the logical memory portion of the Wechsler Memory Scale were not of equivalent difficulty. Because they were administered in a preset rather than random order, a TBI group appeared to have deteriorated on the third administration, when in truth, the form used was more difficult.

Disabilities

Forer (1985) has noted that rehabilitation evaluators are continually searching for better methods of assessing functional gains. In a review of 18 functional assessment instruments pertinent to TBI, he noted that the content of items includes self-care and ADL, vocational status, communication, psychosocial adjustment, and other activities such as leisure. Except for the DRS, no scales have been designed for TBIs, and only a few, such as the Patient Evaluation Conference System (Jellinek, Torkelson, & Harvey, 1982) and the Rehabilitation Indicators (Jacobs, 1984;

Mayer, Keating, & Rapp, 1986), have been applied to TBIs.

In general, the strength of disability evaluation is that it samples behaviors that occur in natural environments or in therapeutic activities. This is the logic behind the adoption of ADL in medical rehabilitation, work samples in vocational rehabilitation, and learning assessments in special education. In TBI, the central issue is that competence may not be solely a matter of the correct performance of an activity. Rather, the style or organization of behavior may reduce the usefulness of a traditional pass/fail criterion. Mayer et al. (1986) provided a framework for teaching ADL skills in a context specific to TBIs. The framework is illustrated in the way toothbrushing skills are taught as the performance of organized, discrete tasks, from picking up the toothpaste to discarding a towel.

Ben-Yishay et al. (1987) and Hart, Plenger, Helffenstein, and Hayden (1985) have developed rating systems for scaling the behaviors of persons with TBI who are undergoing occupational trials. Conventional vocational rehabilitation programs have adapted work sample approaches to populations with disabilities because of the inadequacies of standard vocational tests. These approaches, however, may miss the most salient behaviors of clients with TBIs that make vocational placement difficult. A checklist of 12 areas such as attitude toward occupational trials, attitude toward tasks, and initiation of tasks has been found to be reliable for predicting employability (Ben-Yishay et al., in press). In the cognitive domain, the River Mead Behavioral Memory Test (Wilson, 1986) was developed; it is comprised of a series of memory tasks, including items such as carrying out commands and recalling previous instructions in a quasinaturalistic setting, as well as some standard tests of memory used in clinical testing. Preliminary data suggest that performance correlates with ratings of memory by occupational therapists.

Handicaps

Vocational Outcomes   References to more than 40 studies on vocational outcomes in clients with TBI may be found in Oddy (1984) and Kay, Ezrachi, and Cavallo (1986). From an outcome measurement standpoint, the following are some issues in characterizing the employment status of persons with TBIs.

Work versus No Work   This criterion, which has been used in many reported studies, is too simple. Ben-Yishay and co-workers (1987) have developed an Occupational Rating Scale that describes work levels from unemployable to fully employed at the premorbid occupation. The scale combines assessment of the patient's present overall work competence compared to the preinjury level of employment with assessment of competitive versus noncompetitive employment. Although devised as a measure of employability of individuals participating in clinical occupational trials, it also is useful as a measure of actual employment.

Holding a Job   The high incidence of cognitive and behavioral problems in persons with TBI results in attempts to return to work that are followed by failure or moves from one job to another. For example, in a follow-up of 40 persons with TBIs, approximately 20% were working at the end of 2 years. The individuals still working at the end of 1 year were not always the same as those working at the end of the second year (Diller & Ben-Yishay, 1983). In a follow-up of individuals who completed an outpatient program and were placed vocationally, the Occupational Rating Scale was used to assess employment status at 6-month intervals for periods up to 36 months. This scale enabled the identification of individuals who showed fluctuations in employment and the isolation of three major reasons: 1) social isolation in a poorly structured environment, 2) forgetting to apply consistently acquired "rehabilitation algorithms" and/or use compensatory mnemonic "props," and 3) financial disincentives to work (Ben-Yishay et al., 1987).

Other Dimensions   The types of support that may be needed to secure placement or to maintain employment of persons with TBI have not been examined. In specifying suitable supports or levels of assistance, common descriptors for grades of functional abilities would be useful. Wages earned, a natural marker of employment, has not yet been documented for this population.

Prediction of Employment   There have been numerous attempts to predict employment as an outcome in TBI. The most frequently used measure has been the GCS. The multidetermined nature of employment following TBI may be seen by the fact that Oddy (1984) reported lack of a relationship between cognitive impairment and employment in a group of persons with TBIs who did not sustain major physical damage. It appears that individuals with physical impairments requiring intensive treatment have a lower incidence of employment than those without such impairments (Oddy, 1984). The GCS scores for untreated TBI populations appear to be related to return to work (Hart, Plenger, Helffenstein, & Hayden, 1985; Rimel & Jane, 1983). Although such statements may be adequate for groups of people, they are not justified for individual management because of the large overlap between groups.

When designing the methodology of vocational studies, the following precautions should be taken:

1. Carefully delineate "independent" variables, such as age, severity of injury, time since injury, and premorbid function. The firmest marker at this point appears to be the GCS.
2. Different combinations of variables may be pertinent for predicting employment in different settings. For example, Ben-Yishay et al. (in press) found that a combination of measures from many domains, including cognitive, interpersonal, and demographic, predicted employment in a holistic outpatient program. Kay et al. (1986) found that a measure of word fluency predicted employment at 1 year in individuals who did not receive an intervention, but who were examined at 3 months and 6 months after discharge from acute care.

Living Arrangements The three most important dimensions are the patient's role in the family, the family members as observers of the patient's behavior, and the family as a human environment for the patient.

Role in the family accounts for a great deal of variance in daily behavior. Behavioral sequelae of TBI are expected to impact on role-related be-

havior. Thus, Rosenbaum and Najenson (1976) reported that the wives of TBI war veterans, compared with the wives of paraplegic war veterans, stated that their husbands were more childish, self-centered, and dependent, took less part in running the household, and forced an alteration in family contact and use of leisure time. Despite a general impression that role relationships tend to be more strained between spouses than between parents and children, supporting evidence is inconclusive at this time (Brooks, 1984a).

Finally, there have been no studies of the effects of the family on the patient. Whereas architectural features of the environment have been the major focus in studies of individuals with other physical disabilities, the family is the most salient aspect of the environment for persons with TBI. The importance of the family must be considered in connection with the incidence of disturbed family relations existing before the occurrence of TBI.

Families have been used as observers in outcome studies perhaps more often than as study subjects in their own right. For the most part, this is because the intimacies of daily living in a household, and the fact that outcome studies occur when the person with TBI has returned to the community, place families in a unique position to note the consequences of personality alterations. Several approaches have been used. Jacobs (1984) used a questionnaire. Prigitano et al. (1986) used the Katz Adjustment Scale—Relatives Form (Katz & Lyerly, 1963), which has been well standardized and validated with other populations. A more frequent approach has been the development of rating scales and checklists for relatives to report their observations of the disabled family member (Bond, 1983).

The effects of TBI on the family have been approached by attempting to measure the degree of family burden (Brooks, 1984a). Family burden is conceived in two ways. The first is objective burden, which can be subdivided into two types: 1) changes in family income, household routines, health status, housing conditions, and social-leisure activities; and 2) changes in the brain-injured individual's personality and symptoms. The second is subjective burden, the stress experienced by the family from objective burdens. It was noted, for example, the deficits in emotional control and stability and subjective complaints of slowness, tiredness, and concentration problems posed a greater burden than disturbed physical, language, self-care, memory, and behavioral changes. Furthermore, these burdens tended to persist over time (Brooks, 1984b). No studies have examined family responses in terms of family systems theory—for example, family problem solving, communications, management of household responsibilities—nor have they examined the effect of family interventions. Consequently, the effects of TBI on the family is the least developed area of measurement.

Activity Patterns   Many observers (Bond, 1983; Brooks, 1984a) have noted declining social contacts and increasing passive behaviors in TBI populations. The activity pattern indicators (APIs; Brown et al., 1984), designed to measure how time is used, have been applied in a number of ways. Time usage, a measure reflecting quality of life, can reveal social contacts as well as active versus passive behavior.

Mayer et al. (1986), stressing a context-specific approach to interventions, examined behavior following rehabilitation in terms of time usage.

By modifying APIs, they divided time usage into nine specific categories: self-care, housekeeping, leisure, personal business and finance, consumer activities, community activities, school, work, and special and rare events. In a case study, they demonstrated that a housewife who sustained a severe TBI reduced housekeeping activities from 63% to 46% at discharge, and to 45% upon 6-month follow-up. She also increased leisure time activities from 19% to 35% at discharge and to 42% upon 6-month follow-up. A major part of the increase reflected passive leisure activities, such as napping during the day. Studies using the APIs by O'Shaughnessey, Fowler, and Reid (1984) and Jacobs (1984) pinpointed social isolation as a problem following TBI.

CONCLUSIONS

Assessment of outcomes in TBI is occurring amidst expanding knowledge in three fields— assessment of recovery following TBI, changes in service delivery practices, and functional assessment in rehabilitation. The tools in each of these fields must be adapted to address results generated by the others.

REFERENCES

Ben-Yishay, Y., Silver, S. L., Piasetsky, E., & Associates. (1987). Vocational outcome after intensive holistic cognitive rehabilitation: Results of a seven year study. *Journal of Head Trauma Rehabilitation, 1*, 90.

Bond, M. R. (1983). Effects on the family system. In M. R. Rosenthal, E. R. Griffiths, M. R. Bond, & J. D. Miller (Eds.), *Rehabilitation of the brain injured adult* (pp. 209–216). Philadelphia: Davis.

Braunling-McMorrow, D., Lloyd, K., & Fralish, K. (1986). Teaching social skills to brain injured adults. *Journal of Rehabilitation, 52*, 41–48.

Brooks, D. N., Deelman, B. G., Van Zomeran, A. H., Van Dongen, H., Van Harskamps, F., & Aughton, M. E. (1984). Problems in measuring cognitive recovery after acute head injury. *Journal of Clinical Neuropsychology, 6*, 71–85.

Brooks, N. (Ed.). (1984a). *Closed head injury: Psychological, social, and family consequences.* New York: Oxford University Press.

Brooks, N. (1984b). Head injury and the family. In N. Brooks (Ed.), *Closed head injury* (pp. 123–148). New York: Oxford University Press.

Brown, M. E., Gordon, W. A., & Diller, L. (1984). Rehabilitation indicators. In A. S. Halpern & M. J. Fuhrer (Eds.), *Functional assessment in rehabilitation* (pp. 187–203). Baltimore: Paul H. Brookes Publishing Co.

Cole, J. R., Cope, N., & Cervelli, L. (1985). Rehabilitation

of the severely brain injured patient: A community based low cost model program. *Archives of Physical Medicine and Rehabilitation, 66*, 38–41.

Conkey, R. C. (1938). Psychological changes associated with head injuries. *Archives of Psychology, 232*, 1–62.

Corrigan, J. D., Arnett, J. A., Houcks, L. J., & Jackson, R. D. (1985). Reality orientation for brain injured patients: Group treatment and monitoring of recovery. *Archives of Physical Medicine and Rehabilitation, 66*, 626–632.

Dikmen, S., Reitan, R. M., & Temkin, N. R. (1983). Neuropsychological recovery in head injury. *Archives of Neurology, 40*, 333–338.

Diller, L., & Ben-Yishay, Y. (1983). *Severe head trauma: A comprehensive medical approach to rehabilitation* (Final Report GT #13-P-59082, National Institute of Handicapped Research). New York: New York University.

Fiske, D. W., & Shewder, R. A. (1966). *Pluralisms and subjectivities in social science.* Chicago: University of Chicago Press.

Forer, S. (1985). Rehabilitation outcomes and evaluation systems for traumatic brain injury. *Journal of the Organization of Rehabilitation Evaluators, 5*, 52–74.

Hagen, C., Malkmus, D., & Durham, P. (1979). *Levels of cognitive functioning in rehabilitation of the head injury adult: Comprehensive physical management.* Downey, CA: Ranchos Los Amigos Hospital, Inc.

Hall, K., Cope, N., & Rappaport, M. (1985). Glasgow Outcome Scale and Disability Rating Scale: Comparative usefulness in following recovery in traumatic head injury. *Archives of Physical Medicine and Rehabilitation, 66,* 35–37.

Hart, T., Plenger, P. M., Helffenstein, D. A., & Hayden, M. E. (1985). Neuropsychological correlates and qualitative features of vocational performance after severe closed head injury. *Journal of Clinical and Experimental Neuropsychology, 7,* 148.

Heaton, R. K., Chelune, G. J., & Lehman, R. A. W. (1978). Using neuropsychological and personality tests to assess the likelihoood of patient employment. *Journal of Nervous and Mental Disorders, 166,* 408–416.

Hook, O. (1976). Rehabilitation. In P. J. VinKen & G. W. Bryan (Eds.), *Handbook of clinical neurology* (Vol. 24, pp. 683). Amsterdam: North Holland Publishing Co.

Jacobs, H. E. (1984). *The family as a therapeutic agent: Long term rehabilitation for traumatic head injury patients* (Final Report, Mary Switzer Research Fellowship). Washington, DC: National Institute of Handicapped Research.

Jellinek, H. M., Torkelson, R., & Harvey, R. (1982). Functional abilities and distress levels in brain injured patients at long-term follow up. *Archives of Physical Medicine and Rehabilitation, 63,* 160–162.

Jennett, B., & Bond, M. R. (1975). Assessment of outcome after severe brain damage: A practical scale. *Lancet, 1,* 480–487.

Katz, M. M., & Lyerly, S. B. (1963). Methods of measuring adjustment and social behavior in the community: Rationale, description discriminative validity and scalle dcvelopment. *Psychological Reports, 13,* 503–513.

Kay, T., Ezrachi, O., & Cavallo, M. (1984). *Annotated bibliography of research on vocational outcome following head trauma.* New York: New York University Research and Training Center on Head Trauma and Research.

Kay, T., Ezrachi, O., & Cavallo, M. (1986). Plateaus and consistencies: Long term neuropsychological changes following head trauma. In *Proceedings of the 94th Annual Convention of the American Psychological Association,* p. 175.

Levin, H. S., Benton, A. L., & Grossman, R. G. (1982). *Neurobehavioral consequences of closed head injury.* New York: Oxford University Press.

Levin, H. S., Eisenberg, H. M., Handel, S. E., Kalisky, Z., Amparo, Z. G., Goldman, A. M., McArdle, C. B., Williams, D., & High, W. M. (1986). Magnetic resonance imaging and correlated neuropsychological findings in long term survivors of severe closed head injury. *Journal of Clinical and Experimental Neuropsychology, 8,* 123.

Levin, H. S., High, W., Williams, D., & Eisenberg, H. M. (1985). Automatic versus effortful processing in long term survivors of severe closed head injury. *Journal of Clinical and Experimental Neuropsychology, 7,* 166.

Levin, H. S., O'Donnell, V. M., & Grossman, R. G. (1979). The Galveston Orientation and Amnesia Test: A practical scale to assess cognition after head injury. *Journal of Nervous and Mental Disorders, 167,* 675–684.

Lezak, M. D. (1983). *Neuropsychological assessment* (2nd ed.). New York: Oxford Press.

Mandelberg, I. A. (1975). Cognitive recovery after severe head injury: Wechsler Adult Intelligence Scale during post traumatic amnesia. *Journal of Neurology, Neurosurgery, and Psychiatry, 38,* 1127–1132.

Mayer, N. H., Keating, D. J., & Rapp, D. (1986). Skills, routines and activity patterns of daily living: A functional nested approach. In B. P. Uzzell & Y. Gross (Eds.), *Clinical neuropsychology of intervention* (pp. 205–273). Boston: Martinus Nijoff Publishers.

McLean, A., Temkin, N. R., Dikmen, S., & Wyler, A. R. (1984). The behavioral sequelae of head injury. *Journal of Clinical Neuropsychology, 5,* 361–375.

Meeder, D. L. (1982). Cognitive perceptual motor evaluation research findings for adult head injuries. In L. Trexler (Ed.), *Cognitive rehabilitation: Conceptualization and intervention* (pp. 153–171). New York: Plenum Press.

Nagele, D. A. (1985). Neuropsychological inferences from a tooth brushing task: A model for understanding deficits and making interventions. *Archives of Physical Medicine and Rehabilitation, 66,* 58.

Najenson, T., Sazhon, L., Fiselson, J., Becker, E., & Schechter, I. (1978). Recovery of cognitive functions after severe prolonged trauma. *Scandinavian Journal of Rehabilitation Medicine, 10,* 15–21.

National Head Injury Foundation. (1984). *National directory of head injury rehabilitation services.* Framingham, MA: Author.

Oddy, M. (1984). Head injury and social adjustment. In N. Brooks (Ed.), *Closed head injury: Psychological, social and family consequences* (pp. 108–122). New York: Oxford University Press.

O'Shaughnessy, E. J., Fowler, R. S., & Reid, M. (1984). Sequelae of mild closed head injuries. *Journal of Family Practice, 18,* 391–394.

Panikoff, L. C. (1983). Recovery trends of functional skills in the head injured adult. *American Journal of Occupational Therapy, 37,* 735–743.

Prigitano, G. P., Fordyce, D., Zeiner, H. K., Rouecke, I. R., Pepping, M., & Wood, B. C. (1986). *Neuropsychological rehabilitation after brain injury.* Baltimore: Johns Hopkins University Press.

Rappaport, M., Hall, K., Hopkins, K., Belleza, T., Berrol, S., & Reynolds, G. (1977). Evoked potentials and disability in brain damaged patients. *Archives of Physical Medicine and Rehabilitation, 58,* 333–338.

Rimel, R. W., Giordani, B., Barth, J. T., & Jane, J. A. (1982). Moderate head injury: Completing the clinical spectrum of brain trauma. *Neurosurgery, 11,* 344–350.

Rimel, R. W., & Jane, J. A. (1983). Characteristics of the head injured patient. In M. R. Rosenthal, E. R. Griffiths, M. R. Bond, & J. D. Miller (Eds.), *Rehabilitation of the brain injured adult* (pp. 9–20). Philadelphia: Davis.

Roberts, A. H. (1979). *Severe accidental head injury.* London: McMillan.

Rosenbaum, M., & Najenson, T. (1976). Changes in life patterns and symptoms as reported by wives of severely brain injured soldiers. *Journal of Consulting and Clinical Psychology, 44,* 881–888.

Rusk, H. A., Block, J., & Lowman, E. (1969). Rehabilitation of the brain injured patient: A report of 157 cases with long-term follow-up of 118. In A. E. Walker, A. F. Caveness, & E. M. Critchley (Eds.), *The late effects of head injury* (pp. 327–332). Springfield, IL: Charles C Thomas Publishers.

Scherzer, B. P. (1986). Rehabilitation following severe head trauma: Results of a three year program. *Archives of Physical Medicine and Rehabilitation, 67,* 366–373.

Sehgal, V. (1986, May). *Outcome of medical rehabilitation in brain damaged patients.* Paper presented at the annual meeting of the National Association of Rehabilitation Research and Training Centers, Kansas City, KS.

Stover, S., & Zeiger, H. E. (1976). Head injury in children and teenagers: Functional recovery correlated with duration of coma. *Archives of Physical Medicine and Rehabilitation, 57,* 201–205.

Strub, R. L., & Block, F. W. (1981). *The mental status exam in neurology.* Philadelphia: Davis.

Teasdale, G., & Jennett, B. (1974). Assessment of coma and impaired consciousness: A practical scale. *Lancet, 2,* 81–84.

Tobis, J. S., Puri, K. B., & Sheridan, J. (1982). Rehabilita-

tion of the severely brain injured patients. *Scandinavian Journal of Rehabilitation Medicine, 14,* 83–88.

Wilson, B. (1986). *Rehabilitation of memory.* New York: Guilford Press.

World Health Organization. (1980). *International classification of impairments, disabilities, and handicaps: A manual of classification relating to the consequences of disease.* Geneva: Author.

Chapter 17

Outcome Analysis in Spinal Cord Injury Rehabilitation

Gale G. Whiteneck

To the casual observer, the rehabilitation of persons with spinal cord injury (SCI) appears to produce remarkable outcomes. This positive global assessment, however, conceals considerable need within the SCI rehabilitation community to clarify objectives and quantitatively demonstrate positive outcomes to the more careful and critical observer. The current pressures of accountability, competition, and alternative reimbursement systems all focus attention on desired outcomes and their measurement. This chapter builds a conceptual model of SCI rehabilitation on the theory of disablement offered by the World Health Organization (WHO), reviews various efforts to assess SCI rehabilitation outcomes from the perspective of that model, and proposes future outcome assessment strategies suggested by the model.

A MODEL OF SCI REHABILITATION

Diverse outcomes from SCI rehabilitation have been proposed. Everything from greater independence in daily tasks to a better quality of life has been promised. To aid in understanding these various perspectives, a conceptual model of SCI rehabilitation is proposed in Figure 1.

The Disablement Process

The model of SCI rehabilitation builds upon the WHO model of disablement (1980). The conse-quences of disease in the model are impairment at the organic level, disability at the personal level, and handicap at the societal level.

Impairment is defined as "any loss or abnormality of psychological, physiological or anatomical structure or function" (p. 47) in the WHO model. For SCI, the primary impairment is spastic paralysis of more than one limb (code I72) under the general category of skeletal impairments.

Measurement of impairment from SCI has been standardized by the American Spinal Injury Association (1982) with a high degree of specificity. This detailed assessment separately identifies for each side the lowest neurological segment with normal sensory function and the segment with normal motor function. Motor index scores are computed for each side (and a total score) by summing a 0 to 5 grading system on each of 10 key muscles. On the basis of motor and sensory testing, patients are categorized as having either a complete or incomplete SCI. Finally, the zone of injury (up to three segments) is provided for complete injuries and the functional and anatomical classifications are provided for incomplete injuries.

In the WHO model (1980), *disability* is defined as "any restriction or lack (resulting from an impairment) of ability to perform an activity in the manner or within the range considered normal for a human being" (p. 143). Impairments

The preparation of this chapter was partially supported by The Rocky Mountain Regional Spinal Cord Injury System at Craig Hospital (Grant No. G008535132).

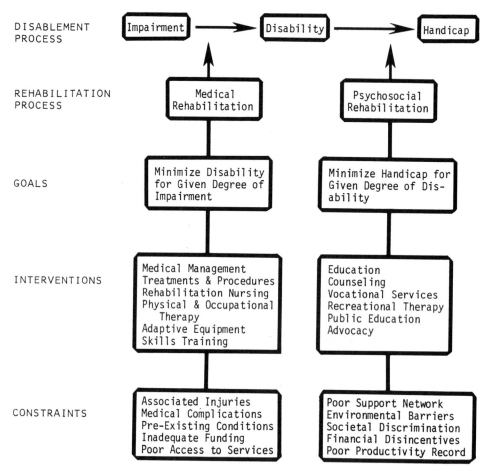

Figure 1.   Model of spinal cord injury rehabilitation.

from SCI can result in disabilities in any of the nine major categories outlined by the WHO. In particular, disabilities in the major categories of personal care, locomotion, body disposition, and dexterity will result to some degree from SCI.

Measurement of disability in the SCI population is not as standardized as the measurement of impairment. Early efforts to measure disability focused on activities of daily living (ADL) scales such as the Barthel Index (Mahoney & Barthel, 1965). Gresham et al. (1980) developed the Quadriplegic Index of Function (QIF) to compensate for the failure of the Barthel and other ADL scales to detect functional changes in quadriplegics. Other recent efforts to broaden the range of activities assessed include the Rehabilitation Indicators Project (Brown, Gordon, & Diller, 1984; Diller et al., 1983; Gordon et al., 1982) and the Longitudinal Functional Assessment

System (Rintala et al., 1984). The role of these instruments in assessing disability among the SCI population is reviewed later in the chapter.

Handicap in the WHO model is defined as "a disadvantage for a given individual, resulting from an impairment or a disability, that limits or prevents the fulfillment of a role that is normal (depending on age, sex, and social and cultural factors) for that individual" (p. 183). The first handicap categorized in the WHO model, orientation handicap, is less relevant to SCI than the other dimensions of handicap since orientation handicap primarily result from language, hearing, and vision impairments and speaking, listening, and seeing disabilities. The other five major categories of handicap are directly relevant to SCI. They are handicaps in physical independence, mobility, occupation, social integration, and economic self-sufficiency.

Measurement of handicap in the SCI population is less developed than either impairment or disability assessment. Often the only attempts to document handicaps are to record employment status as an indicator of an occupational handicap and to record living situation and attendant care as indicators of a physical independence handicap. The tracking of a wide variety of actual behaviors and activities in the community is one methodology that shows promise for assessing handicaps. Two previously mentioned approaches, Rehabilitation Indicators and the Longitudinal Functional Assessment System, incorporated variations of this technique in following SCI populations. Another recent approach to outcome assessment that is directly relevant to measuring handicap grows out of the Independent Living (IL) movement. To measure IL outcomes among persons with SCI, DeJong, Branch, and Corcoran (1984) and DeJong and Hughes (1982) placed value judgments on behavioral measures to produce outcome scales. These techniques and their application to handicap assessment are reviewed later in this chapter.

The application of the WHO model of disablement produces an increasingly broader view of SCI at each stage of the process. Impairment focuses on the consequences of severe trauma to the spinal cord and nervous system. Disability focuses on the consequences to the individual in terms of performing tasks and physical functions. Handicap focuses on the consequences to the member of society in terms of performing roles and social functions.

The Rehabilitation Process

Trieschmann (1980) suggested that SCI rehabilitation has traditionally followed the medical model, with emphasis on dispensing treatments and therapies to a passive recipient in order to improve functioning. She also suggested, however, that growing attention has been paid to a learning model, which emphasizes educating an active participant to live in his or her own environment.

Alexander and Fuhrer (1984) also dichotomize rehabilitation into two models, which they label medical rehabilitation and psychosocial rehabilitation. Medical rehabilitation is described as the delivery of services by a variety of medical disciplines, coordinated by a physician, in order to ameliorate physical impairments, preserve health status, and reestablish behavioral functioning. Psychosocial rehabilitation is described as an educational process, more concerned with addressing handicaps than disabilities or impairments, designed to assist individuals in their environments and enlarge their opportunities to lead meaningful lives.

Rather than considering these as competing models of rehabilitation, the proposed model of SCI rehabilitation diagramed in Figure 1 treats the two models as distinct elements of the overall rehabilitation process. The terms "medical rehabilitation" and "psychosocial rehabilitation" used by Alexander and Fuhrer (1984) are adopted to label the complementary emphases of the two approaches.

Medical rehabilitation concentrates on the disablement phase from impairment to disability, with the goal of minimizing disability for a given degree of impairment. In SCI rehabilitation, this means minimizing disabilities in personal care, locomotion, body disposition, and dexterity for individuals with a given level and extent of neurological lesion.

Psychosocial rehabilitation concentrates on the disablement phase from disability to handicap with the goal of minimizing handicap for a given degree of disability. In SCI rehabilitation, this means minimizing handicaps in physical independence, mobility, occupation, social integration, and economic self-sufficiency for individuals with given degrees of disability in personal care, locomotion, body disposition, and dexterity.

Although much can be learned from the conceptual distinction between medical and psychosocial rehabilitation, they need not be separated in time. In fact, Alexander and Fuhrer (1984) reported a growing trend toward integrating the two models and efforts throughout the entire comprehensive SCI rehabilitation program.

Interventions and Constraints

As illustrated in Figure 1, the two SCI rehabilitation processes require different interventions and operate under different types of constraints. The typical interventions of medical rehabilitation are treatments managed by physicians and delivered by a variety of specialists and allied health professionals. In addition to medical management of the spine and other organ systems, considerable ADL and mobility skills training is provided along with adaptive equipment.

Conversely, the interventions of psychosocial rehabilitation are primarily education and counseling directed toward long-term adjustment in the community. These interventions are interactive and encourage the active participation of clients in decision making. Vocational services and recreational therapy are examples of identifiable services directed toward specific areas of handicap. The targets of psychosocial rehabilitation interventions frequently extend beyond the client. Families as well as individuals are counseled, the general public is encouraged to abandon stereotypes and discrimination, and policymakers are lobbied for legislative change.

Constraints operating in medical rehabilitation are those factors that make minimizing *disability* more difficult. In addition to the basic limiting factor of impairment, several other constraints operate at the organ level. These include associated injuries received at the time of the SCI, medical complications resulting from the injury or occurring after the injury, and conditions existing before the injury. Other constraints include factors that limit access to service or equipment, such as inadequate funding. All these factors act to slow or limit the process of minimizing disability.

Constraints operating in psychosocial rehabilitation are those factors that make minimizing *handicap* more difficult. These factors are characterized by poor interaction between the individual and the environment. Examples include poor family and social support networks, environmental barriers, societal discrimination, financial disincentives to employment, and poor preinjury productivity records.

Outcome Analysis

Making a conceptual distinction between medical and psychosocial rehabilitation helps clarify outcome analysis. The desired outcome of medical rehabilitation is minimal disability. (Note that impairment is viewed as an input to the medical

rehabilitation process rather than an outcome because current medical practice offers little ability to eliminate or substantially reduce impairment). In psychosocial rehabilitation, the desired outcome is minimal handicap.

The desired goals of minimal disability and minimal handicap, however, should not be assessed in a vacuum. The accomplishments of medical and psychosocial rehabilitation should be judged relative to: 1) the respective degrees of impairment and disability brought to the process, 2) the character and extent of interventions applied, and 3) any other constraints on rehabilitation impact. To assess effectiveness, the definitive question becomes, "What interventions produce the best results under certain conditions and constraints?" To assess cost efficiency, the definitive question becomes, "How can impact be maximized while resources are minimized?"

Currently, outcome prediction is substantially more precise in medical rehabilitation than psychosocial rehabilitation. Given a patient with a known degree of impairment (level and extent of lesion) entering an SCI rehabilitation facility, much can be predicted about the degree of disability (tasks that cannot be performed independently) likely to be present at discharge. Authors such as Greb and Mueller (1982) have specified the functional goals expected for each level of neurological impairment. Constraints to medical rehabilitation are more likely to increase the intervention required or delay the intervention than to limit the eventual outcome. Fine (1985) has demonstrated that much of the variability in lengths of stay for SCI rehabilitation, representing quantity of intervention, can be predicted if the level and extent of neurological impairment combined with the specific associated injuries and medical complications are known.

Conversely, disability is not as good a predictor of handicap as impairment is of disability. In the psychosocial rehabilitation process, constraints are more numerous and powerful, interventions are less certain and potent, and the whole process is barely understood. In time, however, greater knowledge of disabilities, handicaps, interventions, constraints, and their interactions will improve outcome prediction in psychosocial rehabilitation.

Economic Consequences of SCI for Society

The model proposed in Figure 1 examines the outcomes of rehabilitation from the perspective of the spinal cord–injured person. At least one other perspective must be overlayed on this model before it is complete: that of society. From this perspective, the major concerns are economic.

The Bureau of Economic Research (1985) reduced a detailed economic model to two primary economic consequences of SCI for society: 1) the increased resources devoted to providing medical goods and services for persons with SCI, and 2) the lost social contribution due to the reduction in gross earnings by SCI persons. Estimates of 1977 costs to society were over one-half billion dollars for rehabilitation and care of SCI persons and over two billion dollars for their lost earnings. Clearly these costs to society are very high and must be continually examined as outcomes of SCI and its rehabilitation. Although programs that prevent SCI are likely the most effective method of cost containment, cost–benefit analysis should be applied to various medical and psychosocial rehabilitation interventions as well.

A critique of cost–benefit studies by Johnston and Keith (1983) concluded that, although definitive proof had not been offered, considerable evidence suggests that comprehensive, multidisciplinary SCI centers are cost-effective compared to unspecialized care for severely impaired SCI patients. Specialized centers improved outcomes, often for less initial hospitalization expense, and consistently produced higher long-term earnings and lower long-term nursing expenses. Johnston and Keith (1983) suggested that future studies should compare the costs and benefits of alternative types or intensities of rehabilitation, as well as techniques of social adjustment.

REVIEWS OF SCI REHABILITATION OUTCOME ASSESSMENT

The National SCI Database and five other systems of outcome assessment either have been developed specifically for SCI populations or have used SCI populations during the development and testing phases of instrumentation. The literature on outcome assessment is replete with interesting examples of additional measures that have, at times, been used in SCI rehabilitation, but these are beyond the scope of this text.

The National SCI Database

The National SCI Database was first established at the National Spinal Cord Injury Data Research Center (NSCIDRC) and later transferred to the National Spinal Cord Injury Statistical Center (NSCISC). It is the largest repository of longitudinal data on SCI cases in existence. As of August 1985, the National SCI Database contained initial rehabilitation and annual follow-up information on 9,647 SCI persons who received their initial rehabilitation in one of the federally designated regional model SCI systems since 1973 (NSCISC, 1985a). These comprehensive care systems are designed to serve SCI persons from the time of injury through acute and initial rehabilitation services to a lifetime of follow-up care. Although the National SCI Database cases represent only a fraction of the total SCI cases (Trieschmann, 1980), they presumably represent the outcome of cases treated in state-of-the-art specialized centers.

The initial list of variables included in the National SCI Database (NSCIDRC, 1975) was ambitious and included substantial information relevant to the model of SCI rehabilitation proposed in Figure 1. Table 1 lists the variables included in the original database that seem to measure aspects of the SCI rehabilitation model. The variables are grouped under labels corresponding to elements of the SCI rehabilitation model, including measures of impairment, disability, and handicap as well as measures of medical and psychosocial rehabilitation interventions and constraints. The column designated "assessment periods" indicates whether data are relevant to conditions at or before onset (O), at initial system admission (A), during initial rehabilitation or at discharge (D), and/or at each annual follow-up period (F). Finally, variables that remain in the current National SCI Database are indicated with an asterisk (NSCISC, 1985b).

As originally designed, the National SCI Database assessed impairment through the category, level, and extent of neurological function measured at several points in time. Disability was assessed using the Barthel Index (Mahoney & Barthel, 1965) as modified by Granger (1972). The Barthel Index was one of the earliest and most frequently utilized ADL instruments in rehabilitation. The modified Barthel Index assessed capability of independence in nine self-care and six mobility tasks on a 4-point rating system from dependent to independent. Items were weighted and summed for self-care and mobility subscores and a total functional index. A variety of information relevant to handicaps was collected at annual follow-ups, including living situation, marital and employment status, hours of physical assistance required, time spent in six types of activities, and time spent outside the home.

Table 1 also indicates the varying amounts of information collected relevant to interventions and constraints. Information about the nature of physical rehabilitation interventions was limited to operations and procedures, urinary and respiratory management, and degree of involvement in follow-up care. The duration and costs of medical care, however, were documented in considerable detail. Full detail was provided on the medical rehabilitation constraints of associated injuries, medical complications, and preexisting conditions. Measures of psychosocial rehabilitation interventions were sparse at follow-up and nearly nonexistent at initial rehabilitation. Only data on educational advancement and Department of Vocational Rehabilitation status and expenses were collected. Measures of psychosocial rehabilitation constraints provided substantial

Table 1. Variables in original National SCI Database[a]

Assessment periods[b]				
				Measures of impairment
A	D	F	*	Category of neurological impairment
A	D	F	*	Anatomical level (R&L) of last normal neurological function
A	D	F	*	Degree of preserved neurological function (Frankel class)
				Measures of medical rehabilitation intervention
	D	F		System vs. nonsystem patient
A				Time to first medical attention and type and expense of emergency transport
	D	F	*	Number of admission days in system and nonsystem hospitals
A	D	F	*	Method of urinary management and use of respirator
	D	F	*	Category of follow-up care provided by system
A	D	F	*	Operations and procedures
	D	F	*	Expenses for hospitalization
	D	F		Expenses for physicians, equipment, and other medical care
	D			Total expenses injury to home (with presystem and system subtotals)
		F		Outpatient expenses for therapies, medications, supplies, and other
		F	*	Attendent care utilization
		F		Expenses for attendent care and custodial care
		F		Average hours/week and wage of hired attendent care
		F	*	Days in nursing home
		F		Total annual medical, maintenance, and rehabilitation expenses
				Measures of medical rehabilitation constraints
O			*	Associated injuries
A	D	F	*	Medical complications and diagnoses
A	D	F	*	Pressure sores (27 locations and 4 grades)
O			*	Preexisting medical conditions
				Measures of disability
	D	F		Modified Barthel Index (15 items, subscores, and total)[c]
				Measures of psychosocial rehabilitation interventions
		F		Vocational rehabilitation expenses
	D	F	*	DVR client and caseload status
		F	*	Increased level of education postinjury
		F	*	Business, trade, or technical courses completed postinjury

continued

Table 1.   (continued)

Assessment periods[b]			Measures
			Measures of psychosocial rehabilitation constraints
O			Preinjury residence and living with whom
O		*	Preinjury marital status
O			Preinjury number of marriages, divorces, and children
O		*	Preinjury occupational/educational status
O			Preinjury occupational DOT code and time devoted
O			Personal salary or wages preinjury (annual)
O		*	Educational level preinjury
O			Business, trade, or technical courses completed preinjury
O		*	Demographics (age, race, sex, etiology)
			Measures of handicap
	F		Living with whom
D	F	*	Place of residence
D	F	*	Marital status
	F		Number of marriages, divorces, and children
	F	*	Occupational/educational status
	F		Occupational DOT code
	F		Personal salary or wages (annual)
	F	*	Comparison of employment pre- and postinjury
	F		Average hours of actual physical assistance required per day
	F		Average hours per week spent in:
	F		Housekeeping activities
	F		Hobbies, sports, and recreation
	F		Reading for pleasure, TV, radio, etc.
	F		Education and other self-improvement activities
	F		Community service
	F		Paid employment
	F		Average total number of hours/week spent outside of home

*Indicates variable remains in current database.

[a]Sources: NSCIDRC (1975) and NSCISC (1985b).

[b]Assessment periods: O, prior to or at onset; A, at system admission or injury to admission; D, at system discharge or injury to discharge; F, at annual follow-up or during follow-up year.

[c]Currently the Barthel instrument has been replaced by a functional assessment of self-care independence and ambulation.

background on preinjury living situation and marital, educational, and employment history.

From the beginning, the longitudinal character of the National SCI Database has increased the potential for outcome assessment. In addition to annual follow-up of impairment, disability, and handicap, medical complications and care required during follow-up periods can be measured to assess the effectiveness of initial SCI rehabilitation training.

Over the last decade, however, the extensive data collection efforts originally begun by the National SCI Database became a practical burden for the regional model systems as the number of cases being followed increased. Various questions were also raised regarding the reliability, validity, and intercenter standardization of several variables. This has resulted in the discontinuation of many measures from the National SCI Database over the years.

Table 1 indicates the variables currently remaining in the database with an asterisk. Although all measures of impairment have been retained, the Barthel Index measuring disability was deleted. In addition to the time and resources required to administer the Barthel Index annually, the appropriateness of the index for SCI populations, particularly quadriplegics, was questioned. The Barthel Index has been replaced by two simple dichotomous functional assessments of self-care and mobility: 1) Is the person independent in performing self-care activities or is assistance required?, and 2) Is the primary mode of mobility ambulation or a wheelchair? Furthermore, the addition of more suitable disability measurement is being considered. A likely candidate is the Functional Independence Measure (FIM) of the proposed Uniform National Data System for Medical Rehabilitation (see Chapter 10), and initial testing is underway.

Among the first areas of information dropped were the hours spent in six specific categories of activities, the total hours spent outside the home, and the hours of actual physical assistance required. The indicators of social role fulfillment (handicap) are now limited to residence, marital status, and employment status. Other variables discontinued include all cost data (except initial hospitalization expenses) and some preinjury background information.

In the National SCI Database, energies have focused on improving the quality of information collected on a smaller set of measures. It is clear, however, that the present list of variables does not adequately measure all components of the SCI rehabilitation model, particularly the all-important outcomes of disability and handicap. The National SCI Database reflects the medical rehabilitation model far more adequately than the psychosocial rehabilitation model; its main contributions to SCI knowledge follow the traditional medical model of describing patients and their problems and judging outcomes on the basis of mortality, morbidity, and length and costs of (re)hospitalization.

The Quadriplegia Index of Function (QIF)

The National SCI Database is the most massive attempt to collect an array of longitudinal data on persons with SCI, but other research efforts have also focused on improving outcome assessment. The QIF is one such project that specifically targeted an SCI subpopulation—quadriplegics (Gresham, 1981; Gresham et al., 1980).

The QIF is an ADL measure of disability similar to the Barthel Index, but is designed to provide a more sensitive index of functional improvements in quadriplegics. Independence in 46 separate tasks is rated on a 5-point scale. The tasks cover transfers, grooming, bathing, dressing, feeding, wheelchair mobility, bed activities, bladder program, and bowel program, but substantial weight in scoring is given to wheelchair activities and bowel and bladder management. In addition, 20 multiple-choice questions form a test for understanding personal care that comprises 10% of the total score. When the same patients were assessed at admission and discharge using

the QIF, the Barthel Index, the Kenny Self-Care Evaluation (Schoening, Anderson, & Bergstrom, 1965), and the Katz Index of ADL (Katz, Ford, & Moskowitz, 1963), the QIF indicated a substantially greater percentage of improvement in admission to discharge scores than any of the other measures (Gresham et al., 1980). The items on the QIF more closely match the content of ADL skills training for quadriplegics than the items in other ADL instruments.

Rehabilitation Indicators

The Rehabilitation Indicators Project is directed at assessing behavior in the community (Brown et al., 1984; Diller et al., 1983; Gordon et al., 1982). For measuring disability, the project specifies hundreds of skills indicators (SKIs) that can be rated. For example, "using a wheelchair" is broken into 42 separate SKIs. For measuring handicap, the project specifies detailed activity pattern indicators (APIs) within the broader social role activities of work, school, personal care, child care, housework, household business, quiet recreation, active recreation, socializing, telephoning, writing/receiving letters, travel, and quiet. The frequency of each API or the time spent in each API is recorded from an interview, questionnaire, or diary.

Although the use of SKIs and APIs is intended for all rehabilitation populations, the techniques have been applied to persons with SCI in the development and testing phases of the project. Using SKIs to assess skills in individuals with SCI at admission, discharge, and follow-up, major differences were found between paraplegics and quadriplegics and both groups showed distinctly different changes in performance over time (Diller et al., 1983). Using APIs to compare the activities of paraplegics, quadriplegics, and the able-bodied, Gordon et al. (1982) found no differences among the three groups on some activities (e.g., social) but did find differences in other activities (e.g., quiet recreation).

Self-Observation and Report Technique

Rintala et al. (1984) have developed an assessment methodology similar to APIs called the Self-Observation and Report Technique (SORT). Focusing on actual behaviors in the environment,

SORT asks subjects to report all activities (of more than 5 minutes' duration) in a diary format. The time involved in the activity, a description of the activity, assistance required, and companions are all recorded. These data are then content analyzed and coded into categories that are used to produce scaled indicators such as independence, diversity of activities, level of activity, and mobility. The SORT, in combination with wheelchair odometers, timers to record time in bed and time in wheelchair, and an environmental negotiability survey, constitute the Longitudinal Functional Assessment system, which is designed to repeatedly monitor rehabilitation progress.

Like Rehabilitation Indicators, SORT is applicable to all populations, but SCI persons have been used for much development and testing. Case studies demonstrate the usefulness of SORT in following the progress of individual SCI patients (Rintala et al., 1984). Data gathered by the SORT during the initial hospitalization of paraplegics and quadriplegics have been found to be highly predictive of functional behavior after discharge (Rintala et al., 1984). Another application of the SORT has been the comparison of SCI persons at various phases of rehabilitation with able-bodied individuals.

Independent Living Outcomes

DeJong and Hughes (1982) have suggested a somewhat different method of assessing outcomes, particularly handicaps. Starting with the theoretically desired outcomes of the IL movement—a person's ability to live in the least restrictive environment and live productively—the authors combined the value judgments of experts with behavioral observations of persons with SCI to develop indices of these two abstract outcomes. Panels of experts in IL ranked the relative desirability of various residential arrangements in order to produce a scale of restrictiveness of living arrangement. Similarly, experts ranked the relative productivity of various combinations of activities (e.g., employment was viewed as more productive than school and homemaking was judged more productive than participating in organizations). Combinations of these activities were thereby converted into a scale of productivity.

Results of this assessment methodology were then successfully used as the dependent measures in a multivariate analysis of SCI outcomes (DeJong et al., 1984). A combination of variables—including marital status, education, transportation barriers, economic disincentives, and severity of disability as measured by the Barthel Index—predicted approximately 63% of the variance in IL outcomes.

Mississippi Methodist Rehabilitation Center System

The Spinal Injury Team of the Mississippi Methodist Rehabilitation Center (MMRC) has attempted to combine measures of impairment, disability, handicap, and treatment constraints into a system of tracking weekly progress during rehabilitation (Vise et al., 1986). The MMRC system consists of a 100-item ADL instrument developed at MMRC, the 100-point American Spinal Injury Association (ASIA) motor index (ASIA, 1982), a 5-point system of grading medical and pulmonary constraints, and a 100-point subjectively rated psychosocial index.

The MMRC system has also been used to set rehabilitation goals for SCI persons by relating their impairment (ASIA motor index) with their disability (ADL index). For example, Vise et al. (1986) suggested that a quadriplegic should obtain an ADL score of twice his or her ASIA motor index score.

STRATEGIES FOR ASSESSING SCI REHABILITATION

The model of SCI rehabilitation proposed in this chapter identifies the major concepts requiring measurement in a comprehensive assessment system. The brief review of available instruments highlighted areas of considerable strength in measurement and offered some promising methodologies for addressing current deficiencies in measurement. The instrumentation needed for the complete assessment system suggested by the model is outlined below.

Adequate methodology for the measurement of impairment among SCI individuals has been provided by ASIA (1982). The process of specifying motor levels, sensory levels, motor scores,

Frankel class, zone of injury, and anatomical classification includes extensive detail regarding impairment.

Better measurement of disability, the outcome variable for medical rehabilitation, may be provided by the FIM of the proposed Uniform National Data System for Medical Rehabilitation (see Chapter 10). The FIM evolved from the established tradition of ADL indices, but the task items included are somewhat more appropriate for persons with SCI (attention was paid to the QIF in selecting FIM items). The FIM assesses functional capability in a controlled setting, which is consistent with the medical rehabilitation model. Although much technical development and validation is still required, the FIM seems a viable strategy for achieving a summative index of disability.

Measurement of handicap, the outcome variable for psychosocial rehabilitation, is in its infancy. However, promising avenues of investigation have been mapped by the APIs, the SORT, and IL outcomes. The focus of these techniques on measuring actual behavior in the "real world" home and community environments is consistent with the psychosocial rehabilitation model. The use of expert panels in the IL outcomes project to rate or assign value judgments to behaviors provides a methodology for converting objective descriptive information into scaled indices of handicap.

The most straightforward application of these procedures would be in developing an index of occupational handicap. This dimension reflects an "individual's ability to occupy his time in the manner customary to his sex, age, and culture" (WHO, 1980) and is quite similar to the IL goal of a productive life. Building on the list of APIs and SORT activity categories, a category of possible ways to spend one's time could be developed. A panel could then apply normal social criteria to rate the productivity or appropriateness of each activity. Once the time distribution in each activity was known for a given individual, the proportion of time in each activity could be multiplied by the value rating for that activity and summed across all activities to yield that person's index of occupation. A person spending a lot of time working or going to school, taking care of children and housework, and participating in organizations and active recreation would receive a high occupation score. A person who spent most of the day watching TV would receive a low score.

Scaled indices for the other dimensions of handicap could be developed using similar methodologies. A mobility index could be created by rating behaviorally based mobility factors such as time out of bed, time away from home, use of transportation alternatives, activities requiring mobility in home and community, and travel. A social integration index could be created by rating whom the person lives with (significant other, family, nonrelatives, alone) and rating various types of contacts with various types of people in different situations. A physical independence index might include categories of physical and mechanical assistance rated in a variety of situations. An index of economic self-sufficiency could be organized around rated consumer behaviors and resources.

Well-developed measures of impairment, disability, and handicap are necessary, but not sufficient, for a complete evaluation system. Good measures of medical and psychosocial rehabilitation interventions and constraints, as well as measures of costs and economic consequences, are also needed. Knowing an outcome is of little value if the interventions that caused it, the situation in which the intervention was used, and the costs of the intervention are not known.

Particularly needed is a taxonomy of psychosocial rehabilitation interventions and meaningful units of both medical and psychosocial services. The development of objective measures of rehabilitation constraints is a massive undertaking and the gathering of cost information requires great diligence.

The effort required to bring a complete SCI rehabilitation evaluation system to fruition would be duly rewarded. The proposed model could integrate both patient evaluation and program evaluation with a common focus on outcome assessment; the system could serve as a model for other rehabilitation specialties; and the growing emphasis on very long-term outcome assessment as the SCI population ages would be an integral feature of the system.

REFERENCES

Alexander, J. L., & Fuhrer, M. J. (1984). Functional assessment of individuals with physical impairments. In A. S. Halpern & M. J. Fuhrer (Eds.), *Functional assessment in rehabilitation* (pp. 45–59). Baltimore: Paul H. Brookes Publishing Co.

American Spinal Injury Association. (1982). *Standards for neurological classification of spinal injury patients*. Chicago: Author.

Brown, M., Gordon, W. A., & Diller, L. (1984). Rehabilitation indicators. In A. S. Halpern & M. J. Fuhrer (Eds.), *Functional assessment in rehabilitation* (pp. 187–203). Baltimore: Paul H. Brookes Publishing Co.

Bureau of Economic Research, Rutgers University (M. Berkowitz, Ed.). (1985). *Economic consequences of spinal cord injury*. New Brunswick, NJ: Rutgers University.

DeJong, G., Branch, L. G., & Corcoran, P. J. (1984). Independent living outcomes in spinal cord injury: Multivariate analyses. *Archives of Physical Medicine and Rehabilitation, 65*, 66–73.

DeJong, G., & Hughes, J. (1982). Independent living: Methodology for measuring long-term outcomes. *Archives of Physical Medicine and Rehabilitation, 63*, 68–73.

Diller, L., Fordyce, W., Jacobs, D., Brown, M., Gordon, W., Simmens, S., & Orazem, J. (1983). *Rehabilitation indicators project*. Final report to the National Institute of Handicapped Research. New York: New York University Medical Center.

Fine, P. R. (1985). *Summary of American Spinal Injury Association, spinal cord injury/average length of stay study*. Presentation at Model Systems Project Directors Meeting, Washington DC.

Gordon, W. A., Lehman, L., Sherman, B., Brown, M., Simmens, S., Orazem, J., & Diller, L. (1982). *Psychological adjustment and characteristics in recent spinal cord injuries*. Final report to the National Institute of Handicapped Research. New York: Department of Rehabilitation Medicine, New York University Medical Center.

Granger, C. V. (1972). *A System for management of selected data in medical rehabilitation* (Monogr. No. 7). Boston: Medical Rehabilitation Research and Training Center, Tufts University School of Medicine.

Greb, M., & Mueller, J. M. (1982). *Functional goals at specific levels of spinal cord injury*. Denver: Craig Hospital.

Gresham, G. E. (1981). *Quadriplegia index of function (QIF)*. Buffalo, NY: Spinal Cord Injury Unit, Erie County Medical Center.

Gresham, G. E., Labi, M. L., Dittmar, S. S., Hicks, J. T., Joyce, S. Z., & Phillips, M. L. (1980). Quadriplegia index of function. *Archives of Physical Medicine and Rehabilitation, 61*, 493.

Johnston, M. V., & Keith, R. A. (1983). Cost-benefits of medical rehabilitation: Review and critique. *Archives of Physical Medicine and Rehabilitation, 64*, 147–154.

Katz, S., Ford, A. B., & Moskowitz, R. W. (1963). Studies in illness in the aged. The index of ADL: A standardized measure of biological and psychosocial function. *Journal of the American Medical Association, 185*, 914–919.

Mahoney, F. I., & Barthel, D. W. (1965). Functional evaluation: The Barthel Index. *Maryland State Medical Journal, 14*, 61–65.

National Spinal Cord Injury Data Research Center. (1975). *National Spinal Cord Injury Data Base Syllabus*. Phoenix: Author.

National Spinal Cord Injury Statistical Center. (1985a). *Common data base model systems' spinal cord injury program syllabus*. Birmingham, AL: Author.

National Spinal Cord Injury Statistical Center. (1985b). *Annual report 3*. Birmingham, AL: Author.

Rintala, D. H., Uttermohlen, D. M., Buck, E. L., Hanover, D., Alexander, J. L., Norris-Baker, C., Stephens, M. A. P., Willems, E. P., & Halstead, L. S. (1984). Self-observation and report technique (SORT): Description and clinical applications. In A. S. Halpern & M. J. Fuhrer (Eds.), *Functional assessment in rehabilitation*, (pp. 205–221). Baltimore: Paul H. Brookes Publishing Co.

Schoening, H. A., Anderson, L., & Bergstrom, D. (1965). Numerical scoring of self care status of patients. *Archives of Physical Medicine and Rehabilitation, 46*, 689–697.

Trieschmann, R. B. (1980). *Spinal cord injuries: Psychological, social and vocational adjustment*. Elmsford, NY: Pergamon Press.

Vise, W. M., Hays, K. L., Crump, J. C., Bodie, R. B., Keller, B. A., Black, R. A., Kliesch, W. F., McCaffrey, D. T., & David, I. J. (1986). *Activities of daily living (ADL) index for spinal cord injury (SCI) patients*. San Francisco: Poster presentation at the twelfth annual meeting of the American Spinal Injury Association.

World Health Organization. (1980). *International classification of impairments, disabilities, and handicaps: A manual of classification relating to the consequences of disease*. Geneva: Author.

SECTION IV

Implications of
Rehabilitation Outcome Analysis

Chapter 18

The Relationship between Interagency Linkages and Rehabilitation Outcomes
Implications for Policy and Practice

Donald J. Dellario

$\mathbf{W}$hy have rehabilitation professionals contributed so little to the study of disability policy questions? Stubbins (1985) attributed this lack of attention to ideological differences among rehabilitation professionals and conflicting values among the numerous groups with vested interests in particular handicapped populations. Another plausible explanation, however, is the ambiguous relationship between research and policymaking. Caplan (1976) discovered in a comprehensive survey of 204 persons holding various executive positions in the United States government that the use of social science information was predicated somewhat arbitrarily upon the nature of the issues under consideration, the values of the policymakers, and the political and administrative networks in which they were operating. In other words, there was no guarantee that policymaking would reflect data-based research, and the probability that such information would be used in policymaking was contingent upon the values of the policymakers themselves. Without a clear sense that research will be used systematically in the policymaking process, researchers are left with the hope that the results of research efforts will somehow filter into the policymaking process. According to Rein and White (1977), "Although research may not influence any specific policy, it can help shape the climate of opinion and contribute to the interchange of ideas" (p. 136).

Majchrzak (1984) defined policy research as the "process of conducting research on, or analysis of, a fundamental social problem in order to provide policy makers with pragmatic action-oriented recommendation for alleviating the problem" (p. 112). Without a distinct mandate and adequate resources to conduct studies that are designed to provide information about specific policy questions, the issue becomes one of incorporating existing data from ongoing rehabilitation research efforts into the policymaking process. Rehabilitation researchers can provide policymakers with critical information to make informed judgments about those courses of action that are most beneficial for persons with disabilities. The following discussion is offered with the hope of shaping a climate of opinion such that policy decisions concerning the role and function of interagency linkages in service delivery will be based upon informed judgments.

Findings from a conference on improving interagency collaboration between mental health (MH) and vocational rehabilitation (VR) services suggest (Cohen, 1981) that VR/MH interagency collaboration has a history of both positive and negative experiences. However, there was a consensus about the necessity for collaboration, which spawned the following recommendation:

> The VR and MH systems have unique capabilities for offering work-related services to some common

client subgroups within the CMI population. A systematic plan for the integration of the services provided by both the MH and VR systems to the shared client population needs to be jointly developed. The plan needs to specify the shared target population, desired client outcomes, unique MH/ VR practitioner activities, inservice and preservice training, and work-related rehabilitation system and policies. (p. 19)

Despite the history of cooperative relationships involving VR and MH services and the current existence of multiple linkages, little research has been done to examine, describe, and evaluate the characteristics and the effectiveness of interagency linkages (Baumheier, Welch, & Cook, 1976). This is especially true of MH/VR interagency linkages and their impact on the outcome of the chronic mentally ill population.

Ultimately, the success of interorganizational linkages in ensuring adequate service delivery depends upon the extent to which autonomous service providers are willing and able to integrate their services with those of other organizations whose goals, mandates, and structures may differ from their own. A clear understanding of the factors that create viable linkages can yield information that supports the role of interagency linkages in policy development and strategic planning.

In the past few years, the basic strategy for improving human service programs in the United States has shifted in a fundamental way. During the 1960s and early '70s, the primary approach used to address major social and health problems such as mental illness was to initiate new programs requiring the infusion of large amounts of federal monies. In the mental health field, the national Community Mental Health Centers (CMHCs) Program was the major tangible product of this approach. First passed in 1963, CMHC legislation continued until its repeal in 1980, resulting in the funding of 798 CMHCs and involving the expenditure of over $2 billion in federal funds and many millions more in state and other monies. However, a decade of recession and inflation in the 1970s, combined with a climate of growing social and fiscal conservatism, eroded public support for such major interventions, ultimately making them no longer feasible.

Recent efforts to address major continuing social and health problems, more modest in scope, are designed to improve the performance of existing systems of service without significant additional resources. Currently, many community mental health programs are concerned not only with improvement of their services, but also with survival. Federal support for mental health services is diminishing rapidly, and there is realistic pessimism concerning the ability and willingness of state governments to fill the gaps created by the decline in federal funding. In this context of scarcity, some argue that interorganizational linkages with other human service provider organizations such as VR may be an important tool for ensuring adequate service delivery to the chronically mentally ill population (Broskowski, O'Brien, & Prevost, 1982).

Why Link Mental Health and Rehabilitation Services?

The most fundamental reason to consider linkages of MH and VR services for chronically ill persons is that many of these people require both types of services. Many chronically mentally ill persons have multiple service needs that cannot be filled adequately in the community by any one service agency. Because of their severe disabilities, these people frequently require a wide range of services, including mental health treatment, medical and dental care, housing income, legal protection and advocacy, leisure and recreational services, and rehabilitation (Talbott, 1980). Meeting their needs in the community requires a coordinated network of services involving linkages among a variety of human service agencies, including MH and VR. In addition, there are potential advantages to the provider organizations themselves, including: 1) increased efficiency and avoiding duplication of services, 2) improved effectiveness of services to patients, and 3) the potential for survival and growth through joint action to maintain or increase resources (Woy & Dellario, 1985).

Linkages between MH and VR fields can occur either by developing linkages between MH organizations and VR organizations (Baumheier et al., 1976) or by incorporating models or technologies from one field into the organizations of the other field. This paper focuses primarily upon issues in interorganizational linkages, but it should be noted that there are active efforts underway to apply VR approaches to a variety of MH settings (Anthony, 1979).

Variables Affecting Interorganizational Linkages

Recent reviews of the literature on interorganizational relationships (Broskowski, 1980; Broskowski et al., 1982) identified 31 variables that can inhibit or facilitate linkages between organizations. These variables were categorized into three distinct areas: environmental factors, intraorganizational factors, and interorganizational factors. These areas, although considered independent, interact in complex and poorly understood ways. Nevertheless, these three areas and their corresponding variables do provide a useful framework for analyzing and understanding the complexities of an interagency linkage.

Several environmental factors may be expected to affect interorganizational relationships. An environment with scarce resources as well as organized and systematic access to those resources in settings with intermediate levels of complexity, predictability, and change tends to facilitate linkages (Broskowski et al., 1982).

Characteristics within an organization can also affect the ability of an organization to form linkages with others. The leadership style of the organization is important, with an exploratory, innovative style most likely to lead to linkages. Strong, well-coordinated internal management systems and an advanced capacity to collect, analyze, and use information also facilitate linkages.

The relative abundance or lack of resources and extent of control over resources are also important variables in linkages. When an organization has complete control over abundant resources, it is not likely to seek linkages, nor is an organization that has limited control over very few resources. Linkages are facilitated when there are intermediate levels of resources and control.

Interorganizational factors that foster linkages include similarities in size, structure, and core technologies; interdependency; good prior experiences with each other; complementary goals;

supportive, higher level sanctioning agencies; and similar philosophies and values.

Relational factors, that is, conditions that characterize the interorganizational relationship, can also affect the likelihood of developing linkages. Reciprocal and mutual planning, gradual implementation, equal benefits, and commitment from top management tend to promote successful linkages, as do mutual and frequent exchange of information in simple forms at a reasonable number of levels.

The current lack of knowledge concerning interagency linkages between MH and VR led me to conduct a study designed to answer the following questions: 1) Is there a relationship between MH/VR interagency functioning and successful rehabilitation outcome?, and 2) If so, under what conditions are MH/VR interagency linkages most effective? (Dellario, 1985).

METHOD

Sample

Oregon's geography, population, and MH/VR referral patterns were collectively used as criteria for selecting the particular MH/VR agencies to be included in this study. The state is divided geographically into 36 counties, with populations ranging from high-density Multnomah County (562,640) in the western part of the state to very low density Wheeler (1,513) and Wallowa (7,273) counties in the central and western parts of the state, respectively. Each county has at least one CMHC and some counties have several, with a range of referrals from MH to VR from 0 to 446 for fiscal year 1979–1980 and 0 to 201 for 1981–1982. Multnomah County, which includes the city of Portland and has the highest population, was excluded from the study because it contained several CMHCs and the referral patterns were difficult to disentangle. Of the remaining counties, 26 had 10 or fewer referrals, with staff too small for studying service delivery as part of interagency linkage. This left nine MH/VR agencies as potential participants. Of these, seven were selected on the basis of geography, population, and referral patterns.

Instrumentation

A structured interview was developed as the primary instrument for determining interagency linkage functioning. There were three phases in the development of this structured interview: 1) review of the literature on interagency linkage to compile a pool of critical incidents, 2) development of a conceptual framework within which to place the critical incident situations, and 3) integration of the critical incidents into the conceptual framework. The following conceptual framework was used to organize the critical incidents:

I. Interorganizational conditions
   A. Communications
      1. Interstaff communications and relations
      2. Mechanisms for referral and other cooperative arrangements
      3. Existing complementary services
   B. Decision making
      1. Budget
      2. Client programming
      3. Accountability
   C. Resources: joint budgeting
II. Intraorganizational conditions
   A. Communications
      1. Intrastaff communications and relations
      2. Client–staff relations
   B. Decision making
      1. Budget
      2. Programming
      3. Accountability
III. Environmental conditions
   A. Extra-agency communications and relations
   B. Extra-agency decisions about clients
   C. Extra-agency funding agencies

As evident from the conceptual framework, the interview dealt with a number of interagency activities related to the dimensions of Broskowski et al. (1982). These interagency activities were used to structure the responses of staff during the course of a 1-hour interview. For example, one structured interview item related to the interorganizational dimension was: "The MH/ VR requires information about one of your clients. Describe the procedure by which you share client information with MH/VR." Mental health and VR administrators and line personnel from the seven agency dyads who had a history of interaction with the counterpart agency were interviewed.

Data Analysis[1]

The responses to each item of the structured interview were rated by two independent judges on a 5-point scale according to how well or poorly the agency dyad performed the interagency activity, ranging from very well (1) to very poorly (5). The judges' ratings on all items across all dimensions were correlated. The resultant .86 Pearson product-moment correlation coefficient indicated a high degree of interjudge agreement (reliability) on ratings of the structured interviews.

Data taken from the VR R-300 on psychiatrically disabled clients from each agency dyad were used to develop interagency performance indicators. Acceptance rate was operationally defined as the ratio of the quantity status 26 + status 28 + status 30 closures to the number of closures in all statuses. Closure rate was defined as the ratio of 26 closures to closures in all statuses. Closure rate and the ratio of closure rate to acceptance rate served as the interagency performance indicators in the study. In phase two, the measures on MH/VR interagency functioning and the interagency performance indicators were compared. It was hypothesized that those agency dyads that exhibit higher levels on interagency linkage would also exhibit higher levels on the interagency performance indicators.

RESULTS

A significant statistical relationship was obtained between agency dyad ($n = 7$) and closure status (00-08, 26, 28, 30): $\chi^2(18) = 47.9, p < .05$. The results indicate that the two agencies that ranked highest on interagency linkage functioning also ranked highest on the two interagency performance indicators. No statistically significant relationship between interagency linkage functioning and closure rate and the ratio of closure rate to acceptance rate was found. Inspection of the agency dyad rankings on closure rate, however, indicated that the two agencies that exhibited the highest score on the interagency functioning also demonstrated the largest closure rates (50% and 30.8%, respectively). Furthermore, inspection of the agency dyad rankings on the closure rate and acceptance rate ratio also revealed a similar pattern. The two agency dyads that exhibited the highest scores on interagency functioning also demonstrated the largest closure rate and acceptance ratio (50%:80% and 30.8%:76%, respectively). The closure rate and acceptance rate ratios for the remaining dyads ranged from 0%:0% to 12.5%:37.5%. These results suggest that psychiatrically disabled individuals who are referred by agencies with high-functioning interagency linkages have increased probabilities of a successful VR outcome.

To establish an overall perspective within which the results of this study could be interpreted, a descriptive analysis of the pattern of service and referral for the psychiatrically disabled population was conducted.

According to the state formula for estimating the number of psychiatrically disabled persons, there are approximately 8,253 such persons in need of services during a single year. The reported number of psychiatrically disabled persons served in the 2-year period 1981–1983 was approximately 5,431, or 32% (5,431/ 16,506), of the estimated total of psychiatrically disabled persons in need of services. Approximately 16% (904/5,431) of the psychiatrically disabled persons who received services were referred to VR. Approximately 5% (272/5,431) were referred to VR from mental health sources. Of these, approximately 26% were referred from the target agencies in this study, or approximately 1.3% (72/5,431) of the total number of clients served during the period 1981 to 1983 were referred to VR from the target agencies in this study. These findings indicated that there is a great discrepancy between the need for VR services and the number of cases that find their way into the VR system.

In order to determine the conditions under which MH/VR interagency linkages were most effective, a *content analysis* of the structured interviews of the highest scoring agency dyads was conducted. One emergent theme from the responses was that there was a *mutuality of purpose* between the agencies. In other words, agencies shared a common perspective with respect to their responsibility to this population and the interdependent nature of their service delivery systems in meeting this responsibility. Examples of responses that support this theme include:

"We like to think that we have complementary services."

Concerning the coordination of services:

"We have client service meetings weekly . . . and discuss each person in the program. So we are all up-to-date at all times."

"Some services are pre-determined based on established working relationships between the two agencies. . . . We don't have to negotiate on a per client basis."

"They provide the money and we provide the services. It's a team effort. It's very cooperative."

Examples of responses that do not support this theme include:

"At the present, there is absolutely no cooperation with them."

"If they decided to make referrals, that would be an improvement."

"We don't rely on them for anything."

Concerning communication:

"If only it could happen. No cooperation with them at all."

Concerning joint conferences:

"We don't do this."

A significant aspect of this theme of mutuality of purpose is that the MH system must recognize VR intervention and outcome as a legitimate MH service. Furthermore, if the VR needs of the psychiatrically disabled are to be met, then MH agencies must move toward providing VR services. According to Anthony, Howell, and Danley (1983), state divisions of VR simply have neither the staffing nor the mandate to provide the level of VR services needed by psychiatrically disabled individuals. Therefore, MH agencies should consider expanding their treatment services to include intervention in vocational functioning.

A second theme that emerged from the responses to the structured interview was a *mutuality of respect* between the two agencies. In other words, the respective professionals from both agencies felt generally positive about the professionals at the other agency. Examples of responses that support this theme include:

"We have a special relationship with the VR counselor."

"We check our end to make sure we're holding our part of the bargain and help him succeed in holding up his."

"We have a good rapport with them."

"Key issue is to maintain mutual respect of each other's professions and what we do."

"There are no general barriers. Little ones come up, but we've always been able to work them through."

"Because of the overlap of the caseloads and the severe problems of the clients, it's important to share and facilitate the process. That's why we try to help out."

Examples of reponses that do not support this theme include:

"Their thinking is limited."

"An improvement would be if they would *do* something."

"We made a program decision that we would be involved anytime that they made an evaluation of our clients, because it was done in a way that was detrimental to them."

"Although we have had staffing with them, the person has not been able to offer anything; he just smiles, nods and disappears."

DISCUSSION: KEY POLICY ISSUES IN THE LINKAGE OF MH AND VR SERVICES

Based on the findings of our study, it would make sense for MH and VR agencies to increase their efforts to establish effective interagency linkages. The following discussion is intended to identify obstacles to policy initiatives that are designed to improve linkages between MH and VR programs.

The Environment

The environmental characteristics of the two fields differ considerably with respect to services to the chronically mentally ill. In general, the environment surrounding MH programs may tend to inhibit linkages. Sources of funding are numerous and disorganized, and the environment is complex, unpredictable, and rapidly changing at the moment. Repeal of the CMHC legislation and passage of the Mental Health Block Grants to states in 1981 represent a major shift in federal-state roles; the federal role is decreasing while the state role is increasing. All these factors may influence policy involving MH programs. The one environmental factor that may facilitate linkages is the increasing scarcity of resources, which makes meeting their goals more difficult for MH programs, thereby providing incentives for supportive linkages with VR and other programs.

In contrast to the environment of MH programs, the environment of VR programs may tend to encourage linkages. The VR system obtains its relatively scarce resources through an organized system operating in an environment of moderate predictability. All of these factors would encourage linkages by local VR programs.

Intraorganizational Conditions

The intraorganizational conditions of community MH programs serving chronically mentally ill persons are extremely variable, and any characterization would have many exceptions. However, several observations bear mentioning. A number of informed observers recently noted reductions in resources for MH services and reduced control of those resources at the local level (Woy & Mazade, 1982). For many years, community MH programs have demonstrated weaknesses in internal management and the capacity to collect and analyze information (Windle, Bass, & Taube, 1976). Although efforts have been made to upgrade the internal management capabilities of community MH programs (Woy & Mazade, 1982), many of them remain relatively weak. When this is combined with the present scarcity of resources and reduced control over resources at the local level, one can anticipate difficulties in establishing linkages with MH programs.

Vocational rehabilitation programs are perhaps more fortunate in this regard. Although resources are scarce, control of resources at the provider level is high. In addition, the simplicity and uniformity of the system's structures and operations enable stronger internal coordination and better information capability. The result is a greater capacity for linkages with VR programs than MH programs.

Interorganizational Conditions

On the basis of our findings, it is clear that interorganizational conditions vary greatly from one setting to another. The number of entities potentially inolved in MH/VR linkage relationships, prior experience with each other, and support by top management can vary greatly from one local situation to another.

Some factors can clearly facilitate linkage between two types of programs. For example, if the goals and domains of the two fields are complementary, then there is a higher probability of establishing successful linkages. However, at least three key sets of issues may cause difficulties in linkage. The first is a frequent lack of mutual dependency between MH and VR programs. In many localities, there is no history of cooperation and mutual support between the two systems at the service delivery level. Neither is dependent upon the other for resources, and each can operate independently of the other. In many cases, there is even little knowledge about the goals, operations, and services of the other (Cohen, 1981). As a result of this lack of dependency and shared knowledge, the need for linkage often goes unrecognized.

A second potentially inhibiting factor is the relative differences in philosophy and values of the two fields. Because they overlap in many ways, there may be a tendency to assume more similarity than really exists. The MH field tends to conceptualize patients' problems as illness and to concentrate on treatment and amelioration of the illness; the VR field tends to conceptualize problems as functional handicaps and to concentrate on skills training to reduce the effect of the disability on functioning. In addition, the VR field emphasizes vocational placement based on matching the person to the work environment. The bases of accountability also differ, with the MH field accountable for effort and quality of care and the VR field accountable for results in terms of employment or other tangible improvements in client status. These differing bases of accountability in turn imply differing types and degrees of responsibility for the chronically mentally ill. By definition, VR services are inappropriate for mentally ill patients who are not expected to benefit in terms of employability. For those who do have potential for employment and eligibility for rehabilitation services, VR is seen as a time-limited service concluding with transition to gainful employment and termination of the rehabilitation service. The MH field, on the other hand, views itself and is viewed by the public at large as having a continuing responsibility for the chronically mentally ill patient, providing care and support throughout a patient's life if necessary. Sensitivity to these differing conceptions of role and mission may play an important part in developing linkages between providers in the two fields.

Third, the typically differing complexity, size, structure, and technologies of the two systems may be important considerations. The MH system, both nationally and, in most cases, at the local level, is considerably larger and more complex than the VR service system; negotiations between markedly different organizations can be difficult. Unless it is sensitive to the resource limitations of the smaller organization, the larger one may press for more service than the other is capable of providing. At the same time, the smaller organization may resist negotiations out of fear of being subsumed or co-opted by the larger entity. Careful handling of these issues on both sides is crucial.

Despite these inhibiting factors to the establishment of interagency linkages, the findings of our study suggest that, under the proper conditions of intentionality and attitude, interagency linkages can influence the probability of successful VR outcome for persons with psychiatric disabilities.

The results of our study certainly could be challenged with respect to research methodology, measurement limitations, sample representativeness, and other technical considerations. Addressing the question of whether or not imperfect data should be used to guide policy decisions, Grobstein (1984) concluded that the best *available* advice is often needed to make a complex decision and that "we would be remiss to withhold what can be useful because it is not perfect" (p. 664). The current study, although far

from perfect, may provide useful information to policymakers in deciding whether or not interagency linkages between disparate service delivery networks warrant the expenditure of fiscal and other resources. On the basis of the "imperfect" results of our study, we suggest that the establishment of an interagency policy resulting in a significant commitment of resources for developing interagency linkages of MH and VR would be well worth the price. Such a policy would potentially increase the probability of successful rehabilitation outcome for persons with physical, emotional, and/or cognitive disabilities.

REFERENCES

Anthony, W. A. (1979). *The principles of psychiatric rehabilitation.* Amherst, MA: Human Resource Development Press.

Anthony, W. A., Howell, J., & Danley, K. (1983). Vocational rehabilitation of the psychiatrically disabled. In M. Miraki (Ed.), *The chronically mentally ill: Research and services.* Jamaica, NY: Spectrum Publications.

Baumheier, E. C., Welch, H. H., & Cook, C. C. (1976). *Interagency linkages in vocational rehabilitation.* Denver, CO: Regional Rehabilitation Research Institute, Center for Social Research and Development, Denver Research Institute, University of Denver.

Broskowski, A. (1980). *Literature review on interorganizational relationships and their relevance to health and mental health coordination* [Final Contract Report to NIMH, Contract No. 278-79-0030 (OP)]. Rockville, MD: National Institute of Mental Health.

Broskowski, A., O'Brien, G. M., St., & Prevost, J. A. (1982). Interorganizational strategies for survival: Looking ahead to 1990. *Administration in Mental Health, 9,* 198–210.

Caplan, N. (1976). Social research and national policy: What gets used, by whom, for what purposes, and with what effect? *International Social Science Journal, 28,* 351–359.

Cohen, M. (1981). *Improving interagency collaboration between mental health and vocational rehabilitation services.* Conference summary report. Arlington, VA: Boston University Center for Rehabilitation Research and Training in Mental Health, Boston, MA.

Dellario, D. J. (1985). The relationship between mental

health, vocational rehabilitation, interagency functioning, and outcome of psychiatrically disabled persons. *Rehabilitation Counseling Bulletin, 28,* 167–171.

Grobstein, C. (1984). Should imperfect data be used to guide public policy? In R. F. Connor, D. G. Altman, & C. Jackson (Eds.), *Evaluation studies review: A manual* (Vol. 9, pp. 664–666). Beverly Hills, CA: Sage Publications.

Majchrzak, A. (1984). *Methods for policy research.* Applied Social Research Methods Series, Vol. 3. Beverly Hills, CA: Sage Publications.

Rein, M., & White, S. (1977). Can policy research help policy? In T. D. Cook, M. L. Del Rosario, K. M. Hennigan, M. Mark, & W. M. K. Trochim (Eds.), *Evaluation studies review: A manual* (Vol 3). Beverly Hills, CA: Sage Publications.

Stubbins, J. (1985). Some obstacles to policy studies in rehabilitation. *American Behavioral Scientist, 28,* 387–395.

Talbott, J. A. (1980). Toward a public policy on the chronic mentally ill patient. *American Journal of Orthopsychiatry, 50,* 43–53.

Windle, C., Bass, R. D., & Taube, C. A. (1976). PR aside: Initial results from NIMH's service program evaluation studies. *American Journal of Community Psychology, 2,* 311–327.

Woy, J. R., & Dellario, D. J. (1985). Issues in the linkage and integration of treatment and rehabilitation services for chronically mentally ill persons. *Administration in Mental Health, 12,* 155–166.

Woy, J. R., & Mazade, N. A. (1982). Community mental health centers in transition: Report on a national conference. *Administration in Mental Health, 9,* 211–224.

Chapter 19

Return to Work
Policy Implications

Edward J. Hester, Paul Decelles, and Gabriel R. Faimon

Program development, program evaluation, and policy analysis are inexorably intertwined, as shown in Figure 1. Part of what is known as "policy analysis" is identifying the problem to be addressed. To start, we need to develop information regarding the scope and nature of the problem. After the program has been in operation a sufficient amount of time, it should be evaluated to determine if the desired outcomes have been achieved. The results of program evaluation are then fed back into policy analysis, which again can result in program or policy changes.

Implicit in this model is the need for accurate outcome identification and assessment. Equally important is the need for reliable baseline data. Not only must we know the characteristics of the individuals we are attempting to help but, also, how many achieve desirable outcomes without intervention. Those programs involving prevention require even better baseline data than intervention programs. The reason is that measuring what does not happen is very difficult.

Since the Menninger Rehabilitation Research and Training Center has been established to develop programs and suggest policies that will eliminate or reduce the financial dependence of workers who become disabled, the examples used in this chapter are drawn from that research.

DEVELOPMENT OF A MODEL

Prior to beginning any research, we needed to define the type of persons we intended to study. We focused on the individual who was gainfully employed, but because of a disabling condition is unable to engage in remunerative work for at least 5 months. Essentially, this population ranges in age from 16 to 64 years.

Next, we developed a conceptual model of the system targeted for research. The model developed by the Menninger Research and Training Center is shown in Figure 2. Each entrance and exit route was then defined. As illustrated in the model, a worker can become physically disabled by three routes: progressive illness, acute illness, or injury. In this model, a worker can also exit from the system through three routes: employment, retirement, or death.

Entrance Routes

Progressive physical illnesses are those that not only develop slowly, but also do not result in extensive surgery or other treatment requiring immediate hospitalization on first diagnosis. Acute illnesses are those in which the first diagnosis normally results in extensive surgery and/or treatment and prevents the person from working for 5 or more months. We would have preferred to have two injury entrance routes: one for those injured on the job and one for those injured off the job. However, the obtainable baseline data do not distinguish whether or not injuries are work related.

The System

We are defining the disability support and rehabilitation system as that collection of income re-

Supported in part by The National Institute on Disability and Rehabilitation Research, United States Department of Education (Grant #G008301477).

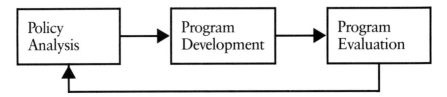

Figure 1.   The relationship between policy analysis, program development, and program evaluation.

placement programs and/or services that exist for those formerly employed persons under the age of 65 who become so disabled that they are unable to work for 5 or more months. The support portion of the system consists of programs such as individual long term disability (LTD), group LTD, social security disability insurance (SSDI), and workers' compensation insurance. The rehabilitation services may be provided by the same organization that provides the support payments, such as the insurance carrier, or by a separate organization such as the state vocational rehabilitation agency.

The worker may be eligible for one or more of the formal support and rehabilitation programs. In some cases, the worker is not eligible for any formal program, but may have to rely on savings or relatives for support. Our primary concern at this time is not the type of support received but, rather, the numbers of disabled workers needing some type of support.

Exit Routes

The first major exit route is through returning to work. The person may return to the same employer in the same job, to the same employer in a different job, or to a new job with a different employer. In any case, the person leaves the disability support system by obtaining a job. At this time, our model does not allow the person to leave the disability system as "recovered but without a job." Therefore, until the individual finds a job after forced unemployment because of a disabling condition, we do not consider the person to have left the disability support system. Persons who leave the system through the retirement route do not necessarily decide to retire at the time they become disabled. Rather, this route indicates that they became 65 years of age without having returned to work. This is consistent with the Social Security Administration's practice of converting SSDI to the Old Age and Survivors Insurance (OASI) benefit at the age of 65. Those who exit the system through death are those who die before returning to work and before the age of 65.

Baseline Data

We were fortunate to find a major insurance company willing to share its data on serious individual LTD claims. Serious claims refer to those claims in which, at the time of assessment, the

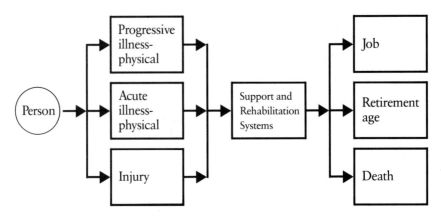

Figure 2.   The different ways a person can pass through the disability support and rehabilitation system.

disabled person appeared unable to return to work for 5 months or more.

This particular insurance company provides individual LTD coverage to hundreds of thousands of workers from coast to coast. Individual LTD refers to policies sold to individual workers, not those sold to employers for their employees. Those holding individual LTD coverage with this company appear to closely approximate the general working population. The vast majority have blue collar, clerical, or service jobs. Slightly more men than women have policies, which approximates the proportion of each in the work force. The majority were between the ages of 25 and 49 at the time the policy was purchased.

The insurance company provided information concerning the entrance to and exit from the disability payment system for 1982 through 1984. Concerning incidence data (i.e., the new cases per year), we included all claimants who began receiving LTD benefits, and were expected to be off work, for 5 or more months. For those leaving the LTD system however, we used the data only for those individuals who had benefits extending for at least 5 years from the date of disability onset. The data were not used from those receiving their last check because they had exhausted the limits of their benefits.

The data presented in Table 1 show the utility of the three entrance routes in the Menninger model. We distinguish how a worker became disabled, whether by injury, progressive illness, or acute illness. For instance, although 48% of all workers who become disabled return to work, this percentage conceals the significant difference between workers who are injured (78% return) and those with an acute illness (32% return).

It has been recognized that age and disability are related (Bowe, 1983); however, for projections, we needed more precise information. Therefore, we looked at the same variables for each 10-year age cohort. These results are shown in Table 2. Because of the small number of persons in the 16–24 age cohort, they were combined with those in the 25–34 cohort. Currently, 5 out of every 1,000 workers per year become so disabled that they are unable to work for 5 or more months. On the other hand, the rate is 9 out of 1,000 for those in the 45–54 age cohort and 19 out of 1,000 for those 55–64 years of age. The differences in the incidence rates for the various age cohorts is very important when considering that the average age of the American work force will increase dramatically over the next three decades. However, the number of disabled workers at any point in time is determined not only by the incidence rate, but also by the amount of time each person spends in the system. An equal concern is that the 45–54 age cohort also contains those workers who tend to stay the longest in the system.

Table 1. Comparison of the entrance routes with respect to some disability variables

| | Entrance routes | | | |
Variables	Progressive illness	Acute illness	Injury	Total population
Newly disabled	36%	28%	36%	100%
Incidence rate[a]	0.18%	0.14%	0.18%	0.50%
Age at incidence				
Average (years)	51.8	54.3	44.7	49.9
Standard deviation	9.31	8.25	10.89	10.43
Years in the system				
Average	4.6	4.0	2.8	3.9
Standard deviation	4.35	3.84	4.42	4.25
Outcomes				
Return to work	38%	32%	78%	48%
Retire	46%	43%	16%	36%
Die	16%	25%	6%	16%

[a]New cases per year.

Table 2.   Comparison of age cohorts with respect to some disability variables

Variables	Age cohorts				Total population
	16–34	35–44	45–54	55–64	
Incidence	0.1%	0.4%	0.9%	1.9%	0.5%
Newly disabled	11.0%	18.0%	28.0%	43.0%	100.0%
Entry route					
Progressive	21.0%	29.0%	37.0%	41.0%	36.0%
Acute	9.0%	15.0%	28.0%	39.0%	28.0%
Injury	70.0%	56.0%	35.0%	20.0%	36.0%
Outcomes					
Return to work	93.0%	87.0%	58.0%	27.0%	48.0%
Retire	1.0%	4.0%	15.0%	60.0%	36.0%
Die	6.0%	9.0%	27.0%	13.0%	16.0%
Average years in the system	2.9	3.2	4.9	3.7	3.9
Standard deviation	1.60	5.63	5.11	2.83	4.25

Attrition Curves

Figure 3 presents a distribution of the population based upon the number of months that former workers spent in the disability system. The average amount of time spent in the system is 3.9 years, with a standard deviation of 4.25 years. Traditionally within the field of vocational rehabilitation, data have been presented in the form illustrated in Figure 3. This representation provides us with useful information about the relationship between disabled workers and time spent in the disability support system. This type of graph, however, does not lend itself to a dynamic analysis of the system. A dynamic analysis of the system is needed because it produces far more accurate projections than does a static analysis. In fact, static analyses of the numbers of disabled workers for the years 1990 to 2020 produce projections that underestimate the population by as much as 30%.

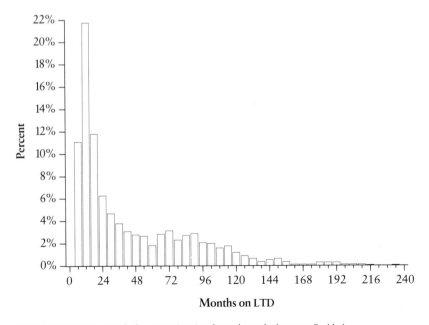

Figure 3.   The number of months spent in the support system by workers who become disabled.

To perform dynamic analyses, we needed to construct attrition curves such as the one shown in Figure 4. The result reflects the same data shown in Figure 3, but arranged differently. For the purpose of constructing this attrition curve, we assumed that all of the people became disabled during the same month. This hypothetical population dwindles over time. Sixty-six percent of the disabled individuals in this group are still in the disability support system after 1 year. At the end of 5 years, 31% remain; the other 69% have left the system through the three exit routes of work, retirement, or death.

Analysis

The model that we have developed is essentially descriptive. According to Greenberger (1976), such "models characterize important features of the reference system" (p. 59) to enable experimentation. The reference system in this case is the total disability support and rehabilitation system.

Based on the input and output rates for this sample, there are an estimated 2,191,000 former workers in the long-term disability support system. Recall that these figures relate only to those persons who were employed at the onset of physi-

cal disability. These data do not allow estimating the number of persons who became physically disabled while temporarily unemployed. Nor are we able to estimate the number of employed or temporarily unemployed persons who became mentally ill.

The model is useful even if it goes no further than this; that is, describing the current inflow and outflow of the system. Those of us in the service delivery system often become so engrossed in our individual clients that we fail to look at the whole picture. Analyzing the structure and parameters of the model reveals where some of the problems exist and where the greatest impact can be made.

Essentially, all strategies or programs are directed toward either prevention or intervention, as we define them. We divide prevention programs into two categories, primary and secondary. Primary prevention programs are directed toward the prevention of the illness or injury. Secondary prevention programs focus on retaining the person in employment after the onset of illness or the occurrence of the injury. We define intervention programs as those beginning after the worker has been totally separated from employment. Typically, public sector rehabilitation services cover the intervention period.

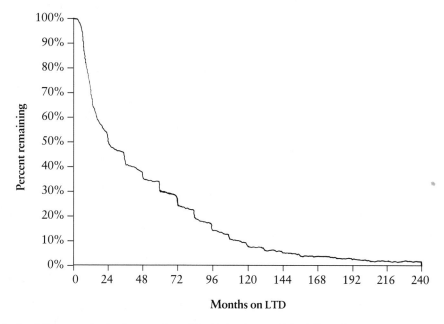

Figure 4.   An attrition curve showing the percentage of disabled workers remaining in the system.

There are major practical problems involved in attempting to evaluate the effectiveness of prevention and intervention strategies and programs upon the total disability support system. The most significant problem is that realizing the full effects of a change on the system can take up to 20 years (Hester & Decelles, 1985). Even if we could afford the luxury of trying a policy and then waiting 20 years to measure the effect, the evaluation would not be valid. That is because so many other uncontrollable factors would intervene during those years that the effect of the policy change would be virtually impossible to isolate. Thus, we need some way of projecting the effects of policy change, new technology, or program innovation upon the disability system over the next 20 years while keeping all other conditions constant.

We believe that we have made a significant step toward this end by developing the Prevention Impact Quotient and the Intervention Impact Quotient.

DEVELOPMENT OF IMPACT QUOTIENTS

Estimating the impact of a new prevention program on the disability support system requires more than merely considering the incidence of a specific illness or injury to be prevented. For instance, if the particular disabling condition accounts for 10% of those entering the disability support system, we cannot say that preventing that condition will reduce the number of persons in the system by 10%. It may, in fact, be greater or less, depending on the rate of attrition for that particular disability or group of disabilities.

A relatively simple way of assessing the impact of a prevention program is through the use of a hypothetical projection. In this analysis procedure, we enter individuals into the system at a steady state equal to the current annual number of new cases. Those who enter the system are then exited according to the attrition curve for that particular disability. If one starts a system from scratch, during the first year the only persons in the system are those who entered that year. However, in the second year, the system contains those persons who entered in the second year as well as those remaining from the first year. Thus, as each year goes by, the number of people in the system continues to increase until a steady state is achieved.

Figure 5 illustrates this projection by using the total disability data presented earlier. The input per year is the 569,000 newly disabled workers we are currently projecting. Thus, during the first year, there were 569,000 disabled workers in

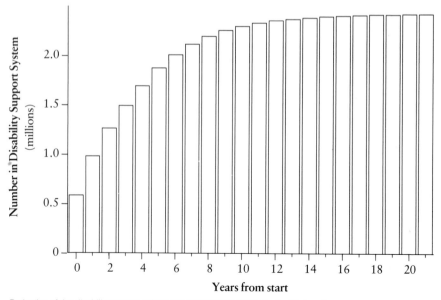

Figure 5.   Projection of the disability system using current estimates of newly disabled workers.

the system. By the beginning of the second year, 36% of the first-year group have left the system. To the remaining 364,160 workers, we add another 569,000, which makes a total of 933,160 persons in the disability system. At the end of 20 years, a steady state is achieved. At that time, there would be 2,365,000 individuals in the disability system.

The astute reader has, no doubt, observed that the steady-state value presented here is 8% more than the 2,191,000 workers estimated to be in the disability system in 1985. In estimating the steady-state size of a system, we have to assume that the input remains constant over time. This of course, is theoretical. In the case of our disability system projection, however, the steady-state value for 1980 was calculated and carried forward to 1985. If we had started with an earlier steady state, the gain in accuracy would have been inconsequential.

This projection, of course, is theoretical and represents an estimate of the number of persons in the disability system in 20 years, assuming that other conditions are held constant. This exercise is done solely to determine the steady-state size of the system based on current incidence and attrition rates.

If we divide the percentage of the target group in the total disability system by the percentage of the group at the time of incidence, that is, the time when they left the labor market because of a disabling condition, we can obtain a measure of impact termed the Prevention Impact Quotient (PIQ) for the given prevention program. For the total disability system, the PIQ is equal to 1.00, since we would divide the 100% in the disability system by the 100% in the incidence. On the other hand, if a disability represents 10% of those entering the system but only 8% of those in the system, the PIQ would be 0.80 (8% divided by 10%). If a condition represents 15% of those entering the disability system but accounts for 20% of those in the system, then the PIQ is 1.33 (20% divided by 15%). We have found PIQs for various disability groups that range from 0.56 to 1.59.

The Intervention Impact Quotient (IIQ) is different from the PIQ in that it does not use the total attrition curve rate, but instead, uses the observed outcomes with their associated attrition

curves. In the development of the IIQ, we assumed that intervention programs will only affect those disabled persons who do not return to work, but live to the age of 65. We also considered that those who currently return to work will continue to do so regardless of the existence of the intervention program. We recognize that this assumption is an oversimplification. Someone who lives until the age of 65 may actually be so severely disabled that return to work is impossible. On the other hand, we assumed that those who die before returning to work or reaching 65 are too severely disabled for vocational rehabilitation services. Again, this is an oversimplification; we presume however, that the errors in each of these assumptions will cancel each other out. We made the additional assumption that those individuals in the current medical/disability retirement group will return to work at the same rate as those who currently return to work.

In order to compute the IIQ, we first have to simulate the disability group under the condition that an intervention program is 100% successful, that is, all of those who now are in the medical/disability retirement group transfer into the return to work group. Figure 6 shows what happens when this simulation is applied to the total disabled worker population. This simulation used the original incidence per year of all disabled workers, but assumed they exited the system only through return to work or death.

The general shape of the incremental annual build-up is similar to that shown in Figure 5, but the steady state is achieved more quickly (18 years) and with a lower final population (1,490,000). This represents a reduction of 874,000, when compared to the steady-state value of 2,365,000. The IIQ is calculated by dividing the number removed from the system through intervention (875,000) by the number of the group in the current estimate (2,365,000). In this case, the IIQ is 0.37 for the total disability group. This means that if a perfect intervention strategy were developed, the number of people in the total disability support system could be reduced by 37% at the present time.

For specific disability groups, we have found IIQs ranging from 0.20 to 0.54. A low IIQ ordinarily indicates that persons in the disability

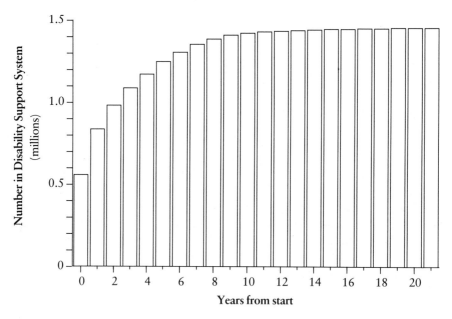

Figure 6. Simulation of the disability system if intervention were completely successful.

group leave the system very rapidly and relatively few remain in the system until retirement age. The opposite is generally true for those groups having a large IIQ.

Note that prevention generally is three times as effective in reducing the numbers of dependent disabled workers as intervention. However, this is without regard to cost.

DISABILITY PROJECTIONS

Because the work force will comprise a higher proportion of older workers in the foreseeable future, more individuals than ever will acquire physically disabling conditions. We have attempted to quantify this result as far as possible using our disability data and the labor force projections of the National Institute on Aging (NIA).

The NIA projects that the labor force participation of those 55–64 years of age will decrease by 12 percentage points, from 57% to 45%, between 1985 and 2020. However, the participation of those 25 to 54 years of age is expected to increase from 77% to 87%. This assumption, of course, limits the full effect of the aging population on the labor force. In other words, although the number of people in the age group 55–64 will increase 68% in the next 30 years, the NIA predicts that this age cohort in the labor force will increase only 39%. Table 3 shows these figures for all the age cohorts.

When we compute the average age of the work force for each year, we find that the average age will increase 1.7 years between 1985 and 2020. In 1985, the average age is 36.5 years. In 2020, it will be 38.2.

Table 3. Numbers of people by age projected by NIA to be in the work force in 2020 as compared to 1985

Age cohorts	Year		Increase
	1985	2020	
16–24	24,291,000	25,506,000	8%
25–34	31,421,000	36,353,000	16%
35–44	24,517,000	33,809,000	38%
45–54	16,500,000	26,346,000	60%
55–64	12,315,000	17,123,000	39%
Total	109,044,000	139,137,000	28%

The projections of the numbers of disabled workers in the disability support system shown in Table 3 were generated by first applying incidence rates of newly disabled workers for each cohort to the labor force projections. This provided the number of newly disabled workers in each cohort for each year between 1985 and 2020.

After the number of workers with a new disability was generated for each cohort for a particular year, the number of workers remaining in subsequent years from that year's input was obtained. Here, however, the population of workers in each cohort at the time of incidence is treated as a separate component of the disability system and the inputs each year are no longer constant, but are derived from the labor force data.

Between the years 1985 and 2020, the number of newly disabled workers per year is expected to increase by 35%, from 569,000 to 770,000, an increase of 201,000 workers per year based only on the aging of the work force. Actually, the greatest number of newly disabled workers per year will be in the year 2015. In that year, 779,000 workers are expected to enter the disability support system, representing a 37% increase over 1985.

The number of workers in the disability support system is only partially related to the annual number of newly disabled workers. The size of the disability support system is also dependent on the amount of time workers tend to remain in the system. Since there are some significant differences in the amount of time age cohorts stay in the system (see Table 2), changes in the number of workers in each cohort will also affect the size of the disability support system.

By combining the changes in the numbers of workers expected to enter the disability support system from each age cohort with the attrition curve for each cohort, we can project the number of persons in the system. Figure 7 shows the results of this projection for the years 1985 to 2020. According to this projection, the number of workers in the system will increase from 2,191,000 in 1985 to 3,297,000 in 2020. This is an increase of 50.5%. During the same time, according to the projection by the NIA, the work force will increase by only 27.4%.

Table 4 lists the variations in the contribution of the different age cohorts to the number of persons in the disability support system. To determine if the eventual outcomes of persons entering the disability system will change, we calculated the annual distribution by eventual outcomes. These results are shown in Table 5. This analysis is based on the outcomes for each of the age cohorts presented in Table 2. It is immediately obvious that during the 1990s there will be a slight reduction of those entering the disability support system who will eventually leave the system through retirement. This is undoubtedly due to the relatively few workers in the 55–64 age cohort during that period.

Despite methodological concerns, these projections appear to be extremely robust. Even when some assumptions are changed, the results are very similar. A case in point is the NIA's projection of the population's work force participation over the next 30 years. They assume the current trends of reduced participation among older workers will continue through the year 2020. However, if we assume that the work force participation by age cohorts will be the same in the

Table 4. Projected contribution quotients of each cohort from 1985 to 2020

Year	Cohort				
	16–34	35–44	45–54	55–65	Total
1985	8%	15%	36%	41%	100%
1990	8%	18%	37%	37%	100%
1995	7%	18%	42%	33%	100%
2000	6%	18%	43%	33%	100%
2005	6%	16%	44%	34%	100%
2010	6%	14%	44%	36%	100%
2015	6%	14%	41%	39%	100%
2020	6%	16%	38%	40%	100%

Table 5. Projected outcomes for those workers entering the disability support system during a given year

Year	Outcome			Total
	Return to work	Retire	Die	
1985	54%	31%	15%	100%
1990	55%	29%	16%	100%
1995	57%	27%	16%	100%
2000	56%	27%	17%	100%
2005	55%	28%	17%	100%
2010	53%	30%	17%	100%
2015	53%	30%	17%	100%
2020	53%	31%	16%	100%

future as it is now, then the projection of the workers in the system is only 7% higher than that shown in Figure 7. That is, if the work force participation rate remains constant, 3,544,000 workers will be in the disability support system.

POLICY IMPLICATIONS

The most obvious implication of this research is that the disability support system as it exists today is going to be greatly overburdened financially, administratively, and operationally in the next 35 years. Current disability wage replacement payments are estimated to be over $100 billion per year. If benefits per person stayed the same, in the year 2020 this country would be paying $150.5 billion in 1985 dollars. However, the benefits are not likely to remain the same. Muller (1983) reported that among SSDI recipients in 1971, only 2% were also receiving private insurance benefits. A recent study conducted by the U.S. Department of Labor (1985) found that currently 47% of persons employed in medium or large firms are covered under group LTD plans. Therefore, the increasing popularity of LTD plans as a fringe benefit and the increasing numbers of persons in the disability support system will drive up disability-related costs tremendously unless offset by effective rehabilitation. The 35% increase in the number of newly dis-

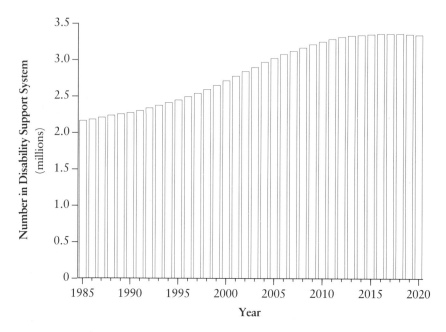

Figure 7. Projection of the numbers of workers in the long-term disability support system from 1985 to 2020.

abled workers will definitely stress those systems providing disability support eligibility determinations.

These projections are based on the assumption that at least the current amount of rehabilitation services are employed to assist newly disabled persons to return to work. If the amount of rehabilitation effort and number of rehabilitation specialists do not increase by 35%, the numbers of persons receiving disability support payments in the year 2020 may be much higher than the 3,545,000 that we are projecting. On the other hand, it seems that increased rehabilitation effort may greatly ameliorate the problem of the disabled worker. Table 6 shows the potential effect of applying intensive rehabilitation services to this problem within the next 35 years.

In this scenario, we assumed that any new initiative for rehabilitating the worker who becomes disabled will take at least 5 years to establish. In addition, realizing the full effect of the effort will take another 5 years. We applied the IIQs to the number of workers projected to be in the disability support system under current practices, in order to show the reduced numbers in support systems if comprehensive rehabilitation services were applied. We believe that the numbers in the right-hand column of Table 6 represent the bottom line number of people that the disability system will have to support.

Obviously, achieving the greatest reduction possible of persons in the disability system will require far more rehabilitation specialists than presently trained to serve older workers who become disabled and to work with public and private employers. Research recently completed by

the Menninger Research and Training Center indicates that only about 6% of workers who become physically disabled are currently receiving either public or private rehabilitation services.

In addition, if the bottom line number of disabled workers is to be achieved through intervention, many more employers will need to establish return-to-work programs, policies, and procedures. According to Hood and Downs (1985), relatively few employers have made a serious commitment to returning the worker who becomes disabled to productive employment. At the current rate of return, there will be a 44% increase between 1985 and 2020 in the numbers of disabled persons returning to work. This increase is necessary just to limit the disability support system to the size we are currently projecting. On the other hand, if over the next 35 years, only the same number of persons per year return to work, the disability support system will increase 88.5% over those years, instead of the 50.5% we are projecting when the percentage of those returning to work remains constant.

New programs for return to work cannot be left only to major corporations. The 1,000 largest corporations employ less than 21% of the labor force. Solving this problem will require a concerted effort in prevention and intervention programs, policies, and strategies by insurance companies, government agencies, medical professionals, and employers.

The majority of the disabled worker problem involves the worker who is 45 years of age or older. Eventually, these workers will represent more than 75% of those in the disability support system. Therefore, if we want to reduce the numbers of persons receiving disability support payments, we must devote more attention to workers 45 years of age and older who become physically disabled. These people are currently largely ignored by the public rehabilitation system. For example, Hester and Faimon (1985) found that, although 68% of the new SSDI beneficiaries are over 49 years of age, Illinois referred only 0.4% of this group to the state vocational rehabilitation agency during a 5-year period ending in 1984.

It is not surprising that 99% of disabled workers who reach 65 years of age without returning to work are persons who become dis-

Table 6.   Number of workers projected to be in the disability support system over the next 35 years, compared to what is possible with rehabilitation

Year	Projected	Possible
1985	2,191,000	—
1990	2,277,000	—
1995	2,430,000	1,604,000
2000	2,673,000	1,791,000
2005	2,965,000	1,957,000
2010	3,297,000	2,143,000
2015	3,483,000	2,229,000
2020	3,545,000	2,233,000

abled after reaching 45 years of age. As a society, we apparently believe that a person over the age of 44 who becomes seriously disabled should not, or will not, return to work. In the next 5 years, before the disability support system begins to go totally out of control, a national commitment is needed to rehabilitate the worker who becomes disabled after the age of 44.

REFERENCES

Bowe, F. (1983). *Demography and disability: A chartbook for rehabilitation*. Fayetteville: University of Arkansas.

Greenberger, M. (1976). *Models in the policy process: Public decision making in the computer era*. New York: Russell Sage Foundation.

Hester, E., & Decelles, P. (1985). *The disability system: A dynamic analysis*. Topeka, KS: The Menninger Foundation.

Hester, E., & Faimon, G. (1985). *The effectiveness of vocational rehabilitation services with the SSDI recipient*. Topeka, KS: The Menninger Foundation.

Hood, L., & Downs, J. (1985). *Return-to-work: A literature review*. Topeka, KS: The Menninger Foundation.

Muller, L. (1983). *Receipt of multiple benefits by disabled worker beneficiaries*. Washington, DC: U.S. Department of Health and Human Services, Social Security Administration.

U.S. Department of Labor. (1985). *Employee benefits in medium and large firms, 1984*. Washington, DC: U.S. Government Printing Office.

Chapter 20

Acute Care Prospective Payment
Impact on Medical Rehabilitation Outcomes

Julia F. Costich

Since the implementation of prospective payment under Medicare using the diagnostic related groupings system (DRGs), acute care hospitals have been under considerable pressure to shorten their inpatient length of stay and intensity of service. With the arrival of Peer Review Organization (PRO) procedures in November 1984, this pressure was compounded by strict surveillance of patient charts for appropriateness of admission and continued hospitalization. The PRO review process applies to all governmental payors and to a variety of other third parties, including both insurance companies and employers who contract with the independent reviewing organization.

Representatives of health care professions and senior citizens' organizations have expressed apprehension regarding the potential effect of these regulations on the quality of care that hospitals can afford to deliver under this payor-driven system (Mickel, 1985a, 1985b). Congressional hearings during 1985 included a number of accounts of problems that have arisen under prospective payment (McIlrath, 1985).

According to Brent England, Director of the American Hospital Association's Center for Rehabilitation Facilities and Services, rehabilitation hospitals report that "they are seeing the sicker, more involved patients" (Burda, 1984). Therapists are having to learn new skills, such as "teaching patients to ambulate when they are still attached to respirators." In the same report, Edward Stein of the Rehabilitation Institute of Chicago added that many patients admitted to that facility "are not stable medically, so the rehabilitation staff has the added responsibility of resolving patients' medical problems."

In the rehabilitation sector, the anecdotal experience of "quicker and sicker" referrals has received some statistical confirmation. The 1985 survey undertaken by the California Association of Rehabilitation Facilities (Cal-ARF) indicated that 28 of the 34 respondents found that their patients were admitted after shorter acute hospital stays. The same number reported that patients were more severely ill on admission. Comments accompanying these data expressed concern regarding patients' medical stability, ability to participate in therapy, and need for acute transfer back to the referring hospital. In the latter connection, 22 of the 34 respondents indicated that patients' rehabilitation programs were more frequently interrupted than previously by medical complications. Those who did not share this experience appear to represent nonexempt units or exempt units in acute care hospitals that have ready access to higher levels of medical service than are available in a freestanding or independent facility (Cal-ARF, 1985).

The balance of this chapter describes a study intended to assess the impact of prospective payment and PRO review in a freestanding, comprehensive rehabilitation facility. The emphasis is on assessment of effects on the functional status of rehabilitation inpatients, as well as the change in other significant patient-related variables under these new systems.

METHOD

Chart reviews were undertaken for all patients admitted for the first time with a diagnosis of cerebrovascular accident to a Kentucky rehabilitation hospital during the first 3 months of 1983 (before DRGs) and the first 3 months of 1985. These periods were chosen to avoid seasonal variation in requests for admission. The study was limited to a single diagnosis to maximize uniformity in the patient population and to reflect the preponderance of governmental third-party payment (86%) in this group. The facility at which the study occurred experienced a high degree of stability in staff and admissions policy during the period in question.

Of the 74 patients admitted for the first time during the 1983 study period, 63 completed their rehabilitation without interruption and were included in the study group. Seventy-one first-admission patients met these criteria in the 1985 group of 93. The rehabilitation courses of the remaining patients were also studied, but their data are not included in the comparative figures.

The average age of patients admitted in the earlier period was 65, a significant difference from the average of 69 for the later group. In comparison, the average age of stroke patients undergoing acute care at the University of Kentucky Hospital was 62 in 1983 and 63 in 1985. The acute hospital length of stay for patients in the two groups declined from 20 days to 18 days; the latter figure is larger than the local area hospital average stay of 11 days for DRG 14 in 1985. (This decline has become more precipitous in 1986: For the 83 patients who completed stroke rehabilitation in the first 3 months of the year, the average acute care length of stay was slightly under 15 days.) These figures suggest that stroke patients referred for inpatient rehabilitation are older and have more complicated inpatient courses than the average.

In keeping with the methodology used by Melvin and colleagues (Melvin & Fiedler, 1985a, 1985b), activities of daily living (ADL) and mobility scores were extracted from therapists' chart notes. The comparison of functional measures at admission and discharge was limited to those patients who completed their rehabilitation course in a single stay.

ADL Measures

Six ADL measures—transfer, drinking/feeding, dressing, grooming, washing/bathing, and bladder management—were coded 0, 1, or 2 on the following basis: $0 =$ full independence; $1 =$ requires assistance; and $2 =$ fully dependent. The six values then were summed to yield a composite score for ADL.

Mobility Measures

Mobility scores ranged from 1 to 5: $1 =$ no ambulation problems; $2 =$ needs assistance with vertical mobility only; $3 =$ minimal requirement for assistance with mechanical mobility; $4 =$ moderate need for mechanical mobility assistance; $5 =$ full dependency in mobility.

Patient endurance was included as a surrogate measure for the degree of impairment upon admission, discharge, and follow-up. As with the mobility measures, these scores ranged from 1 to 5, based on the number of hours per day that the patient was able to be out of bed and participate in daily activities. The specific scores were $5 = 1$ hour or less per day; $4 = 2$–3 hours per day; $3 = 4$–5 hours per day; $2 = 6$–8 hours per day; $1 = 10$ or more hours per day.

RESULTS

Frequency distributions and means for the composite ADL scores at admission of the 1983 and 1985 groups are contained in Table 1. The significantly higher average for the 1985 group indicates a greater need for assistance in these activities ($t = 2.07, p < .05$). Frequency distributions and means for mobility and endurance scores at admission are presented in Table 2. The means for the 1985 group were significantly higher for both mobility and endurance, indicating relatively greater deficiency in both areas. The difference between the groups in mobility was statistically significant ($t = 4.632, p < .001$), and the difference in endurance approached significance ($t = 1.775, p < .10$). In summary, compared to the 1983 group, patients admitted in 1985 were deficient in composite ADL scores and mobility and tended to have less endurance.

Tables 1 and 2 also contain frequency distributions and means for the two groups at discharge. The 1985 group had significantly higher mean values on composite ADL, mobility, and endurance ($t = 2.865, p < .005; t = 3.301, p < .002;$

Table 1.   ADL composite score distribution

| | 1983 | | | 1985 | |
Score	Admission	Discharge		Admission	Discharge
0	0	20		0	8
1	2	9		0	8
2	3	9		2	5
3	3	4		5	6
4	5	9		3	9
5	21	8		14	13
6	15	1		22	12
7	9	1		11	5
8	7	1		11	5
9	1	1		1	0
10	0	0		1	0
12	0	0		1	0
Mean	5.5	2.3		6.0	4.0

and $t = 3.146$, $p < .005$, respectively). Comparisons between the groups at admission and discharge reveal that the degree of difference at admission tended to be preserved at discharge for the mobility and endurance scores, but not for the ADL composite score. The latter mean scores for the 1985 group did not improve between admission and discharge in proportion to the improvement shown by the 1983 group.

Forty-three of the 63 patients in the 1983 group and 46 of the 71 patients in the 1985 group returned to the rehabilitation facility for outpatient follow-up. Their records were reviewed to determine the stability of functional gain achieved during inpatient rehabilitation. The time elapsing between discharge and follow-up varied between 40 and 90 days, the mean being 61 days.

Table 3 contains frequency distributions and means for ADL composite scores at discharge and follow-up for the 1983 and 1985 groups. Comparable data for mobility and endurance scores are provided in Table 4.

The 1985 follow-up subgroup had a poorer mean composite ADL score at discharge than the 1983 subgroup ($t = 5.643$, $p < .001$), but this difference had diminished at follow-up ($t = 1.662$, $p < .10$). This tendency to convergence in the two groups' follow-up scores holds true for

Table 2.   Mobility and endurance score distributions

| | 1983 | | | 1985 | |
Score	Admission	Discharge		Admission	Discharge
Mobility					
1	2	18		0	7
2	5	16		2	20
3	16	21		3	28
4	20	6		17	11
5	20	2		49	5
Mean	3.8	2.3		4.6	2.8
Endurance					
1	8	39		4	29
2	17	22		10	26
3	20	2		28	11
4	10	0		21	4
5	8	0		8	1
Mean	2.9	1.4		3.2	1.9

Table 3. ADL follow-up score distribution

	1983		1985	
	Discharge	Follow-up	Discharge	Follow-up
0	13	26	7	20
1	7	4	4	3
2	7	3	5	9
3	2	1	4	4
4	6	2	8	3
5	7	5	8	6
6	1	1	8	0
7	0	0	2	0
8	0	1	0	0
10	0	0	0	1
Mean	1.4	2.1	1.8	3.5

mobility (discharge $t = 4.497, p < .001$; follow-up $t = 1.03$, not significant), and is present to a lesser extent in endurance scores (discharge $t = 2.612$, $p < .01$; follow-up $t = 2.466$, $p < .05$).

The numbers of acute transfers during the rehabilitation stay were also analyzed. These inpatients were not included in the preceding analysis because they did not meet the criterion of uninterrupted rehabilitation stays. Eleven (14.9%) of the 1983 group developed complications requiring acute transfer, whereas 22 (23.7%) in the later group fell into this category. This difference, although not statistically significant, is suggestive of a higher level of medical instability. Six of the 11 in the 1983 group never returned to complete their rehabilitation; exactly half (11) of the 1985 group were readmitted, and 9 completed rehabilitation programs. An examination of the reasons for transfer reveals a significant increase in cardiovascular complications, a category that includes 4 of the 11 in the earlier group and 12 of the later group of 22.

DISCUSSION

Stroke patients admitted since the onset of DRGs appear to be more severely impaired on admission, especially in mobility. The discrepancy persists at discharge, but becomes somewhat less severe with the passage of time as measured on follow-up visits. Because follow-up information was not available for all patients in the study

Table 4. Mobility and endurance follow-up score distribution

	1983		1985	
	Discharge	Follow-up	Discharge	Follow-up
Mobility				
1	15	20	4	12
2	11	8	14	16
3	12	11	19	12
4	5	3	6	5
5	0	1	3	1
Mean	2.0	2.2	2.3	2.8
Endurance				
1	29	37	22	21
2	12	3	14	20
3	2	2	6	4
4	0	0	3	0
5	0	1	1	1
Mean	1.4	1.4	1.7	1.8

group, no firm conclusions can be drawn from these data. In the absence of any difference in the two groups' acute hospital length of stay, alternative explanations for the greater severity of their impairment must be considered. The most obvious are that 1) referring hospitals are offering a lower level of rehabilitation service during the acute care stay, and 2) patients who previously spent a convalescent period at home or in extended care are now being referred directly from the acute care facility.

In the groups studied, there was a small decrease in the proportion of patients referred from sites other than the acute facility (1983—14%; 1985—10%), but this change is not adequate to explain the difference in outcome measures. Consistent with the first hypothesis, it is reasonable to surmise that the fiscal incentives under prospective payment may encourage lower levels of hospital-based service. The reasons for earlier and less medically stable referrals to rehabilitation under prospective payment are summarized by Cassel in an analysis suggesting that the problem will continue to worsen:

> There is a strong likelihood that hospitals will continue to cut back on services that are not specifically covered by DRGs, such as rehabilitative therapies, psychological testing, dietetics and nutrition, and audiology. . . . Acute and intensive care will continue to be reimbursed urging overutilization of some services at the loss of others which may be more relevant to the patient's needs. For example, functional improvement with physical therapy will seldom be reimbursed, but it will be financially

possible for every elderly person to receive coronary bypass surgery (Cassel, 1985).

The positive change in follow-up measures has a number of possible explanations; greater availability of outpatient services, more effective use of these therapies, and improvement in patient and family education are obvious ones. As pressures increase to shorten inpatient stays, monitoring the ability of patients to retain and improve on the functional gains made in formal rehabilitation will become even more important.

The results of this study appear to confirm the opinions of the respondents to Cal-ARF's 1985 survey, especially the significant increase in number of patients transferred back to acute care facilities during their rehabilitation stay. Single-institution analyses such as this one can be pooled to enhance the advocacy position of the rehabilitation sector in the public sector; this should be encouraged by facility administrators and academic departments.

Refinement and uniformity in outcome measurement will become a matter of urgency for rehabilitation facilities if they are to justify their existence under prospective payment. The "big ticket" items centering on the acute care facility continue to receive the preponderance of federal funding, whereas the potential benefits in improved outcomes available from rehabilitation services continue to be ignored. If rehabilitation is to compete successfully with acute care for its share of the health care dollar, some way of measuring improvement as a function of empirically determined variables will be essential.

REFERENCES

Burda, D. (1984, September 16). PPS has not encouraged formation of large numbers of rehabilitation hospitals. *Hospitals*, pp. 72, 76.

Burda, D. (1986a, January 5). PPS—a risky proposition for rehab hospitals? *Hospitals*, pp. 88–89.

Burda, D. (1986b, January 5). Rehab. not immune to PPS: Survey. *Hospitals*, pp. 89–90.

California Association of Rehabilitation Facilities. (1985). *Impact of prospective payment (DRGs) on the delivery of rehabilitation services* (survey). Sacramento: Author.

Cassel, C. K. (1985). Doctors and allocation decisions: A new role in the new Medicare. *Journal of Health Policy, Politics and Law, 10,* 549–564.

McIlrath, S. (1985, December 27). Effects of PPS on quality of care studied. *American Medical News*, p. 2.

Melvin, J., & Fiedler, I. G. (1985a, August). Prospective payment system for rehabilitation facilities (Abstract). *Archives of Physical Medicine and Rehabilitation, 66,* 555.

Melvin, J., & Fiedler, I. G. (1985b, September). *Prospective payment system for rehabilitation facilities.* Paper presented at the annual meeting of American Congress of Rehabilitation Medicine, Kansas City, MO.

Mickel, C. (1985a, November 1). Long-term care gaps seen plaguing PPS. *Hospitals*, p. 93.

Mickel, C. (1985b, November 16). Premature-discharge allegations intensify. *Hospitals*, p. 31.

Chapter 21

Medical Rehabilitation Outcome Measurement in a Changing Health Care Market

Gerben DeJong

Medical rehabilitation, like most disciplines, is an evolving one that continuously needs to adapt to a changing environment. One of the great changes in medical rehabilitation's present environment is the larger health care market that promises to alter significantly how we deliver and pay for medical rehabilitation services. The purpose of this chapter is to consider how selected changes in health care policy and finance are likely to alter how we think about, and how we measure, outcomes in medical rehabilitation.

Many of the major changes that have occurred in various sectors of the health care economy have yet to affect medical rehabilitation. This delay has given the medical rehabilitation industry a reprieve during which it can anticipate many of the changes that are about to occur. This chapter seeks to identify the economic pressure points likely to affect medical rehabilitation's future by extrapolating from various trends already evident in the larger health care market. More specifically, this chapter will note how these economic pressures are likely to shape, or should shape, medical rehabilitation's approach to outcome measurement.

Before considering the specific changes in health care policy and finance, we need to take a broader and more historical look at outcome measurement in medical rehabilitation. This longer range view can offer meaningful insight into the future of outcome measurement in medi-

cal rehabilitation. Accordingly, this chapter is organized as follows: first, the larger historical context in which outcome measurement has evolved in medical rehabilitation is examined; second, specific changes in health care finance and its meaning for outcome measurement in medical rehabilitation are identified; and third, a future agenda for outcome-oriented research is presented.

THE LARGER HISTORICAL CONTEXT

Outcome Measures Vis-à-Vis Other Medical Specialties

Historically, it has been common practice among medical rehabilitation practitioners to exercise a measure of self-flagellation over the status of outcome measures in their chosen profession. They have criticized their own profession for failing to develop measures that would demonstrate to payors and medical colleagues alike the worthiness of their interventions in ameliorating the consequences of injury and disability. Medical rehabilitation professionals have long sought a definitive set of outcome measures that would provide medical rehabilitation a measure of intellectual respectability and thus place the profession on a more equal footing with other medical specialties. As is argued below, much of the self-

The views expressed in this paper are those of the author and do not necessarily reflect the views or the position of the National Rehabilitation Hospital.

flagellation is based on a distorted perception about the measurement capabilities of other specialties.

Over the years, medical rehabilitation, relative to other medical disciplines, has been handicapped in outcome measurement mainly because its *unit of analysis* is different than that of many other medical disciplines. In other medical specialties, the unit of analysis is an organ, a body system, or a particular type of pathology. In fact, much of medicine is organized around specific organs and body systems (e.g., cardiology, nephrology, and neurology). Within these disciplines, the ultimate goal is cure. Outcome measures in these disciplines follow accordingly.

In medical rehabilitation, the unit of analysis is the individual and the individual in relation to his or her environment. The ultimate goal is not cure but enhanced function, that is, the ability to function as independently as possible within a specific set of activities. Consequently, outcome measures must extend well beyond the performance of a specific organ and the mere absence of pathology.

Simply put, medical rehabilitation is a more holistic discipline. As such, its measurement tools must necessarily address a wider spectrum of activity than most specialties. However, as the spectrum of functional activity broadens it becomes more difficult to achieve a consensus on both conceptual and measurement issues. Moreover, medical rehabilitation is an interdisciplinary enterprise that seeks to integrate perspectives from a variety of disciplines—physical medicine and rehabilitation, physical therapy, occupational therapy, neuropsychology, speech pathology, and others. Medical rehabilitation is enriched because of such perspectives, but it also has greater difficulty in developing a firm consensus around key outcome measurement issues.

Although medical rehabilitation has traditionally been apologetic about its ability to measure outcomes relative to other medical specialties, we also need to take note of how medical rehabilitation is far ahead of other specialties. Most other medical specialties are also becoming more holistic. They too have come to realize that cure is often impossible and that residual function is the paramount issue. For example, as a result of major epidemiological studies, the discipline of cardiology has come to recognize that coronary heart disease is not the product of a specific pathological agent but the result of life-style factors such as diet, exercise, and stress. Interestingly, cardiology is interested not only in how life-style and function affect disease but also how diseases affect life-style and function, such as the person's ability to participate in various activities of everyday living—work, social contact, household chores, sex, sports, and the like (Neill et al., 1985).

The historical irony is that other medical specialties are just now beginning to address outcome issues that have dominated medical rehabilitation for some years. Even a casual review of work in other disciplines will underscore how primitive disability and functional outcome measurement has been in other fields. Other disciplines—perhaps with the exception of gerontology and a few others—simply lack the conceptual tools and the intellectual scaffolding needed to develop or adapt functionally oriented outcome measures (Society for Automotive Engineers, 1986).

The Lag in Outcome Measurement

Another reason why medical rehabilitation has been so self-critical about developing a consensus on a set of outcome measures is the failure to understand that outcome measures tend to lag behind clinical practice and changing circumstances in society at large.

We have only to look at spinal cord injury, medical rehabilitation's model disability. Prior to the introduction of sulfa drugs and antibiotics in the late 1930s and early 1940s, persons with spinal cord injury who made it to the hospital usually did not die because of their injury but because of secondary health problems that could not be controlled. Rehabilitation in most instances was not even considered. The outcome of significance was mere survival.

Even in the late 1940s and early 1950s, most persons with spinal cord injuries were destined to have very limited life-styles, often in an institutional setting. Thus, outcome measurement was limited to very simple physical activities such as range of motion, mobility, and personal care—

all generic to institutional concerns such as levels of nursing care.

The advent of the model spinal injury systems program (see Chapter 17) brought a clinical focus that materially altered postrehabilitation opportunities. Likewise, the independent living movement of the 1970s, perhaps more than any other single force, radically altered our thinking about the range of opportunities potentially available to persons with disabilities such as spinal injury.

More recently, advances in emergency medical service (EMS) systems have created a new population of spinal cord–injured persons who require permanent ventilator assistance. The clinical advances that have made the survival of this population group possible raise new conceptual and outcome measurement issues—often under the rubric of "quality of life."

The point is simply this: Outcome measures have always lagged behind clinical practice, social norms, and the expectations of persons with disabilities. This state of affairs should not always be bemoaned. The gestation period for the development of new outcome measures—including research funding, testing for validity and reliability, and publication—is such that application of outcome measures will tend to lag their conceptual inspiration by as much as 10 years or more. A good example is the Functional Assessment Inventory (FAI) developed by Crewe and Athelstan (1981) in the mid 1970s. The FAI was the product of an effort to develop an assessment tool and an outcome measure that addressed the clinical and management needs of rehabilitation agencies. The FAI has since been tested for reliability and field tested for use in rehabilitation agencies. More recently, it has been programmed for computer use. And now, 10 years after its initial development, the FAI is being marketed by a proprietary research company for use on IBM-compatible microcomputers. The question that remains—and one that I will not attempt to answer here—is whether we can shorten this lag in order to be more responsive to changing circumstances.

The lag observed with respect to changes in clinical care can also be observed in medical rehabilitation's response to changes in health care finance. Once again, medical rehabilitation will have to adapt, extend, or change its outcome measures to accommodate these changes. Interestingly, with respect to changes in health care finance, the medical rehabilitation industry's approach to outcome measurement is much more anticipatory than in the past. This anticipatory mode of thinking is evident in the creation of the Task Force for the Development of a Uniform National Data System for Medical Rehabilitation (see Chapter 10). The Task Force was established, in part, for the purpose of developing standardized data elements and a uniform approach to functional assessment and outcome measurement. The economic incentives for assuming an anticipatory posture are very real since an industry-adopted assessment tool or outcome measure may well become the basis for future reimbursement. In fact, I would argue that much of the quest for a new generation of functional assessment tools and outcome measures is not the product of the industry's search for mere self-improvement; instead, this quest is the product of a search for a more intellectually defensible set of measures that will withstand the scrutiny of service buyers in a more competitively organized health care market.

The next section of the chapter outlines the changes in health care finance most likely to impact on medical rehabilitation and identifies where the pressure points will be for outcome measurement in medical rehabilitation.

CHANGES IN HEALTH CARE FINANCE

At the risk of some oversimplification, one can identify five major trends in health care finance that are likely to shape the future of medical rehabilitation services and its approach to outcome measurement:

1. The development of prospective payment systems based on the use of diagnostic related groups (DRGs).
2. The rise of health maintenance organizations (HMOs).
3. The emergence of preferred provider organizations (PPOs).
4. The emergence of self-insured companies and third-party administrators.

5. The development of multifacility "vertically integrated" health care corporations, both profit and nonprofit.

Other trends can also be discerned. For example, traditional third-party carriers such as Blue Cross/ Blue Shield have lost market share to HMOs and self-insured companies. Since we are mainly concerned about the future of health care finance, this chapter will not address trends such as the diminished role of conventional payment systems or the demise of solo practitioners.

For the most part, medical rehabilitation has been sheltered from many of the major changes in health care finance. Medical rehabilitation comprises only 2% of the health care economy and, as a result, has not captured the attention of third-party payors and health finance analysts. In fact, in the health services research literature, one is hard pressed to find any papers or articles that address medical rehabilitation as a service industry. Medical rehabilitation services are, for the most part, still being paid using the conventional fee-for-service and cost-based reimbursement through Medicare, Medicaid, and mainline commercial carriers.

The chill in medical rehabilitation's spine is that, as the health care market shifts to new methods of payment, the effectiveness of medical rehabilitation services will be subjected to greater scrutiny. Herein lies the concern for outcome measurement.

Diagnostic Related Groupings (DRGs)

With the passage of the 1983 Social Security Amendments (Public Law 98-21), Congress significantly altered the manner in which inpatient services would be paid under the Medicare program. Henceforth, Medicare would pay a fixed sum for each patient stay based on which of 467 DRGs the patient belonged in. In other words, Medicare would no longer simply reimburse hospitals using cost-based hospital charges (Newcomer, Wood, & Sankar, 1985).

With the enactment of DRGs, government signaled the health care market that it was willing to leverage its purchasing power to reshape the terms of the exchange between buyer and seller. Government finally realized that "it was purchas-

ing better than 40% of the hospital industry's product and has attained enough economic power to dictate to hospitals the terms, product structure, and price of their product" (Goldsmith, 1984).

The impact of DRGs extends well beyond the Medicare program: DRGs have been adopted by some states as the basis for inpatient reimbursement in the federal-state Medicaid program. Also, because Medicare pays for a significant portion of all inpatient care, hospital financial systems tend to be driven by the reporting demands induced by the Medicare program.

The 1983 Amendments exempted four types of facilities from DRGs: rehabilitation hospitals and units, psychiatric hospitals and units, long-term care hospitals, and pediatric hospitals. These facilities were excluded for three main reasons: 1) their patient diagnoses do not conform to the DRGs; 2) the mix of services they provide differs significantly from acute care facilities; and 3) the data used to develop DRGs contained little, if any, data from these facilities.

The DRG exemption for rehabilitation facilities was intended to be temporary. The exemption has given the medical rehabilitation industry a reprieve that will allow the industry to develop alternative reimbursement formulas consistent with the intent of the DRG formula. To date, the industry has used the exemption primarily to bolster its argument that the DRGs are inappropriate for rehabilitation. In 1984, the industry, through the National Association of Rehabilitation Facilities (NARF, 1985), acquired the services of Coopers & Lybrand, a public accounting firm, to conduct an industry-wide study documenting current practice and costs. The study concluded, as expected, that DRGs bore no relationship to inpatient service utilization.

The 1983 Amendments required the U.S. Department of Health and Human Services (DHHS) to study the feasibility of developing a prospective payment system for rehabilitation hospitals and units and to report its findings to Congress. As a result, the Health Care Financing Administration (HCFA), the responsible operating unit in DHHS, initiated a second industry-wide study in 1984 through the Rand Corporation and the Medical College of Wisconsin (hereafter,

Rand-MCW study). This study specifically concluded that DRGs did not predict utilization of inpatient services (Hosek et al., 1986).

Although the industry has succeeded in discrediting the use of DRGs as the basis for a prospective payment system in medical rehabilitation, the issue remains as to what should be the basis for such a system (McGinnis, Osberg, DeJong, Seward, & Branch, 1986). One finding of the Rand-MCW study was that an activities of daily living (ADL)-based measure of functional capacity was the only consistent predictor of inpatient resource utilization. As a result, some industry leaders now favor using some type of functional measure as the basis for prospective payment in medical rehabilitation.

Should a functionally based method of prospective payment for medical rehabilitation be adopted, we can anticipate at least three major consequences for functional measurement in general and outcome measurement in particular.

First, functional measurement, which until now has been an optional enterprise among many medical rehabilitation providers, will instead become a fixture in every medical record and will become a routine data element on every patient (Keith, 1984). No longer will researchers and program evaluators have to beg clinical staff for such data. It is remarkable how certain types of data can be elicited when financial reimbursement is tied to them.

Second, a functionally based reimbursement system will force the industry toward some degree of standardization in terminology and measurement. As mentioned earlier, the need for standardization has already been anticipated as noted by the creation of the Uniform National Data System Task Force. The development of a uniform functional measure may, over time, cause the demise of many of the more than 40 known measures of functional performance used in the industry today (Gresham & Labi, 1984; Gresham, Phillips, & Labi, 1980). However, if a new reimbursement formula is based on a watered-down, lowest common denominator functional measure, general dissatisfaction will induce researchers and providers to continue working with their own venerated measure of functional performance.

Third, and most important from the standpoint of outcome measurement, a reimbursement-driven measure of functional performance will simply accustom providers to using functional indices. Once a sufficient level of familiarity and comfort with functional measurement is obtained, the incremental effort to obtain functional outcome data will be relatively marginal. To the extent to which reimbursement is tied to functional outcome or gain—as well as to functional performance at admission—outcome measurement will become routine rather than the exception.

Should functionally based outcome measures become routine, it will be only a matter of time before we develop normative performance guidelines for rehabilitation centers based on functional gains or outcomes. The real reason for developing outcome norms—as we now do for heart transplantation and coronary bypass surgery—is economic: to restrict competition. One by-product of the DRG exemption, as claimed by some long-standing providers, is that the exemption has induced new providers to enter the market. It is alleged that the DRG exemption has encouraged acute care hospitals to convert excess acute care beds to rehabilitation beds that are not subject to DRG reimbursement ceilings. The claim is sometimes made that these new entrants compromise the reputations of existing providers who are still struggling to communicate what rehabilitation is all about to the larger health care industry on whom they depend for referrals. Normatively based outcome criteria, it is thought, may help to squeeze certain marginal providers out of the market and may discourage others from coming into the market in the first place. Thus, outcome norms may become a part of the rehabilitation landscape in a simple effort to restrict unwanted competition.

Health Maintenance Organizations (HMOs)

Health maintenance organizations have been a part of the American health scene since 1942, when industrialist Henry Kaiser started prepaid health plans on the West Coast, which later became the Kaiser–Permanente health plan (Starr, 1982). Health maintenance organizations did not become a routine part of public policy discourse until the HMO concept was adopted by the Nixon Administration as its major health policy initiative. Interestingly, it was the rehabilitation community that introduced the HMO concept to the Nixon Administration when Paul M. Ellwood, Jr., a physician with the American Rehabilitation Foundation, persuaded several administration officials of the merits of the HMO approach.

The key element in the HMO concept is that health services are provided by a health service organization on a capitated basis, meaning that all needed health services are to be rendered for a fixed dollar amount per capita. Expenses below this fixed amount represent profits for the HMO; expenses above this fixed amount represent losses. Theoretically, the task of the HMO is to keep its subscribers healthy and thus avert more expensive health care downstream in the form of hospitalization. The clincher is that the provider, not the payor, assumes the financial risk.

Only in recent years have HMOs become a major force in the American health care economy. In fact, HMOs have become one of the fastest growing elements in health care today. By mid-1985 there were 400 HMOs—a 29% increase in just 12 months—serving 19 million persons nationwide—a 25% increase during the same period. Much of this recent growth can be attributed to the development of multistate or national HMOs (Medical Benefits, 1986b).

Much of this growth has bypassed the medical rehabilitation industry. The irony is that even though much of the intellectual leadership behind the HMO concept during the Nixon years was spawned by elements of the rehabilitation community, HMO plans often exclude the "services of a rehabilitation facility." Medical rehabilitation services are often associated with costly and unpredictable "catastrophic" injuries and illnesses. In an effort to price its products competitively, HMOs often mention rehabilitation services as one of the fine-print exclusions.

Critical to medical rehabilitation's financial survival is its ability to obtain third-party coverage. However, as HMOs increase market share, with their exclusions of rehabilitation services, medical rehabilitation facilities may find their niche in the American health care economy eroding.

The challenge for medical rehabilitation is to demonstrate that its services are not only effective but, in the long run, will also help to avert future medical complications and costs. This is the language HMOs understand. Administrators of HMOs want to know how an expensive investment in rehabilitation will pay off downstream in the form of reduced need for expensive medical services, especially inpatient care. In other words, changing market conditions, as illustrated by the rise of HMOs, will force the medical rehabilitation industry to sell its services on the basis of longer term outcomes. However, outcomes based largely on functional performance in ADL will not be adequate. Third-party payors such as HMOs want to know how functional gains translate into outcomes that have economic significance. They will want to know how functional gain will result in a reduced need for such services as attendant services, home health, institutional care, and inpatient care for which the HMO might be liable.

The implication is clear: HMOs will cover rehabilitation services to the extent to which functional gains eventually translate into outcomes that indicate reduced need for hands-on care and supervision. Only sporadically has medical rehabilitation research attempted to demonstrate the degree to which functional performance is predictive of future resource needs.

We can now bring together the earlier discussion on prospective payment systems (PPS) under Medicare and the present discussion on HMOs. The leading research question with regard to PPS under Medicare is whether functional ability is a good indicator of inpatient resource utilization. The leading research question with regard to HMOs is whether functional performance at discharge is a good predictor of subsequent health care utilization. Both questions are flip sides of the same coin that the medical rehabilitation research community is well equipped to address, but neither question has been adequately researched.

Even with good documentation on outcome impact, HMOs may still hesitate to finance medical rehabilitation services. An HMO usually provides or arranges services only for the period in which the person is actually covered by the plan. If employees becomes disabled and are forced, by circumstance or by their employer, to leave their jobs, those employees also loose their attachment to a specific HMO plan. Knowing this—and knowing that employees sometimes change plans frequently—HMOs may, in many instances, have little incentive to cover services of a long-term nature such as rehabilitation services. Thus, research on the impact of rehabilitation on longer term outcomes of economic significance for HMOs is a necessary, but not sufficient, condition for HMO financing of rehabilitation services.

Preferred Provider Organizations (PPOs)

Preferred provider organizations, also known as preferred provider arrangements, are a more recent phenomenon and not as well known as HMOs. Simply stated, a PPO is an organization of providers such as physician groups and hospitals that agree to make health care services available to specific groups of consumers such as employee groups. Consumers or employees are not "locked in" or required to use the services of a PPO under the terms of their employer-sponsored health plan. However, if the consumer obtains health services from a preferred provider, copayments and deductibles are usually lower or nonexistent. In some instances, consumers can obtain a richer package of benefits by going through a preferred provider.

Preferred provider organizations are growing rapidly. Based on a national survey conducted by Gabel, Ermann, and de Lissovoy (1986), the number of persons enrolled in a health insurance plan with an option of using a PPO increased from 1.3 million at the end of 1984 to 5.8 million in mid-1985. In the spring of 1985, nearly 2.9 million were enrolled in the nation's 10 largest PPOs. Less than a year later that figure increased to 6.2 million (February 1986).

To date, the impact of PPOs on medical rehabilitation is unclear. Because there is a shortage of medical rehabilitation facilities in most mar-

kets, medical rehabilitation facilities have not had to price their services competitively or join a PPO. However, some rehabilitation programs, in order to protect their referral base and ensure adequate third-party coverage, may feel compelled to become part of a PPO. Rehabilitation programs that are departments or units within larger hospitals may become part of a PPO because their parent institution or corporation has become part of a PPO.

What do PPOs portend for the future of outcome measurement in medical rehabilitation? The answer is unclear and will depend, in part, on local market conditions. In order to maintain market share in certain markets, it will become important for some rehabilitation centers to become preferred providers. To do so, rehabilitation centers must be able to document that they can produce outcomes consistent with the interests of the payor, whether a conventional commercial insurer, an HMO, a self-insured employer, or the government.

More than anything else, the emergence of PPOs sends a clear signal that health care is simply becoming a more competitive enterprise. Since it is unlikely that medical rehabilitation will be able to compete much on price, it will have to compete on the quality of its product, that is, outcome.

Self-Insured Companies and Third-Party Administrators (TPAs)

Another trend in today's health care market is the willingness of larger companies to self-insure instead of turning over large sums of money to conventional insurance carriers. Many companies have simply come to mistrust insurance carriers who, year after year, have increased premium charges. To the company, the insurance carrier has become a "black box" or, better yet, a "black hole" into which funds disappeared. Another impetus for becoming self-insured is that companies have become more sophisticated in cash management. "In moving to self-funding, employers can not only decide to time their payments into [benefit trusts and special funds] to meet their unique cash flow cycles but can keep the interest on that float" (Goldsmith, 1984). This was especially true in the early 1980s when interest rates were high.

However, once self-insured, many companies were unable to administer their own health insurance programs and turned to TPAs, of which there are more than 1,000 nationwide. From 1977 to 1984, TPAs and self-administered plans grew from 6% to 23% of the group health market. By the end of 1985, TPAs and self-administered plans were estimated to have a market share equal to Blue Cross/Blue Shield plans (Medical Benefits, 1986a).

The key implication for medical rehabilitation is that self-insured companies tend to scrutinize claims and outcomes more carefully than would a more distant and disinterested insurance carrier with multiple policyholders. The old axiom still applies: One is usually more careful in spending one's own money than someone else's money.

The trend toward self-insurance also means that medical rehabilitation must market its services to many possible payors rather than a few insurance carriers or HMOs. It is more difficult to reach the health benefits managers of several hundred companies in a given market area than a handful of third-party payors. In short, medical rehabilitation is faced with a burden of proof that previous market conditions did not require.

Multifacility Health Care Corporations

The final trend to be noted is the development of multihospital and "vertically integrated" health care corporations, both profit and nonprofit, which are challenging the traditional independent nonprofit hospital. Although this trend has little to do with the trends in health care payment systems noted above, the development of new multihospital health care corporations is a major force in today's health care market. "In 1984, 38% of the nation's hospitals belonged to a multihospital system." The largest and most visible segment of the multihospital sector are the investor-owned chains, which grew at an annual rate of 11% from 1977 to 1984 (Gabel et al., 1986).

A "vertically integrated" health care corporation is a multi-institutional health care system that provides a wide range of services that can accommodate a patient's needs from the onset of a condition to its eventual resolution. For exam-

ple, in a vertically integrated health care corporation, a seriously injured patient may first be taken to the corporation's trauma center, then transferred to an intensive care unit, then admitted to a relevant acute care department, transferred to a rehabilitation unit, discharged to the corporation's transitional living facility, and finally released to a home setting staffed with nurses from the corporation's home health agency. This somewhat theoretical example serves to illustrate how rehabilitation may eventually find itself lodged in a much larger corporate system of health care.

The concept of vertical integration is often promoted with continuity of care in mind. From a marketing and financing point of view, the concept of vertical integration is intended to make sure that scarce patients and revenues are not lost to competitors. The anchor institution in most multifacility health care corporations is one or more acute care hospitals. The multifacility system is often designed to ensure that its anchor institution has a solid referral base that is largely controlled by the parent corporation.

Some vertically integrated multifacility systems seek to include the financing as well as the delivery of care within a single corporate entity. Thus, for example, we see multi-institutional corporations forming their own HMOs.

The challenge to rehabilitation is whether it will find itself inside or outside of such multi-institutional systems. To the extent to which it is part of such a system, its referral base and economic well-being will be largely assured, with some compromise in its economic autonomy. To the extent to which it is outside of such a system, it may have to struggle to maintain referral sources and economic health, especially in competitive markets. From the standpoint of outcome measurement, the demands for documentation will probably be greatest for rehabilitation facilities outside of multi-institutional corporate systems that are more exposed to competitive market conditions.

SUMMARY AND IMPLICATIONS FOR THE FUTURE OF OUTCOME-ORIENTED RESEARCH

The health care market is becoming more competitive (Schlenker & Shanks, 1983). With excess physicians and hospital beds in many markets (Goldsmith, 1984), health care is becoming more of a "buyers' market." This basic shift in demand and supply is altering behavior on both sides of the market. The *demand* side of the market is determining how health services will be paid, as in the case of DRGs. The *supply* side of the market is attempting to position itself to be more price competitive and to lock in its referral sources. In the process, the traditional financial intermediaries that have occupied the middle ground between the demand and supply sides find themselves squeezed out, as can be observed in the diminished role of Blue Cross/Blue Shield and commercial carriers. Instead, buyers and sellers have begun to take on more direct responsibility for the financing of health care, as evidenced by the willingness of buyers to become self-insured and the desire of providers to form their own HMOs.

Input versus Output

This historic shift in the marketplace has major implications for the manner in which we evaluate the delivery of health services, including medical rehabilitation. When the market was a "sellers' market," we were content to measure the *input* side of the production equation (Jette, 1984). Over the years, the health industry has established a mind-boggling array of licensure and accreditation criteria, much of which is industry controlled. "Quality of service"—that eternally hallowed phrase shared by providers and consumers alike—is still largely determined by the extent to which providers measure up to input criteria.

To a large extent, licensure and accreditation criteria are enormously self-serving. They serve to enhance the requirements for professional practice in a manner that lends credibility to service providers and discourages new entrants into the market. Input criteria, however well intentioned, reflect the privileged position that providers historically have had in the health care market.

Now that the market has become more of a "buyers' market," buyers want to examine the *output* or *outcome* side of the production equation. Buyers are interested in licensure and accreditation criteria mainly to the extent to which

these input criteria may serve as indicators of future output and as safeguards against unnecessary human harm.

Beyond ADL

When looking at the outcome side of the production equation, medical rehabilitation has made significant advances in ADL-based measures of outcome. However, such outcome measures are still largely *clinical* tools and do not speak adequately to the concerns of health care buyers and policymakers (DeJong & Branch, 1982; DeJong & Hughs, 1982). The mere acquisition of selected ADL skills is not enough (Labi & Gresham, 1984). Buyers and policymakers want to know how the acquisition of these skills results in social and economic benefits for society, the individual, and the family—approximately in that order.

Rehabilitation needs to listen to its own rhetoric. When selling the merits of rehabilitation to third-party carriers, to HMOs, or to government policymakers, one does not say, for example, that "inpatient rehabilitation will increase a patient's ADL score 16 points or that it will increase a patient's self-esteem index 5 points." Instead we indicate how rehabilitation enables persons to become more *independent* and *productive* members of society. By productive, we mean not only participation in gainful work, but how persons can also make significant contributions to community and family life. Medical rehabilitation's outcomes must reflect these concerns.

As we noted earlier, especially in our discussion on HMOs, buyers and policymakers will be increasingly concerned about how an expensive investment in medical rehabilitation can help to avert costs downstream, especially medical costs. A significant outcome measure largely ignored by medical rehabilitation is the extent of postdischarge use of health care services, particularly inpatient care.

Thus, there are three outcome issues that medical rehabilitation needs to address on a routine basis. All three have significant social and economic implications:

1. The degree to which individuals can live *independently*. In other words: Can individuals be discharged to, and remain in, a rela-

tively unstructured living arrangement that a) provides for the maximum degree of self-direction and b) requires the minimum amount of hands-on care and supervision?

This outcome reflects a perspective offered by the independent living movement. The minimization of hands-on care is not the only issue. Equally important is the ability to become self-directed in a manner that will allow a person to direct and manage his or her own personal care to the maximum extent possible.

2. The degree to which individuals can live *productively* and actively, not only in terms of gainful work, but also in terms of contributions to community and family life.
3. The degree to which individuals can *maintain health* and *avert medical complications* that result in costly medical interventions, especially inpatient care.

These are the outcomes that are convincing and the outcomes that must be advanced in a more competitive health care market. In fact, these are the outcomes suggested by rehabilitation when it goes public in advancing its claim to health care dollars.

Cost Analysis

A claim often advanced by medical rehabilitation specialists is that rehabilitation is cost beneficial (Johnston & Keith, 1983). The argument is that a dollar invested in rehabilitation will yield a positive lifetime return in the form of increased earnings and tax revenues. This argument is impossible to prove and self-defeating.

Cost–benefit analysis is inherently troubling, since no matter how extensive and accurate the raw data, the analysis still pivots on a few key assumptions such as the discount rate that will be used to compute the present value of a future stream of earnings. Cost–benefit analysis is also self-defeating. As medical rehabilitation attempts to serve more severely impaired persons such as those with severe head injury, benefit–cost ratios will look less and less promising.

The more useful tack is to emphasize cost savings: How will an investment in medical rehabilitation help to avert or minimize medical and so-

cial support costs in both the short and long term? This is the language that health care buyers understand. This is the language that should drive our consideration of outcome measures. This is the language that should shape medical rehabilitation's research agenda. It is on these terms that medical rehabilitation can win the credibility battle in a competitive health care market.

Needed Outcome Studies

A question that remains is this: How should the burden of proof regarding medical rehabilitation's effectiveness—or lack thereof—be distributed? Medical rehabilitation should not have to prove itself over and over again. There are certain research questions regarding outcomes that should be answered and then put to rest for a period of time. Medical rehabilitation needs a number of outcome studies—using the outcomes suggested in this chapter—to which it can point with some authority in staking out its claim in a competitive health care environment. In particular, outcome studies are needed in which outcomes of those who received medical rehabilitation services are compared with the outcomes of those who have not received services. Opportunities for a well-controlled comparison group design do exist, although they are rare. A study of this nature is not a short-term effort, should be done prospectively, and requires a substantial level of funding. An understanding funding source needs to be found.

Although major definitive outcome studies are needed, individual medical rehabilitation providers cannot simply defer to the industry's research leadership for a few key studies. Outcome measurement is every provider's responsibility (Keith, 1984). Each provider has to contend with the outcome demands expected of buyers in its own market area. Outcomes of policy significance must be mainstreamed in each facility's program evaluation protocol if a given facility is to demonstrate its effectiveness to the buyers of its services.

Beyond Economic Self-Interest

Even armed to the teeth with excellent data, medical rehabilitation will not be able to overcome certain problems inherent in health care finance. Some buyers of medical rehabilitation services will not be willing to make certain investments in the well-being of disabled persons mainly because they are not going to be liable for certain downstream costs. That is the problem of multiple funding sources, where each source seeks to limit its liability for rehabilitative care and out-of-hospital expenses. The health care market has yet to produce adequate single-source funding mechanisms where all the trade-offs and hard choices can be focused at a single financial decision point.

This observation is made to underscore the fact that even those outcome measures that address the economic self-interest of buyers cannot overcome deficiencies inherent in our system of health care finance. Eventually, the battle for the well-being of disabled persons will be won because the well-being of disabled persons is in the economic interest of society as a whole, not because it serves the interest of a single payor. Ultimately, the battle for the well-being of disabled persons should be won simply because disabled persons have a claim to resources in a society that calls itself humane and just.

REFERENCES

Crewe, N. M., & Athelstan, G. T. (1981). Functional assessment in vocational rehabilitation: A systematic approach to diagnosis and goal setting. *Archives of Physical Medicine and Rehabilitation, 62,* 299–305.

DeJong, G., & Branch, G. (1982). Predicting the stroke patient's ability to live independently. *Stroke, 13,* 648–655.

DeJong, G., & Hughs, J. (1982). Independent living: Methodology for measuring long-term outcomes. *Archives of Physical Medicine and Rehabilitation, 63,* 68–73.

Gabel, J., Ermann, T. R., & de Lissovoy, G. (1986). The emergence and future of PPOs. *Journal of Health Politics, Policy, and Law, 11,* 305–322.

Goldsmith, J. (1984). Death of a paradigm: The challenge of competition. *Health Affairs, 9,* 5–19.

Gresham, G. E., & Labi, M. L. C. (1984). Functional assessment instruments currently available for documenting outcomes in rehabilitation medicine. In C. V. Granger & G. Gresham (Eds.), *Functional assessment in rehabilitation medicine* (pp. 65–85). Baltimore: Williams & Wilkins.

Gresham, G. E., Phillips, T. E., & Labi, M. L. C. (1980). ADL status in stroke: Relative merits of three indexes. *Archives of Physical Medicine and Rehabilitation, 61,* 355–358.

Hosek, S., Kane, R., Carney, M., Hartman, J., Reboussin, D., Serrato, C., & Melvin, J. (1986, March). *Changes and outcomes for rehabilitative care: Implications for the prospective payment system* (working draft). Santa Monica, CA: Rand Corporation.

Jette, A. M. (1984). Concepts of health and methodological issues in functional assessment. In C. V. Granger & G. E. Gresham (Eds.), *Functional assessment in rehabilitation medicine* (pp. 46–64). Baltimore: Williams & Wilkins.

Johnston, M., & Keith, R. A. (1983). Cost-benefits of medical rehabilitation: Review and critique. *Archives of Physical Medicine and Rehabilitation, 64,* 147–154.

Keith, R. A. (1984). Functional assessment in program evaluation for rehabilitation medicine. In C. V. Granger & G. E. Gresham (Eds.), *Functional assessment in rehabilitation medicine* (pp. 122–138). Baltimore: Williams & Wilkins.

Labi, M. L. C., & Gresham, G. E. (1984). Some research applications of functional assessment instruments used in rehabilitation. In C. V. Granger & G. E. Gresham (Eds.), *Functional assessment in rehabilitation medicine* (pp. 86–98). Baltimore: Williams & Wilkins.

McGinnis, G. J., Osberg, S., DeJong, G., Seward, M. L., & Branch, L. G. (1986). *Predicting charges for inpatient medical rehabilitation: Toward a prospective payment system.* Boston: Department of Rehabilitation Medicine, New England Medical Center Hospitals.

Medical Benefits. (1986a). Third party administrators: An industry in transition. *Medical Benefits: The Medical-Economic Digest,* 4–5.

Medical Benefits. (1986b). National HMO firms, 1985. *Medical Benefits: The Medical-Economic Digest,* 1–2.

National Association of Rehabilitation Facilities. (1985). *NARF position paper on a prospective payment system for inpatient medical rehabilitation services and a study regarding a prospective payment system for inpatient medical rehabilitation services: Final report.* Prepared by Coopers & Lybrand. Washington, DC: National Association of Rehabilitation Facilities.

Neill, W., Branch, L. G., DeJong, G., Smith, N. E., Hogan, C. A., Corcoran, P. J., Jette, A. M., Balasco, E. M., & Osberg, S. (1985). Cardiac disability: The impact of coronary heart disease on patient's daily activities. *Archives of Internal Medicine, 145,* 1642–1647.

Newcomer, R., Wood, J., & Sankar, A. (1985). Medicare prospective payment: Anticipated effect on hospitals, other community agencies, and families. *Journal of Health Politics, Policy, and Law, 10,* 275–281.

Schlenker, R. E., & Shanks, N. H. (1983). The private sector and competition in health care markets. *Journal of Health Politics, Policy, and Law, 8,* 598–606.

Society for Automotive Engineers. (1986, February). *Crash injury impairment and disability: Long-term effects.* A compilation of papers presented at the International Congress and Exposition, Detroit, MI.

Starr, P. (1982). *The social transformation of American medicine.* New York: Basic Books.

Index